DID YOU KNOW . . .

Air fresheners are made from neurotoxic solvents and synthetic fragrances that can cause headaches, mood swings, memory loss, and chronic fatigue?

Prepackaged lettuce is washed in a chlorine solution twenty times more concentrated than that found in an average pool?

Mouthwash containing alcohol is associated with an increased risk of throat and mouth cancers?

The artificial sweetener aspartame breaks down into carcinogenic formaldehyde during storage in the body?

Overuse of **antibacterial soaps, detergents, and cleaners** will eventually have the same effect as overuse of antibiotics, producing resistant strains of bacteria that can't be killed?

Eyeshadow has been found to contain unsafe levels of lead, cobalt, nickel, chromium, and arsenic?

Flea and tick control products can expose people to pesticides five hundred times greater than the recommended safe limits?

Microwave popcorn contains a flavoring chemical that is a relative of paint stripper?

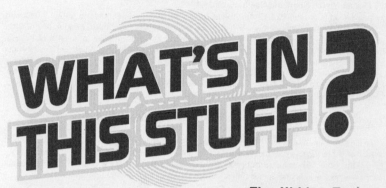

WHAT'S IN THIS STUFF?

The Hidden Toxins
in Everyday Products
and What You Can Do About Them

PATRICIA THOMAS

"In the absence of an effective regulatory system, it's increasingly important that we learn for ourselves what products to trust and what to avoid. Pat Thomas has made that job much easier. Every household should own a copy of this amazing book."
—Zac Goldsmith, Director, *The Ecologist*

A PERIGEE BOOK

A PERIGEE BOOK
Published by the Penguin Group
Penguin Group (USA) Inc.
375 Hudson Street, New York, New York 10014, USA
Penguin Group (Canada), 90 Eglinton Avenue East, Suite 700, Toronto, Ontario M4P 2Y3, Canada
(a division of Pearson Penguin Canada Inc.) • Penguin Books Ltd., 80 Strand, London WC2R 0RL,
England • Penguin Group Ireland, 25 St. Stephen's Green, Dublin 2, Ireland (a division of Penguin
Books Ltd.) • Penguin Group (Australia), 250 Camberwell Road, Camberwell, Victoria 3124, Australia
(a division of Pearson Australia Group Pty. Ltd.) • Penguin Books India Pvt. Ltd., 11 Community
Centre, Panchsheel Park, New Delhi—110 017, India • Penguin Group (NZ), 67 Apollo Drive,
Rosedale, North Shore 0632, New Zealand (a division of Pearson New Zealand Ltd.) • Penguin Books
(South Africa) (Pty.) Ltd., 24 Sturdee Avenue, Rosebank, Johannesburg 2196, South Africa

Penguin Books Ltd., Registered Offices: 80 Strand, London WC2R 0RL, England

While the author has made every effort to provide accurate telephone numbers and Internet addresses at
the time of publication, neither the publisher nor the author assumes any responsibility for errors, or for
changes that occur after publication. Further, the publisher does not have any control over and does not
assume any responsibility for author or third-party websites or their content.

First American edition: January 2008
Originally published in Great Britain in 2006 by Rodale Books International.

Library of Congress Cataloging-in-Publication Data

Thomas, Patricia, 1959–
    What's in this stuff? : the hidden toxins in everyday products and what you can do about them /
Patricia Thomas.— 1st American ed.
        p.   cm.
    "A Perigee book."
    "Originally published in Great Britain in 2006 by Rodale Books International."
    Includes bibliographical references and index.
    ISBN-13: 978-0-399-53388-4
    1. Toxicology—Popular works.   2. Food—Toxicology—Popular works.   3. Household supplies—
Toxicology—Popular works.   4. Environmental toxicology—Popular works.   I. Title.
    RA1213.T46 2008
    615.9—dc22   2007034946

PRINTED IN THE UNITED STATES OF AMERICA

10   9   8   7   6   5   4   3   2   1

PUBLISHER'S NOTE: Neither the publisher nor the author is engaged in rendering professional
advice or services to the individual reader. The ideas, procedures, and suggestions contained in this
book are not intended as a substitute for consulting with your physician. All matters regarding your
health require medical supervision. Neither the author nor the publisher shall be liable or responsible for
any loss or damage allegedly arising from any information or suggestion in this book.

Most Perigee books are available at special quantity discounts for bulk purchases for sales promotions,
premiums, fund-raising, or educational use. Special books, or book excerpts, can also be created to fit
specific needs. For details, write: Special Markets, Penguin Group (USA) Inc., 375 Hudson Street, New
York, New York 10014.

Acknowledgments

I am indebted to all the usual crowd of loved ones, especially my son Alex, who has been patient and supportive while so much was put on hold during the researching and writing of this book.

My eternal gratitude goes out to my agent and partner in crime, Laura Longrigg, for more than a decade of loving care. I am also grateful to all at Rodale, especially Anne Lawrance, who understood the need for a comprehensive look at household toxins and weren't afraid of the subject matter, and to Tom Genrich, for his contributions to the pesticide section. And to Sharyn Wong, my friend and favorite subeditor—another big thank-you.

I am also indebted to all the authors, environmentalists, toxicologists, and scientists whose work is listed in the bibliography for everything they have done in bringing the vital issue of toxic chemicals to the fore.

Finally, with more gratitude than mere words can express, I thank everyone at the world's best magazine, the *Ecologist*—especially Harry Ram, Tyler Moorhead, and Zac Goldsmith—for reeling me into an office full of amazing, inspiring, dedicated, fearless, wildly entertaining, and, above all, warmhearted people.

Contents

INTRODUCTION

We are what we eat. We are what we breathe. We are what we put on our skin. We are whatever we expose ourselves to. And because of all this, we are in trouble.

Today, cheap, mass-produced, and poorly tested chemicals are used to make many of the products we buy every day. The price you pay at the checkout may seem reasonable, but there is a hidden cost—in terms of human health and the ecology of the planet—that may be higher than any of us can imagine.

The food we eat and the products we use to clean ourselves and our homes, as well as those we use in the garden and on our pets, can contain carcinogens (cancer-causing substances), hormone-disrupting chemicals, central-nervous-system disrupters, reproductive toxins, and psychoactive chemicals (substances that alter brain function).

While many of us have gotten into the habit of scanning food labels for unwanted ingredients, it can be hard to keep up-to-date on what is safe and what is not. What's more, intelligent consumers who scan food labels for harmful additives rarely apply the same critical faculties to the other products they buy and use.

Today, scientists have grave reservations about the witches' brew of chemicals we are regularly exposed to. It's not just that the individual chemicals are harmful. New data are coming in all the time to show that mixtures of chemicals can often react in unexpected ways, or combine to produce entirely new compounds that are harmful to human health. Through such a combination of everyday foods and household products, we are conducting chemical warfare against our own bodies.

The bigger picture of chemical toxins and the threat they pose to our health can be difficult to take in—even when all the evidence is in front of you. Nevertheless, several large studies have concluded that, because of the chemicals in the products you buy, the environment inside your home may be more seriously polluted than the air outdoors, even in the largest and most industrialized cities. Considering that we spend as much as 90 percent of our time inside our homes, the health risks from these indoor pollutants are much greater than from those we encounter outside.

Many of us rely on the fact that the chemicals we use every day have been fully tested and found to be safe for humans. But the reality is that there are about seventy thousand chemicals currently in use, with one thousand new chemicals coming on the market each year. There are no basic safety data for 43 percent of all chemicals in use today, and full safety information is available for only 7 percent. Among the compounds commonly used in household products, there are full safety data for only a quarter of them.

While it is easy to assume the role of a victim and to think of environmental toxins as things we consume involuntarily, not all toxins come from "out there." Many are found in what we allow into our homes and our bodies without a second thought.

Nowadays, we ingest dozens of harmful and largely unevaluated chemicals when we eat conventionally grown produce; fertilizers, herbicides, pesticides, and fungicides all combine to make so-called fresh food a significant source of poisons. When we eat conventionally reared meats, we are ingesting growth hormones and a myriad of just-in-case medications given to conventionally farmed animals—not to mention the pesticides, herbicides, fertilizers, and fungicides contained in their feed. As the bovine spongiform encephalopathy (BSE, or mad cow disease) saga has shown us, we are also sometimes ingesting deadly microorganisms.

In addition, when manufacturers try to reassure us that potentially harmful chemicals are used only in small amounts in their products, they are glossing over some relevant facts. Each day, we are exposed to many different chemicals. For example, we don't just use a shampoo once in our lives; we use it regularly, sometimes daily, and we use it in hot showers and baths, so that the chemicals become vaporized and are absorbed in greater quantities into our bloodstream.

We also use a shampoo in combination with other products, such as conditioner, hair gel or mousse, hairspray, toothpaste, deodorant, body wash, air fresheners, and furniture polish—each of which contains "minute" amounts of the same harmful chemicals. Add up all these "minute" amounts of chemicals and the potential exposure becomes disturbingly high.

Given these facts, you may wonder how we manage to stay healthy at all. The reality is, we don't. Even though we are now living longer than ever before, we are strikingly unhealthy. Chronic conditions are on the rise. Respiratory problems, such as asthma and bronchitis, have doubled in recent years, with young people being the most affected. Vague disorders like sinusitis and allergic rhinitis are becoming major problems, especially in inner-city areas. Heart disease, diabetes, and thyroid problems are all on the rise, too. Infertility, in both men and women, is becoming more common, as are other hormonally linked disorders. Cancer continues to be a persistent disease across all cultures, age groups, and genders, with still no medical solution in sight.

This is not an encouraging picture. But what's worse is that we have allowed ourselves to believe that such unhealthy conditions are a normal part of being human and an inevitable result of aging.

There is nothing normal about disease. The human body is a robust and remarkable organism that is oriented toward survival and wellness. Without our even being aware of it, our bodies work hard every day to keep themselves in balance and to eliminate the toxic by-products of modern life. But even this most perfect automatic system can't function indefinitely without some help from its owner.

While *What's in This Stuff?* focuses on the chemical onslaught to which our bodies are subjected through the products we buy, we can't make the mistake of assuming that we buy these things in a vacuum. Often, we are coerced by high-pressure sales tactics into believing that we simply can't live without the modern conveniences of everything from bagged salad to wet wipes to antiwrinkle creams, and that our lives would be diminished without these modern miracles.

The supermarket has become one of the primary sources of such beliefs. Much has already been written about the way supermarkets have changed our diets, our communities, and our landscapes—and not always for the better. Because of their "pile it high, sell it cheap" philosophy and persuasive advertising campaigns that entice us to buy and use cheaply produced products laden with chemicals, supermarkets have also become the main pushers of most of the poisons we put into our bodies and our homes.

Supermarket shopping forces us to switch off. In fact, supermarkets actively pursue the ideal of the "switched-off consumer." By encouraging such a mind-set, the supermarket can encourage even the smartest shopper to make dumb choices over and over and over again. This book is about us switching on again, about being aware of what's for sale, of what its real value is, and of what illusions, limitations, and risks are attached to all the stuff we buy, week in and week out.

Not everything you read here will be easy to take in. Not everything you read will motivate you to change. But make no mistake. The next revolution in consumer spending is an anti-chemical revolution, as more and more of us begin to realize that there may well be a darker meaning to the phrase "shop till you drop" and begin to say no to products that contain harmful chemicals.

The premise behind *What's in This Stuff?* is simple. Readers will find, as they become more aware of the ingredients in the stuff they buy, and of the damning evidence of harm attached to some and the unacceptable uncertainties concerning the safety of many others, that these products will rapidly lose their appeal and more of us will feel able to join this revolution.

Science may be slow to deal with issues of harm and uncertainty, but this book offers a commonsense approach that anyone can implement. When you feel uncertain as to what to believe or how best to go forward, follow what is known as the precautionary principle—in other words, it's better to be safe than sorry.

Some of the alternatives included in this volume are practical and simple, whereas some require a bit of effort or a complete change of habits and lifestyle. Some may seem part of a utopian ideal, but other individuals are making them work—and so can you. As a first step, pick five or ten—or, if you're really ambitious, twenty—of the many suggestions in this book and make a commitment to doing them. The more you are able to implement the alternatives suggested here, the more noticeable and beneficial will be the changes you'll see in your day-to-day health.

If *What's in This Stuff?* has any goal at all, it is to help you, the reader, to make more healthy choices, more conscious choices, more compassionate choices, and more ecologically sound choices. In addition, the information here aims to help you feel confident about buying less and using less, and, when you do decide to put something into your shopping cart, to feel reassured that it will sustain your life rather than detract from it.

A Note to the Reader

Where the names of chemicals and additives appear in italic type, it indicates that the terms are included in the glossary at the back of the book. In addition to providing definitions for these chemicals and additives, the glossary contains information on their use in food and household products, their potential to harm your health, and their relation to other chemicals and additives, where applicable.

1. WHAT'S IN STORE?

You are about to be taken on a journey . . . and it begins in your local supermarket.

If you are like most people, supermarket shopping has become a regular part of your weekly routine. Well stocked, competitively priced, and with all the amenities laid on, these "cathedrals of modern commerce" issue a friendly and open invitation to come on in, linger, and spend.

These days, for more than 90 percent of us, a supermarket is the main or sole place of shopping; and the weekly excursion to the supermarket is a central event in our lives. And as much as weekly shopping is a chore, it has also become a ritual—and, for some families, the only weekly outing together.

Clever advertising and marketing help to paint a picture of the supermarket as a place you can go to fulfill all your needs to excess cheaply and regularly. The supermarket has become positioned in our minds as a necessary part of life, as part of the extended family, and as able to respond to all our needs and desires.

Yet, while supermarkets promote themselves as helpful friends, the relationship is not one of equals. Supermarkets are powerful "friends" that have become so central to our lives that we are barely aware of the power they wield over us, how they direct and limit our shopping choices and disconnect us from the origins of the things we buy. Many of us are completely unaware of how they shape and destroy communities by closing down local shops and establishments, how they change the physical landscape of the places where we live, and how they pollute the environment, including our homes and bodies.

The Big Weekly Shopping Trip

Bringing home life's essentials has always been a challenge. Certainly, these days we don't have to dodge tigers and bears to put food on the table, and the majority of us in the West don't have to walk miles to meet our other daily needs, such as obtaining clean water, or to rely on what food we can grow ourselves. Nevertheless, providing for a family is still complicated, and sometimes just plain hard work.

In the modern world, the task is made even more difficult by the fact that we have drastically altered our idea of what is necessary. These days, most families' lists of basic requirements—most of which need to be purchased somewhere— have become unmanageably large. The larger the list gets, the more urgent the need becomes to find a way of getting the things we want quickly, easily, and cheaply. The alternative—buying what we need at a succession of specialty shops, such as butchers, bakers, greengrocers, shoe and clothing shops, hardware stores and liquor stores—seems unthinkable and old-fashioned.

Enter the Modern Supermarket

While much has been made of the way supermarkets have changed how we eat, their influence stretches well beyond food consumption. Consumption of all kinds has expanded, thanks to the convenience factor of today's supermarkets, which provide an all-encompassing, one-stop solution to meeting our "basic" needs. In addition to food and drink, most supermarkets now sell a huge variety of nonfood items—and, at the biggest superstores, you can outfit your entire home in one trip. Surveys show that, in a typical supermarket, you can now buy:

- alcoholic beverages
- baby foods and products
- beauty products
- bed linens and towels
- breakfast cereals
- car-care products
- cell phones

- cleaning products
- clothing and footwear
- computer and small-office goods
- confectionery
- dairy products
- diet foods
- dry cleaning

- DVDs, CDs, and videos
- electrical items (from toasters to freezers)
- feminine hygiene products
- flowers
- frozen foods
- fruits and vegetables
- greeting cards and stationery
- housewares
- international money orders and wire-transfer services
- lottery tickets
- luggage
- meat
- medicines and first-aid items

- newspapers, books, and magazines
- nonalcoholic beverages, such as juice, mixers, and water
- personal financial products (including mortgages, credit cards, and savings accounts)
- personal hygiene and grooming products
- pet foods and products
- photo processing
- snacks
- toys and games
- travel goods
- video rentals
- vitamins

The goal of the supermarket is simple: to encourage customers to buy more of these things and more often. And several aspects of our weekly shopping experience help them accomplish this objective.

First is the clarion call of good value. In most supermarkets, there are regular announcements and product advertisements to guide shoppers to special offers. The promise of permanently low prices, bargains, buy-one-get-one-free and three-for-two offers, blue light specials, and discount days are all designed to give the impression that we are saving money with every item we buy.

But giant supermarket chains sell little more than the illusion of value, wrapped up in the seductive creed of convenience. Over and over again, studies have shown that—from fruit and vegetables to the Sunday roast—smaller, independent local shops can offer much better value. At the supermarket, only a few key items are sold at value prices, while the store maintains a huge profit margin on everything else, especially household goods, over-the-counter drugs, and DVDs.

With so many goods in store, supermarkets make a huge effort to make us linger. As you walk down the aisles, strategically placed lighting creates an atmosphere of warmth, soothing music plays in the background, tempting scents waft through the air, and brightly colored product displays entice you to pause, reach out, and put yet another item into the cart.

In addition, the more facilities a supermarket has, the more time we spend there. Play areas for children mean moms can browse the aisles at a more leisurely pace. One-hour photo-processing counters can double the time you might otherwise spend pushing your cart around, and cafés invite you to linger over coffee before or after you shop.

Whatever your approach to supermarket shopping—whether you go in with a list and get only what you want, or float along the aisles browsing, picking items up out of interest and inspiration—the big weekly shopping trip is an investment of both time and effort.

Whatever we choose to believe before we enter the supermarket, and however seductive the process of cruising the aisles is, reality hits hard at the checkout, where long lines and the final total make us realize that, for all the ads reassuring us that food is cheaper than ever, the weekly shopping trip still takes a huge bite out of our monthly income.

Another persuasive factor is the illusion of control. The more a supermarket

The Expanding Shopping Cart

Shopping cart sizes have grown exponentially over the last thirty years. Consumer advocate Ralph Nader was the first to notice the growing-shopping-cart phenomenon, offering it as a prime example of how consumers are manipulated by the system. Bigger carts, he said, served the straightforward purpose of shaming consumers into making bigger purchases.

Other explanations have been put forward to explain the expanding-cart phenomenon—for instance, changes in women's lives. As more and more women chose to work, trips to the supermarket went from every one or two days to once a week. This led to the tendency to buy more per (less frequent) trip.

As supermarkets have grown, the width of their aisles has grown with them— and once you have the wide aisles, you might as well have the bigger carts.

Whatever the reason, today's average shopping cart is almost three times as large as its 1975 counterpart. It's also used for much more than just putting things in. New high-tech carts are being designed with display screens that will allow shoppers to scan items as they shop, show the purchase price of each item, and keep a running tally of what they have spent.

These new "smart carts" can advertise specials appropriate to whatever aisle you are in and can even remind regular customers of what they might have forgotten. And it's here that privacy issues emerge: once a shopper logs on to the shopping cart, it can make suggestions based on previous visits to the supermarket. So, is it a time-saver, a brainwasher, or Big Brother on wheels?

stocks, the more it invites you to spend time there, to ponder and make comparisons and choices. Thus, shopping requires decision-making abilities—do you go to the fresh-foods aisle first, or get the heavy stuff like canned goods and bottles first? It also requires perseverance—for instance, to push along a cart that has a mind of its own and to endure the long lines at the checkout—and a sense of adventure. For some, finding a parking space as near to the door as possible has become a point of principle.

The supermarket also represents freedom of choice, although, in reality, the choice is limited to what the supermarket is willing to offer. Ironically, studies show that no matter how we approach weekly shopping, most of us reach the checkout with the same basic goods in our shopping carts. That's because, along with the illusion of value, supermarkets can only ever offer the pretense of choice.

Witness the six-foot-wide display of toothbrushes found in most supermarkets. There is no basic difference in the way these brushes function. But by presenting them to shoppers in a range of sizes, shapes, colors, and bristle strengths, supermarkets create the illusion of personal choice and control.

Once again, the reality is rather different. Most of the brands we buy are largely interchangeable. Whatever your heart may tell you, your head knows that, apart from the packaging style and occasionally the price, there are no major differences between the ten brands of laundry detergent on the shelf, or the twelve brands of toothpaste, the twenty varieties of shampoo, or the six brands of potato chips. But, by pricing some higher than others, they can also claim to offer luxury.

This democratization of luxury is another important aspect to the allure of the supermarket. When we shop in a supermarket, we enter a world of beautifully displayed luxury items, of shelves continually stocked to give the impression of plenty. The supermarket also flatters us that it is classless: everyone gets to spend time there, and is temporarily freed from the limitations of geography and season. Even if you live in the middle of a large city, you have access to fresh produce, and even if you live in the North Atlantic, you can still have fresh mango for breakfast.

How Supermarket Shopping Changes Us

Our increasingly hectic lifestyles are having a major impact on the goods we choose to buy. We want our food to be fast, our cleaners to be spray-and-wipe, and our toiletries to be wash-and-go.

Many of our day-to-day decisions are made on the basis of what's convenient at the time or in the immediate future. If something is quick, easy, and painless, we are far more apt to do it than if it requires forethought, the weighing of options, planning, and effort.

Today, entire industries are built around the objective of making life simpler, easier, and more efficient, and the convenience credo now dominates many facets of our lives—from how much sleep we get to our personal-hygiene habits, what we might eat for lunch or dinner on any given day, and how we choose to raise our children.

In the name of convenience, we now buy things because we desire them, not because we need them. Retail therapy has become an increasingly common way to counter stress and dissatisfaction in our lives. Seemingly unnecessary commodities are given value by their perceived ability to make life happier and easier, to solve problems, and/or to change the customer into a more desirable person. Through shopping, we actively seek magic-bullet solutions to the most insignificant human dilemmas—everything from the occasional upset stomach or pimple to the disinclination to peel and chop a carrot or mend a hole in a sock ourselves.

The enormity of the dissatisfaction we feel with our lives has helped turn markets into supermarkets, and supermarkets into superstores. By piling it high and selling it cheap, these edifices distract us from what should be the central point of supermarket shopping—to provide healthy food for the family and a safe, effective means of meeting life's other demands, such as cleaning, child and pet care, and gardening.

We now buy and use—and throw away—more goods than ever before. Frivolous and highly packaged goods—like microwave popcorn or the latest cheap T-shirt with a novelty image or slogan on it—bring short-term satisfaction and are then tossed away when they are no longer novel or fashionable, or convenient. As a result, the majority of us are buying more products than ever before, and living increasingly wasteful and overburdened lives.

Sometimes, the price we pay is just more money, but, increasingly, science is showing us that the true cost of supermarket convenience can be marked out in incremental declines in human health and well-being, and the poisoning of the environment.

Convenience at a Price

When we buy into the convenience culture, we buy into a whole set of values and ways of life that, for the most part, remain hidden beneath the glitz, the democratized luxury, and the hard sell. The convenience culture is a one-dimensional way of living, devoid of spiritual or otherworldly concerns. It encourages us to be lazy, to live beyond our means, to overindulge and spoil ourselves and our children, to ignore our pasts, and to block out all thoughts of the future.

Like the wider consumer culture of which it is a part, it celebrates the body but is not attentive to its true needs. Thus, we can satisfy our hunger with microwaveable meals and never once concern ourselves with the fact that this "food" contains nothing that actually nourishes the body. Likewise, we can attack the signs of aging with antiwrinkle creams and never once think about what it is about our lives and lifestyles that is making us look and feel so old and tired.

Let's consider just some of the fallout from a convenience culture. It can, for instance:

- **Skew our values.** We no longer expect excellence. We expect things to break, we expect them to fail, we expect them to disappoint, and we expect claims for them to be exaggerated.

- **Discourage discernment.** We take all the advertising and manufacturers' claims for products at face value.

- **Disempower the individual.** We forget how to do things for ourselves; we have lost the ability to make value judgments that go beyond price and convenience when we shop.

- **Cause us to abdicate responsibility.** When things go wrong or we get sick, we blame others rather than ourselves. A litigation culture is an offshoot of a convenience culture.

- **Change our social interactions.** We are more likely to talk to each other about the stuff we buy than about what we are feeling, or our thoughts or spiritual concerns. In addition, we no longer communicate with the people who make, supply, or even sell the products we buy.

- **Make us lose basic skills.** These days, many people don't know how to make basic repairs around the house, and can't sew or mend clothing. Some younger people don't know how to prepare or cook fresh foods.

- **Waste resources.** Convenience goods are highly packaged, so you pay for and throw away packaging made from nonsustainable and often toxic materials.

- **Encourage overconsumption.** We buy things in bigger "value packs," use more than we need to get the job done, eat more than we need to be nourished, and/or throw away whatever we can't use.

- **Encourage a "live for today" attitude.** Too many consumers have stopped asking questions about goods, such as where they come from, who made them, and what they are made of. Living for today fails to protect us as well as our future generations.

These things impact every individual, but there are global consequences as well. Convenience consumerism is in and of itself wasteful, and increased levels of waste and industrial pollutants in our water, air, and food are the inevitable by-products of our love affair with this increasingly unsustainable way of life.

Manufacturers are more than happy to meet our demands for cheap goods. To meet our price expectations and keep their profit margins high, they inevitably make or grow these products somewhere else—usually in developing countries—and then fly them halfway across the world. The resulting air miles cause considerable environmental pollution and drain depleted petroleum reserves. They promote a system of unfair trade and low wages for workers while taking work away from local areas. When it comes to food, intensive farming practices to speed up the journey from farm to table mean an increased use of pesticides, flirtations with unsafe technologies to create GM (genetically modified) foods, increased productivity at a cost to animal health, and unsafe eggs, meat, and fish.

The Human Cost

There are many ways in which we humans are hoist by our own petard by the convenience culture. For instance, according to Harvard researchers in 2004, cheap convenience foods are the driving force behind the rising rates of obesity in the West. Partly based on food diaries kept by the study's participants, a surprising picture emerged of American eating habits. People are not consuming any more calories at mealtimes than they did twenty years ago, but they have nearly doubled their consumption of calories from snacks and sodas between meals.

Food companies, seeking an outlet for the glut of cereals and other raw food-stuffs in the 1980s and 1990s, developed literally hundreds of new products that increased the demand for food beyond previously imagined levels. The industry took advantage of the burgeoning science of chemical flavoring, and new technologies for processing and preserving foods, to create high-fat, high-sugar, and high-taste foods. In just a few years, processed foods grew cheaper, more convenient, and, more important, tastier.

At the same time, snacking was legitimized as American culture celebrated the practice of "grazing" as a supposedly healthful alternative to heavy meals at mealtime.

Some could reason that the convenience and pleasure of snack foods is worth carrying a few extra pounds, but, of course, obesity carries with it a high risk of developing type 2 (non-insulin-dependent) diabetes, hypertension, heart disease, and other serious illnesses, such as cancer.

The results from this Harvard study could easily have come from Britain or Australia or anywhere else where the free market rules the food industry, where regulatory systems are lax and allow almost any amount of additives to be put into foods, and where snacking, and, as a result, obesity, are on the rise.

While changes in agricultural and manufacturing processes and in consumer habits are the most obvious examples of the problems of a convenience-obsessed society, examples abound from every corner of the marketplace.

Just half a century ago life was very different. Our milk was delivered in bottles by the milkman, we wrapped our lunches in waxed paper, and we cooked our food in cast-iron skillets. When it rained we donned rubber boots, coats, and hats. Today, we buy ready-made meals and snacks in plastic boxes that can be popped in the microwave. To help spread the heat and keep food from sticking at high temperatures, fast-food containers are often lined with nonbiodegradable Teflon. On rainy days we slip on coats coated with Gore-Tex—a relative of Teflon—to help keep us comfortable and dry.

The common thread running through all these things is man-made chemicals. Most convenience goods are mass-produced, and the ability of manufacturers to make vast quantities of identical goods at dirt-cheap prices has increased enormously since the end of World War II. Since that time, manufacturers have created, overproduced, and then looked for new uses for a glut of waste chemicals, including organochlorines, plastics, and other petroleum-derived substances.

Many of these chemicals were the result of wartime research and development. When the war ended, the dovetailing of excess production of these substances with the spirit of enterprise and a desire to expand our personal horizons created an unprecedented appetite for the selling and consuming of "stuff."

The advantage of the chemical society is that these cheap industrial chemicals can be used to produce cheap everyday goods. Added to food, they give us ready meals that can be made a long time in advance and stocked on the shelves for ages. In cosmetics, they promise professional results without ever stepping inside a salon or spa. And why call an exterminator when you can buy a spray can of powerful insecticide at the supermarket that will make the bugs go away? Our cars are now lighter, cheaper, and more energy-efficient because they are made from an astonishing array of metals and plastics. At night, we can pull dinner out of the refrigerator in plastic containers that can go straight from the freezer to the microwave without cracking or burning.

The chemical advances that have made these things possible may, on the one hand, seem miraculous. But every one of these products has a carry-over effect on our health since their use increases our exposure to potentially toxic chemicals. For instance:

• Around 90 percent of us are carrying trace amounts of a chemical called perfluorooctanoic acid (PFOA) in our blood. That's because PFOA or its by-products are used in the making of Teflon and Gore-Tex, and can be released from products with stainproof coatings, such as those treated with Scotchgard or Stainmaster carpet. PFOA is an industrial chemical, and, in 2006, the U.S. Environmental Protection Agency (EPA) recommended that it be classified as a potential human carcinogen. PFOA has also been shown to be toxic to the kidneys, while, in animals, it causes reproductive problems and growth retardation.

- Numerous studies have shown that a commonly used ingredient in plastic called *bisphenol A* causes abnormal pregnancy in mice and could cause reproductive problems in people, too.

- Likewise, studies have found that polybrominated diphenyl ether (PBDE), a flame retardant used in TV sets, computer circuit boards and casings, foams, and fabrics is rapidly accumulating in the breast milk of women in Sweden and the United States. The chemical has been shown to cause thyroid cancer and neurodevelopmental problems in test animals.

These are by no means the first examples of innovative new technologies we've taken and run with, only to find out years later that we've unwittingly been endangering ourselves as well as our planet.

The pesticide *DDT* was touted as revolutionary in the 1940s before it became apparent that it caused the eggshells of predatory birds, such as the bald eagle, to become too thin, lowering their numbers dramatically. Soon after, DDT was found to cause cancer in humans and is now banned in most developed countries. *Chlorofluorocarbons*, or CFCs, were prized for their chemical stability until scientists discovered they eroded the ozone layer. *Polychlorinated biphenyls*, or PCBs, were the darling of manufacturers until their toxicity to people and wildlife became evident.

At the dawn of the twenty-first century, the question many are asking is whether the short-term convenience we gain from all these new materials is worth the trouble they cause us in the long run. We also need to ask whether the time has come to insist upon more stringent testing rules to avert future human and environmental catastrophes.

Quick Fixes

The wide availability of convenient prepackaged foods and other quick fixes is something that most of us believe makes our lives a little easier. Science is only too happy to oblige us in our pursuit of such things. So if you want to get a jump on your day, you can now use soap with caffeine in it, which is absorbed into your skin as you wash. Soon, it may even be possible to fix sugar cravings with a shampoo that sends chemicals to your brain to mimic the effects of a sugar rush. It's only a matter of time before cigarette companies start putting vitamin C or calcium in cigarettes so that you can get your vitamins while destroying your—and other people's—lungs.

Buying convenience goods has become such an ingrained habit for most of us that we can't imagine life without them. Most of us never really question whether such goods are good for us, whether they actually save us significant amounts of time, or what impact they may have on our health or our planet over the longer term.

Some innovations, such as vacuum cleaners and washing machines, do genuinely save us hours of backbreaking work. Imagining life without them is almost impossible. But along with these devices are thousands of false conveniences that we buy into every day without thinking. Thanks to clever marketing, we have genuinely come to believe that the mere seconds we save by buying prepackaged lettuce or pregrated cheese buy us even more extra time to live better, fuller lives.

In your heart of hearts, you know this isn't true, and, what's more, every convenience item you buy or use has a hidden cost. Sometimes you are simply paying more, but often the cost is to your own health and well-being, and to the environment. Consider the true cost of some well-known convenience and quick-fix items, and, whenever you can, try to get out of the quick-fix habit.

ITEM/QUICK FIX	TRUE COST	TRY THIS INSTEAD
Air fresheners Cover up bad smells	• Effect is temporary • Made from neurotoxic solvents and synthetic fragrances that can cause headaches, mood swings, memory loss, and depression • Strong perfumes trigger asthma and allergies • Spray varieties contain ozone-depleting propellants	• Open a window • Don't smoke in the house (in fact, don't smoke at all!) • Use a ventilator when cooking • Keep bathroom surfaces clean and dry
Aspartame Allows you to consume sweet foods without consuming calories	• Breaks down into carcinogenic formaldehyde during storage and in the body • Other breakdown products—such as phenylalanine and aspartic acid—damage and destroy brain cells • Women, children, and those with poor immune function are particularly vulnerable to its effects • According to the U.S. FDA, common adverse effects from regular use of aspartame include headaches, memory loss, skin rashes, seizures, heart palpitations, disorientation, dizziness, hives, joint pain, sore throat, and impaired vision	• Use the real thing, but use it less often—sugar only contains 15 calories per teaspoon

continues on following page . . .

ITEM/QUICK FIX	TRUE COST	TRY THIS INSTEAD

Dryer sheets / fabric softeners
Soften clothes and eliminate static cling
	• Surfactants in dryer sheets can irritate skin
	• Contain more synthetic fragrance chemicals than any other household item, including:
	  –*benzyl acetate*, linked to pancreatic cancer
	  –*benzyl alcohol*, an upper-respiratory-tract irritant
	  –*ethanol*, linked to central-nervous-system disorders
	  –*limonene*, a known carcinogen
	  –*alpha-terpineol*, can cause respiratory problems and central-nervous-system damage
	  –*ethyl acetate*, a narcotic
	  –*camphor*, causes central-nervous-system disorders
	  –*chloroform*, a neurotoxin, anesthetic, and carcinogen
	  –*linalool*, a narcotic that causes central-nervous-system disorders
	• Heated in the dryer, they release toxic vapors onto clothes and into the air
	• Scents used in fabric softeners are designed to stay in your clothing for long periods of time; when you wear "softened" clothes, your body heat helps to release chemicals into the air for you to inhale and onto your skin for you to absorb
		• Add baking soda to your wash cycle *or*
		• Add vinegar to your wash cycle (don't add both)

Microwave popcorn Tasty popcorn in a jiffy	• Artificial butter flavoring is made from a caustic chemical, diacetyl, a relative of paint stripper • Heating diacetyl produces vapors that irritate the skin, eyes, mucous membranes, and respiratory tract • Long-term exposure to diacetyl can permanently damage your airways • Packaging is lined with Teflon, which releases lung-damaging and cancer-causing microparticles into the air when heated • Many brands of microwave popcorn contain tartrazine (FD&C Yellow No. 5), a synthetic dye linked to hyperactivity, asthma, and other health problems	• Use an air popper and add real butter

ITEM/QUICK FIX	TRUE COST	TRY THIS INSTEAD
Prepackaged lettuce You don't have to cut the lettuce yourself	• More expensive than a regular head of lettuce • Standards are improving, but some brands are washed in a chlorine solution twenty times more concentrated than in the average swimming pool—to prevent deterioration • Ingesting chlorine raises the risk of liver, kidney, heart, and neurological damage, is harmful to unborn children, and is a trigger for cancer • Chlorine destroys the taste of the leaf • Bacteria on lettuce become resistant to chlorine so washed lettuce can still contain virulent strains of *Listeria* and E. coli • Packed in modified-atmosphere packaging (MAP), in which normal levels of oxygen and carbon dioxide are altered to maintain the appearance of freshness • MAP destroys many vital nutrients, such as vitamins C and E, polyphenols, and other micronutrients	• Buy a fresh head of lettuce and tear it up yourself
Standby electronics Your computer, TV, DVD player are ready to use at any time	• Pump millions of tons of carbon into the atmosphere each year • Electrical goods on standby in all the G8 nations waste the equivalent of the electricity generated by twenty power stations each year • Many appliances use as much power on standby as when turned on • Accelerate climate change • Can add as much as $350 a year to your energy bills	• Unplug electrical items when not in use • Buy products that allow you to choose whether or not you will use a standby function
Wet wipes A quick wash without water	• Once opened, they are a breeding ground for bacteria • Contain lots of preservatives and antibacterial ingredients that can cause skin rashes and encourage bacterial resistance • Detergents and perfumes can also irritate the skin, especially as they are not washed off • Made from plastic, cellulose, and polyester fibers, so are not biodegradable	• Use soap and water • Carry a washcloth in a plastic bag for a quick wipe when with kids • See also p. 160

continues on following page . . .

ITEM/QUICK FIX	TRUE COST	TRY THIS INSTEAD
	• Highly perfumed, so can cause neurotoxic effects, such as headaches, agitation, forgetfulness, mood swings, depression • Chemicals can be transferred to food during cooking and eating	

Supermarkets as Sources of Mass Poisonings

Most of us are so busy with the challenge of getting the shopping done that we never stop to analyze what's actually in our carts. And because we buy so much from the supermarket, it has become the most significant source of pollutants in our homes. This may seem an incredible statement, yet, as subsequent chapters will show, almost all the toxic chemicals we are exposed to on a daily basis—solvents, aerosols, food additives, plastics, pesticides, heavy metals, GM organisms, and antibiotics—are brought home from the supermarket. The true extent to which our bodies have become polluted by these man-made chemicals is shocking, and the effects of living with a polluted body are wide-ranging.

Many of us are so used to feeling below par that we no longer even question why we suffer from regular headaches, stomachaches, skin rashes, pain, fatigue, breathing problems, or poor memories. "That's life," we say, as we pop another pill or eat something or turn up the plug-in air freshener a notch and carry on regardless.

Throughout the world, supermarket shoppers have become part of an unregulated experiment that involves the buying and consumption of a whole range of toxic and contaminated products.

Supermarkets may have revolutionized certain aspects of our lives, but most people, when encouraged to dig deeper and to ask questions about the direction this revolution has taken, find that they cannot shop in supermarkets with the same level of enthusiasm and blind faith they once did. There are just too many unanswered questions related to the pollution of our bodies and our planet, the destruction of genuine communities, and the poor quality of food and other goods purchased in supermarkets to feel as easy as we once did, pushing our supersized shopping carts up and down the aisles.

Is There a Way Out?

Our lives may have been made somewhat more convenient by the chemical revolution, but they have also been made inexorably more complicated, too. The more goods we buy, the more government controls are necessary to regulate those goods. Agencies are established and overseen by the government to regulate and supervise economic activity, and to protect the consumer from exploitation and health damage from other sources, but also from ourselves.

The more government agencies there are involved in the regulation of commercial goods, the more manufacturers spend on lobbying and influencing regulators to keep their goods on the shelf. The more lobbying that goes on, the more corruption there is, and the more corruption there is, the greater the need for consumer groups and whistle-blowers to guard the guards.

Historically, in the West, a risk-benefit analysis—that is, assessing whether the potential benefits of a new technology outweigh the potential risks—has been the yardstick, and most businesses still evaluate their products on this basis.

But consumer advocates are increasingly turning toward a theory that is both more sophisticated and more simple. It's known as the precautionary principle. This is based on the notion of the *Vorsorgeprinzip*, literally "the forecaring principle," which emerged in Germany when laws were enacted to save forests by reducing the power-plant emissions causing acid rain. It was considered an act of forecaring, or precaution, because, at the time, there wasn't 100 percent scientific certainty that power-plant emissions were in fact the cause of acid rain.

The concept was defined in 1998 as: "When an activity raises threats of harm to human health or the environment, precautionary measures should be taken even if some cause-and-effect relationships are not fully established scientifically."

In ordinary language: better safe than sorry.

The precautionary principle doesn't mean that we have to go back to living in the Stone Age, but it does provide regulators—and ordinary people—with a framework that encourages them to act before disaster strikes and so avoid what could be called the "ooops! factor"—which we so often experience when a product that has been on sale for years is suddenly found to cause widespread and irreversible damage to human health.

By applying the precautionary principle to your own life, you can also avoid the "ooops! factor" linked to so many of the products we buy and use on a regular basis.

New Ways to Shop

If you believe that supermarket shopping is just the way things are, then you have been seduced into believing in a world where maximizing the production and consumption of goods is the only worthy goal. We all have the power to do something different. We can rethink weekly shopping, and rethink what we buy and why we buy it. We can begin to change the way we shop to reduce our exposure to toxic chemicals, to make an investment in our local areas, to ensure we are getting more nutrients per mouthful, and even to spend less.

It's all too easy to point the finger of blame at supermarkets for their misleading advertising and abuse of power, and at industry for polluting the planet. Such things are a given. But as consumers, we are also part of the problem. Our thoughtless demands for more throwaway stuff—plastic containers, aerosol sprays, wet wipes, and ready-made everything—are damaging the planet and adding to the pollution. If we stopped buying unnecessary stuff, there would be no reason for manufacturers to produce it, and without public demand, the convenience culture would collapse. You have the power to change things. If you are ready to apply the brakes on a toxic modern lifestyle that is accelerating out of control, consider taking these first simple steps.

Buy less. We buy and eat too much food; we buy and often use only half of too many toiletries and cosmetics; we buy too much stuff for babies in the belief that the investment in wipes and plastic toys makes us good parents. Get off the treadmill; ignore all those two-for-one offers that supermarkets use to offload products they have a surfeit of. Think about what you really need, about what is essential to your life, and stick to that.

Reuse, repair, recycle. Sometime after World War II, the concept of doing without, making do, and sticking to the necessities became practically unpatriotic, and somewhere along the way the personal freedom that had been fought for got confused with the freedom to buy things, to have things, to show off the things to others and be envied for them. As a result, many of the skills that sustained our forefathers fell out of fashion. It's not just that we don't know how to build our own barns or grow our own food anymore. Many of us don't know how to repair clothing or make a meal from scratch or fix a clogged drain. Frugality, too, has gone out of fashion, but, in a world rapidly running out of resources, it's time to resurrect it.

Shop locally. It can be hard to shop if you have no local retailers or a car but, remember, supermarkets are the reason for this, and the way most of us shop these days has fostered the demise of the local shopkeeper. There are plenty of online stores you can now order quality food from. Farmers' markets are popping up in more places, and organic farms make weekly deliveries. Now's the time to ask yourself: How well do I know my local area? Are there people who offer goods and services that I can and should be taking advantage of? And if there are, use them.

Forget brand loyalty. When you are buying food or toiletries, brand loyalty may mean that you are getting poor value for money, and you may even be exposing yourself to more chemicals than you have to. By learning to read labels and make comparisons, you will find that there is often little difference between brands, that cheaper brands are just as good, and that there are low-chemical options for almost everything you buy.

Voluntary simplicity. Many of the toxins we encounter every day are the result of our unbridled consumerism, so choose not to buy into this unhealthy addiction. The fact is, the less stuff you have in your life, the less likely you are to come into contact with environmental toxins.

If you only use the microwave to heat up coffee or bake potatoes, perhaps the time has come to get rid of this significant source of radiation in your home altogether. If you declutter your home, chances are you will not need so many plastic boxes to store things, thereby reducing the amount of *formaldehyde* gas in the air. Likewise, if you use fewer cosmetics, toiletries, air fresheners, and harsh household cleaners, you will be lowering your exposure to solvents and other volatile organic chemicals (VOCs), as well as environmental hormone mimics.

Cultivating simplicity in your life is not some vague hippie ideal. These days, it requires an iron will to resist advertising pressure to buy more stuff and consume more than you need. Dig down deep and see if you can find that will in yourself.

2. NOT EVERYTHING GIVES YOU CANCER . . . BUT LOTS OF THINGS DO

It would be easy, while reading this book, to believe that it's simply not safe for any of us to live in the modern world. Conclusive evidence that our chemicalized society is damaging our health is accumulating rapidly, and if we don't take action to protect ourselves, the prospect of living long and healthy lives gets slimmer with each and every compromise we make in the name of convenience and quick fixes.

Even in the face of all the evidence, those who shine a light on the problems associated with environmental chemical exposure and who advise caution are often derided or portrayed as scaremongers or killjoys. They are continually challenged with objections along the lines of, "Well, everything gives you cancer these days, doesn't it?" or "Why worry when I could get hit by a bus tomorrow?"

Yes, you could get hit by a bus tomorrow. But would you deliberately throw yourself in front of that bus? Not making the effort to understand which toxins you are exposing yourself to every day is very much like throwing yourself in the path of an oncoming vehicle. You know that it's coming, you know that it will harm you, and you know that doing nothing to get out of the way is an act of profound irresponsibility to yourself, your family, and all those whom you love and who love you.

Not everything gives you cancer, but a great many things do. Indeed, according to the U.S. National Toxicology Program, around two hundred chemicals encountered every day are either known or potential human carcinogens. There is no established safe dose for any carcinogen, so why are we continually surprised when cancer rates soar? In the same vein, not everything causes infertility or birth defects or dementia or migraines or allergies, but many hundreds of chemicals that we encounter every day do—and again, it is hardly surprising to see rates of these conditions rising rapidly among the general population. Why invite these risks into your home if you have the power to keep them out?

How Polluted Are You?

It is impossible to say how many different chemicals we each carry in our bodies. This is because beyond the chemicals that are added to food or used as drugs, there is no requirement for manufacturers to disclose how their chemicals are used or to keep track of the various routes through which people may be exposed. Neither are they required to understand the fate of their chemicals in the environment, to measure concentrations of their products in either the environment or people, or to develop and share methods of analysis that would allow other scientists to gather this kind of information independently.

In the largest study of chemical exposure ever conducted on humans, the U.S. Centers for Disease Control and Prevention (CDC) showed that most American children and adults are carrying in their bodies more than one hundred substances that aren't supposed to be there, including pesticides and the toxic compounds used in everyday consumer products, many of them linked to potential health hazards.

Many toxicologists and environmental scientists reviewing the report expressed grave concerns that in studies of animals and, in some cases, of people, most of these compounds could affect the brain, hormonal balance, the reproductive system or immune system, or were linked to cancer.

The report documented the fact that many children are carrying much higher levels of these chemicals than adults. These include *pyrethroids*, which are found in virtually every household pesticide, and *phthalates*, plasticizers that are found in nail polish and other beauty products, as well as in soft plastics.

Throughout the world, the phenomenon of polluted people is becoming more commonplace. For instance, to reveal more about how much toxic material we carry around in our bodies, the World Wildlife Foundation (WWF) environmental group conducted a series of blood tests on people from all walks of life in the U.K. In 2003, they tested the blood of individuals across the country and found an average of twenty-seven chemicals in every one of them. These compounds included such long-banned chemicals as the organochlorine pesticide DDT (dichloro-diphenyl-trichloroethane), and PCBs from old electrical equipment and building materials, as well as more common chemicals found in such everyday materials as paints, glues, toys, electrical goods, furniture, carpets, and clothing.

The following year, they tested the blood of environment ministers from thirteen European Union countries and found a total of fifty-five different chemicals in the ministers' blood. The lowest number of chemicals found in any one minister's body was thirty-three and the highest was forty-three. These chemicals were pollutants commonly found in sofas, pizza boxes, and pesticides.

Most recently, in 2005, the WWF tested the blood of a handful of British celebrities and found, on average, twenty-four chemicals in each one. The chemicals they found included DDT and PCBs, brominated flame retardants found in furniture and electrical equipment, phthalates found in perfumes, cosmetics, and flexible plastics, perfluorinated chemicals found in the Teflon used on nonstick pans and Scotchgard used for stainproofing.

In 2005, a Canada-wide study by the group Environmental Defence tested for a broad range of chemicals in average Canadians and found toxic chemicals such as DDT, PCBs, stain repellents, flame retardants, mercury, and lead in every person sampled.

What these unique surveys show is that no matter where you live, you are unlikely to be able to avoid the kind of chemical exposure that can lead to chemical overload.

Total Body Load

As research in the field of chemical exposure has advanced, two pivotal concepts have emerged: the total body load and the low-dose effect. Essentially, these measures allow scientists to study and determine how much of any given chemical we carry in our bodies, and the level at which this is likely to be harmful.

Many of the chemicals we are exposed to each day are persistent—that is, instead of breaking down, they remain intact, and dangerous, in the environment and in our bodies for years, even decades. Small regular doses can and do build up to health-harming levels over time.

Scientists refer to the accumulation of such chemicals as an individual's body burden or total body load—the consequence of lifelong exposure to industrial chemicals used in thousands of consumer products and that linger on as contaminants in our air, water, food, and soil.

These chemicals come from household products like detergents, cosmetics, fabric treatments, and paints, as well as upholstery, computers, and TVs. They accumulate in the fat, blood, and organs, or are passed out of the body via breast milk, urine, feces, sweat, semen, hair, and nails. Over time, if the total body load is high, the likelihood of the body breaking down under the weight of it becomes higher.

Quiz

Your Total Body Load

It's not always easy to gauge what your daily exposure to toxic chemicals is. Take this simple quiz to help you get an idea of how much you might be carrying in your body.

About You

____ Do you have children?

____ Are you a woman?

____ Are you of retirement age?

____ Do you work with chemicals?

____ Do you have pets?

About the Products You Buy

____ Do you read and understand the ingredients labels on the products you buy?

____ Is the greater proportion of your diet made up of preprepared or convenience foods?

____ Do you buy your cleaning products at the supermarket, hardware stores, or other mainstream outlets?

____ Do you regularly use air fresheners?

____ Do you use bleach in your laundry?

____ Do you use fragranced household cleaners and cosmetics?

____ Do you use disinfectants or antibacterial products?

____ Do you use a commercial oven cleaner?

____ Do you use commercial carpet cleaners?

____ Do you use mainstream commercial bath, tile, and toilet cleaners?

___ Do you store a number of partially used cleaning products from commercial sources under your kitchen sink?

___ Does your furniture polish say "flammable"? Do you spray a commercial dusting product?

___ For all-purpose cleaning, do you use a mainstream commercial product?

About Your Health

___ Are you sensitive to chemicals, car fumes, odors, perfumes, or fragrances?

___ As you get older, are you becoming increasingly sensitive to caffeine, alcohol, or medications?

___ Do you have bad reactions to *monosodium glutamate* (MSG); foods containing sulphites, such as wine and dried fruit; salad-bar food; beverages that contain caffeine; or diet sodas?

___ Do you suffer from fibromyalgia (widespread musculoskeletal pain and fatigue), chronic fatigue syndrome (CFS), cancer, or an autoimmune disease?

___ Do you have acne, eczema, hives, or unexplained itching?

___ Do you suffer from fatigue, lethargy, joint pain, muscle ache, or weakness?

___ Are you subject to irritability, mood swings, anxiety, depression, poor concentration, a "spaced-out" feeling, or restlessness?

___ Do you get headaches, a stuffy nose, frequent sinus infections, or allergies?

___ Do you suffer from nausea, bad breath, foul-smelling stools, a bloated feeling, or intolerance to fatty or starchy foods?

___ Do you keep getting sick "for no reason"?

___ Do you drink more than two alcoholic beverages a day?

___ Do you use over-the-counter, prescription, or recreational drugs on a regular basis?

If you answered yes to five or more of these questions, you may be exposing yourself to harmful chemicals on a regular basis, and these may be building up in your body. Follow the advice in this book to help you decrease your total body load.

Small Doses, Big Effects

The low-dose effect suggests that even small doses of certain chemicals can have big repercussions on health in both the short and long term. What constitutes a low dose is not always clear, although it's generally defined as a dose much lower than would normally be expected to have an effect.

The idea that small doses can have big effects is beginning to receive a great deal of serious attention from scientists throughout the world, some of whom have found that chemicals in amounts as diluted as only a few parts per trillion (ppt) can have profound biological effects. Worryingly, these low-dose effects are often seen at levels well below those that have been deemed safe by regulatory authorities.

This phenomenon has been particularly well researched in the field of hormone disruption, where even minute quantities of different estrogen mimics present in the environment can produce an effect on the body that is many times greater than would be expected.

For instance:

- **Phthalates.** Extremely low levels of these estrogen-like chemicals can be found in most everyday items, including soft toys, plastic water bottles, household paints, toiletries, and perfumes. Studies link phthalates to sperm damage in men, and reproductive abnormalities, asthma, and allergies in children.

- **Bisphenol A.** Minuscule doses of this compound, which is used in polycarbonate plastic baby bottles, in resins that line food cans, and in dental sealants, have been found to cause health effects at levels twenty-five hundred times lower than the EPA's "lowest observed effect" dose. Exposure to low levels of bisphenol A can alter brain structure, neurochemistry, behavior, reproduction, and immune responses in animals.

- **Atrazine.** This weed killer unbalances a number of hormones necessary for the normal development and functioning of the reproductive system, including estrogen, prolactin, luteinizing hormone, and follicle-stimulating hormone. It has been linked to gross sexual malformations in frogs that were exposed to water containing just 1/30 of the concentrations that the EPA regards as safe for use in drinking water.

There are several reasons why low doses can be dangerous. One is that some people are simply more sensitive than others to some chemicals. Allergy specialists understand this problem well. If a person becomes sensitized to an allergen—for example, peanuts or cat dander—then exposure to even the tiniest amounts can set off a dramatic reaction. In chemically sensitive individuals, exposure to even small amounts of certain chemicals may be all that is required to start their health spiraling downward.

The timing of an exposure is also influential. With many chemicals, a low dose to a baby in the womb or during childhood can produce potentially much more serious toxic effects than similar exposures as an adult. Good examples of this can be seen with the heavy metals lead and mercury, where low-dose exposures in utero and during infancy cause permanent brain and nervous system damage, while the same doses appear to have no observable effects in adults. Similar problems have been found with exposure to certain pesticides in babies and infants.

The Cocktail Effect

Another way that low doses of chemicals can become dangerous is through what is known variously as synergy, the cocktail effect, or the additive effect.

This happens when two toxic, or potentially toxic, chemicals are combined either in a product or in the human body, and produce a toxic effect much greater than would be predicted by the sum of their individual effects.

As with low-dose effects, most of the research into synergy has so far centered on the cocktail effect of hormone-disrupting chemicals. British research published in the journal *Environmental Health Perspectives* in 2002 found that combinations of minute levels of eleven environmental estrogens, including genistein (one of the main estrogens in soy), resorcinol monobenzoate (a protective coating commonly found on plastic items, such as computer mice, sunglasses, hearing aids, and ballpoint pens), phenyl salicylate (a sunscreen agent), and bisphenol A had more than double the estrogenic effect on living cells than would have otherwise been predicted.

While the number of estrogen mimics—"xenoestrogens," or estrogens produced outside the body—used in this study may seem high, it's worth remembering that most of us are exposed to many more than this number each day simply through household products, cosmetics, and toiletries. It's also worth bearing in mind that estrogen in amounts higher than those naturally produced by the body can cause cancer.

The authors concluded: "Considered in isolation, the contribution of individual environmental estrogens, at the concentrations found in wildlife and human tissues, will always be small. However, such reasoning cannot be used to support claims of negligible health risks from weak xenoestrogens, because the number of xenoestrogens present in wildlife and humans is unknown but likely to be very large . . . by not taking combination effects into account, significant underestimations of the effects associated with exposure to xenoestrogens are likely."

This kind of synergy occurs with many different classes of chemicals and, in the real world, we are exposed to multiple chemicals every day. Yet, such chemicals as food additives, pesticides, and cosmetic ingredients are still tested for safety in the laboratory one at a time, with no allowance being made for cocktail effects.

The effects of synergistic interactions are not widely reported in the press, so many consumers remain unaware of the dangers of exposure to more than one chemical at a time. The notion is hardly new, however. In the 1960s and early 1970s, Dr. Samuel Epstein, then with the Children's Cancer Research Foundation in Boston, and Dr. Keiji Fujii, with the National Institute of Hygienic Sciences in Tokyo, published a series of papers highlighting the increased carcinogenicity of everyday pesticides used in combination, even at very low levels, or when applied as far apart as two hundred days. Epstein has since gone on to become the chairman of the Cancer Prevention Coalition, and is a recognized expert in the way chemicals in everyday products can harm health.

Most of us, however, only became aware of the idea of the cocktail effect after the Gulf War, when soldiers who returned from their tours of duty complained of numerous chronic illnesses. Gulf War soldiers were given an extraordinary mixture of drugs in preparation for life in the region, and the interactions among these compounds was the suspected cause of a range of health problems, especially the abnormal neurological function experienced by so many veterans.

Animal research has suggested that this suspicion is correct. Researchers at Duke University Medical Center and Texas Southwestern Medical School reported in 1996 that the simultaneous exposure to the topical insecticides *DEET* (N,N-diethyl-meta-toluamide) and *permethrin*, and pyridostigmine bromide, a drug taken as a prophylaxis (just in case) against toxic gas-warfare agents, can cause nervous-system damage in chickens.

The researchers found that the many symptoms experienced by Gulf War veterans, including headaches, fatigue, muscle aches, decreased attention, and rashes, were similar to the symptoms seen in exposed chickens.

Chickens given any two chemicals became lethargic, unable to fly, lost weight and their coordination, and demonstrated tremors. For those administered all three chemicals, paralysis and death were common outcomes.

Because of the inadequacies of chemical testing, we have little concrete knowledge of the way the cocktail of chemicals we are exposed to each day will impact our bodies and/or minds. The failure of regulatory authorities to acknowledge and allow for the synergism that occurs within just a single product, or in the human body due to exposure to several chemicals at once, is one of the greatest failures of modern health regulation.

3. HOW YOUR BODY REACTS

Our bodies are miraculous. In spite of all the man-made pollutants we are exposed to each day, we seem to stay healthy—at least in the short term. This is because our bodies are equipped with numerous biological mechanisms that aid the process of defending and repairing our cells, tissues, and organs.

These mechanisms work quietly in the background minute by minute and day by day. Skin, for example, is the largest excretory organ in the body. It helps to rid the body of toxins through sweat. It also protects us from dehydration and from external temperature variations. The immune system protects us from foreign bodies, such as bacteria, that can make us ill. The kidneys eliminate waste products; the liver detoxifies the blood; the respiratory system enriches the blood with oxygen as well as filters out irritants and toxins.

There are, however, limits to what the body can do without support, and certain lifestyle factors can make it considerably harder for the body to provide 24/7 protection. For example, a person may be eating foods laced with pesticides or to which they are sensitive; exposing themselves daily to chemical toxins in the home or office; allowing emotional and psychological stress to build up; not be exercising regularly; not getting enough sleep; not allowing themselves to recover fully from illness before going back to work; taking too many painkillers; drinking too much; and smoking cigarettes. This person's body is overloaded and will eventually break down.

Who Is Vulnerable?

Each of us has some vulnerability or weakness that makes exposure to toxic chemicals risky. Some of these weaknesses are mediated by gender or age. Women, the very young, and the elderly are, for instance, much more likely to experience health problems from daily exposure to toxic chemicals and pollutants. Other types of vulnerability are genetic; if you have symptoms of illnesses that run in your family, you may have this kind of constitutional weakness.

Where you fall on the socioeconomic ladder is another factor. Lack of education and a very low income can often dovetail with lifestyle risk factors, such as excess alcohol intake, broken families, inadequate diet, older housing with lead paint and aging water pipes, drug abuse, smoking, and exposure to industrial pollution, as well as inadequate prenatal health care and high rates of bottle-feeding babies with artificial milk. This means that the poorest urban populations are already at the highest risk of health and behavioral problems. Adding exposure to toxic chemicals to the mix can often quickly tip these people over into ill health.

The relatively affluent should not consider themselves immune to toxic effects, however. Our consumer-oriented society encourages us to buy and use a wide range of products that contain toxic chemicals, endocrine disrupters, and heavy metals, all of which can cause similar health problems in the longer term.

All of us are vulnerable to a greater or lesser extent. The unique vulnerability of children is discussed in chapter 4. Nevertheless, there are some things that make women and the elderly more likely to be harmed by exposure to toxic chemicals.

It's Different for Girls

Women are more likely to use a greater number of toxic products while carrying out everyday grooming and household cleaning. Many women also work in jobs that expose them to toxic substances. This higher rate of exposure is one significant reason why women are more likely to suffer health problems from chemical exposures.

As is the case with children, women tend to have smaller body frames, so their exposure per pound of body weight will also be greater than men's. In addition, women naturally carry more body fat than men and, as many toxic substances are stored in fat, this means that women carry potentially more toxins in their bodies.

Once again, trends in health and behavior tell us something about how women are likely to be affected by these toxins. Rates of such disorders as diabetes, arthritis, and systemic lupus erythematosus (SLE, or lupus) are rising, as are such reproductive disorders as endometriosis, polycystic ovarian syndrome (PCOS), and infertility.

Many cancers, including those of the breast, endometrium (lining of the womb), lungs, and skin are becoming more common in women, too. Because cancer is a multifactorial disease, it can be difficult to pinpoint its origins. But an examination into the rise in once-rare cancers, such as non-Hodgkin's lymphoma (NHL), may shed an entirely different light on the subject.

The term "non-Hodgkin's lymphoma" is a catchall phrase used to cover several different cancers that develop from the lymphatic system, a complex network of tissues and organs that runs throughout the entire body. Scientists admit that they are baffled by the steady rise of this immune-system cancer, which now accounts for around 3 percent of all cancers. Yet, in the last twenty years, the incidence of NHL has increased by about 73 percent. A large proportion of that increase occurred between 1973 and 1987, when the incidence of NHL rose by a massive 51 percent. Most victims are women.

To understand how important the link is between toxins and immune-system cancer, it is helpful to know that the primary function of the lymphatic system is to clear debris and help defend the body. A cornerstone of the immune system, the lymphatic system is made up of fine vessels that branch out like veins into all parts of the body and carry lymph, a watery colorless fluid, to the lymph nodes—small bean-shaped nodules found in clusters in the neck, armpits, pelvis, and abdomen. The lymph nodes produce infection-fighting cells, such as lymphocytes and antibodies, and also act like a filter and drain, sifting out foreign matter into the lymph fluid.

A number of significant associations between NHL and solvent exposure have been reported in the medical literature. In 1976, the accidental release of large quantities of poisonous industrial by-products called *dioxins* in Seveso, Italy, resulted in the exposure of more than five thousand local residents. Follow-up studies revealed elevated rates of NHL and soft-tissue sarcomas—cancers of the muscle, fat, blood vessels, or any of the other tissues that support, surround, and protect the organs—among exposed individuals.

But chemicals such as those used in everyday pesticides are also implicated in raising the risk of NHL by 50 percent or more. One investigation by the U.S. National Cancer Institute (NCI) in 1986 found that farmers who used the pesticide *2,4-D*—a common ingredient in garden "weed and feed" products—on more than twenty days a year were six times more likely to develop NHL compared with unexposed persons. Another found that people who frequently mixed or used herbicides themselves were eight times more likely to develop this type of cancer.

Increased exposure to PCBs (polychlorinated biphenyls; found in flame retardants, plastics, and insulation materials, as well as in some detergents, hairspray, and other personal-care items) has also been linked to the continuing rise in NHL. Similarly, those exposed to the flame retardant tetra-BDE (bromodiphenyl ether), such as professional car, bus, and truck drivers, are also at an increased risk (and it's important to note that this same flame retardant is used in all vehicles).

NHL, however, is not just an occupational hazard. Women who use hair dye (particularly dark brown, black, and red) may be increasing their risk of rare cancers, including NHL and multiple myeloma (a progressive blood disease), by anywhere from two to four times over nonusers.

Rare cancers, of course, are not the only effect of toxic exposures. Women are also at greater risk of menstrual disorders, mood swings, headaches, allergies, and chronic fatigue. Women, of course, also have the responsibility of bearing children, and decades of research show that a woman's fertility can be affected by pollution. Should she conceive, her child's level of health will be largely dependent on her own. Many of the environmental illnesses that children suffer from have their roots in toxic exposures in prenatal life—in other words, in the womb.

The Elderly at Risk

There are a number of reasons why older people may be at an increased risk from environmental toxins. Natural aging, for instance, involves decreases in bone mass and blood flow through the heart, and diminished pancreatic, thyroid, and lymphatic functioning. These changes make the body less effective at clearing toxins. Other factors that can add to the risk include:

- A lifetime of environmental stress, which can lead to increased stress hormones, such as corticosteroids, that, in turn, can lead to immune suppression and a diminished healing capacity.

- The accumulation of free-radical damage, cellular "garbage," and DNA damage due to environmental toxins, which can result in mutations that make cells less resilient and more prone to disease.

- The development of such diseases as atherosclerosis (clogged arteries) that prevent the elderly from exercising regularly and staying active, which then has the subsequent effect of exacerbating any other health problems they may have.

It is also widely acknowledged that the elderly are generally overmedicated. Doctors who prescribe unnecessary drugs to the elderly are not only compromising these patients' health, but also adding to the toxic burden of their bodies. Even more worrisome, some medications and environmental toxins interact with each other, making their individual effects on the body even more powerful (see "The Cocktail Effect," page 28).

What to Look For

Because everyone is different, the first symptoms of toxic exposure in some may be in the digestive system, whereas for others it may be the skin or immune system. Others may get headaches, mood swings, or symptoms of depression when exposed to certain chemicals.

Certain conditions—such as pregnancy or breast-feeding, or if you're trying to conceive—and particular illnesses can also make you more susceptible than others to the adverse effects of toxic chemicals. If any of the following conditions apply to you, you may find that lowering the total toxic load on your body may be beneficial for your health in both the short and long term:

- constant tiredness, chronic fatigue syndrome

- autoimmune diseases, such as osteoarthritis, diabetes, multiple sclerosis

- a family history of cancers

- respiratory problems, such as asthma or chronic bronchitis

- sinusitis or hay fever

- frequent colds or susceptibility to flu

- watery, itchy eyes or eyes that produce excess mucus

- skin problems, such as dermatitis or eczema

- regular headaches or migraines

- mental symptoms, such as depression

- menstrual problems, such as PMS, irregular periods, and anovulatory cycles

- parasitic infestations

- overweight or underweight

Most of us would not automatically look for chemical causes of these conditions, but, while no one is suggesting that chemical overload is the sole cause of such problems, it cannot be ruled out as a contributing factor. What's more, diseases that do not appear to respond to conventional treatment often do respond once your environment and your body are cleared of toxins.

Taking a look at some of these conditions in greater depth may help to clarify the role of chemical exposure in your day-to-day health.

Stress

Feeling stressed is a common experience of modern life. Most of us equate stress with the physical and emotional experiences of everyday life. But, as humans have evolved, so have our sources of stress. Today, we can come under physical, chemical, electromagnetic, nutritional, traumatic, and even psychospiritual stress—and, in all cases, the body's reaction is the same.

The body does not differentiate between emotional and environmental stress. Anything that threatens to unbalance or harm the body can trigger our primitive fight-or-flight responses and trigger the release of a flood of stress hormones.

In the right proportions, stress hormones help to keep our bodies healthy; too much or too little of them, and they become a form of slow poison, depressing our immune systems and leading to a staggering list of stress-related disorders, including:

- allergies
- anorexia nervosa
- arthritis
- asthma
- atherosclerosis
- cancer
- constipation
- depression
- diabetes
- diarrhea
- eczema
- fatigue
- headaches
- high blood pressure
- indigestion

- infections
- insomnia
- irritability
- irritable bowel syndrome
- loss of appetite
- muscle tension
- neck and back pain
- nutritional deficiencies
- peptic ulcer
- premenstrual symptoms
- psoriasis
- psychological problems
- sexual problems
- weight changes

Stress, whatever its origin, can also follow a circular pathway. For instance, physical stress can lead to emotional stress and vice versa. Whatever the origin, a stressed-out body is simply less able to deal with poisons in the environment, and, therefore, is one that may be more likely to become overwhelmed and less efficient at defending and repairing itself.

Chronic Fatigue Syndrome

When a person has chronic fatigue syndrome (CFS), several body systems are affected. These include the immune, the endocrine, the hematological (responsible for the formation of new red blood cells), and the nervous systems.

Severe fatigue is the most common symptom of CFS. In some cases, it can be so overwhelming that just minor exertion, such as a short walk or light housework, can be debilitating. While many sufferers try to curtail their normal daily activities and rest more, this doesn't appear to help.

CFS produces other symptoms as well, including headaches, low-grade fever, swollen lymph nodes, sore throat, depression, poor concentration and decreased mental acuity, muscle and joint aches and pains, allergies, digestive complaints, weight loss, and skin rashes.

Mental and emotional symptoms are also common. CFS sufferers often have trouble remembering specific names or places, or doing complex mental work, such as bookkeeping, administrative tasks, or teaching.

Many CFS sufferers have a history of extreme and prolonged emotional stress, anxiety and depression, and a history of poor nutritional habits, which are thought to contribute to the disease. But environmental pollutants and contaminants are also thought to play a significant role. The body, having been run down, becomes much more susceptible to the viruses known to trigger CFS.

Perhaps not surprisingly, given their higher rate of chemical exposure and increased vulnerability, 70 percent of CFS sufferers are women.

Autoimmune Diseases

Chemical overload and autoimmune diseases often go hand in hand. A good example of this is the role that toxic exposures and allergic reactions often play in the development of arthritis. Studies where arthritis patients have been exposed to various pollutants, such as natural gas, car exhausts, perfume, hairspray, insecticides, and tobacco smoke, have shown a clear link between such exposure and the worsening of symptoms.

Likewise, there is good evidence to show that the autoimmune disease systemic lupus erythematosus (SLE) can be made worse by *fluoride*. Lupus is a connective tissue disorder, and connective tissue is around 30 percent collagen. Fluoride, which is added to water supplies in many places and to most commercial toothpastes, disrupts the synthesis of collagen and leads to its breakdown in skin, muscle, tendons, ligaments, bone, lungs, kidneys, cartilage, and elsewhere.

While we have always assumed that diabetes, another common autoimmune disorder, is linked solely to diet, this may not be the case. There is evidence that exposure to pesticides during pregnancy may raise a child's risk of developing juvenile diabetes. Such findings have opened the door to the possibility that other types of chemical exposure may also be contributing factors to both juvenile and late-onset diabetes.

Most recently, exposure to small amounts of bisphenol A have been shown to increase the risk of diabetes. This synthetic plasticizer is used to make dental sealants, sturdy microwavable plastics, linings for metal food and beverage containers, and baby bottles—to name but a few products. Bisphenol A can leach into food and water from these products, and, not surprisingly, it's widely found in human blood. In animals, repeated exposure over several days provoked insulin resistance, a prediabetic state in which tissues lose their sensitivity to normal levels of insulin.

Cancer

Cancer rates are on the rise. In the U.K., the number of cases diagnosed each year has increased by a massive 50 percent in the last twenty-five years. Researchers say it's not just because the population is getting older, or because we are getting better at detecting the disease in its early stages. So why is this happening?

Cancer doesn't just suddenly appear. It is generated in two steps: initiation and promotion. The initiation process is what triggers the development of cancer. This is the factor(s) that interacts with cellular DNA to start the process of producing abnormal cells. Initiators can be carcinogens, viruses, radiation, oxygen, and cell-destroying free radicals and hormones, particularly estrogens.

While none of your daily exposures to these toxins may be significant on their own, added together their action is cumulative, challenging the immune system and damaging cells over a long period of time until, eventually, cancer develops.

Many of the ingredients in consumer products—volatile organic compounds (VOCs) and solvents, surfactants, formaldehyde, nitrosamines, plastics, and preservatives—can act as initiators either because they are directly cancer-causing or because they disrupt hormonal or other normal bodily functions.

Several lifestyle factors can also become disease-causing agents, working away silently for years and damaging body cells. For instance, a low-fiber diet means that waste products remain in the gut longer than they should, giving the body ample time to absorb more toxins. Toxins in the body can interrupt the process of cellular repair and cause cells to replicate too quickly or to mutate.

After initiation, the disease may lie dormant for many years until something comes along that signals it to grow. Promoters, which cause the disease to develop, are factors that damage the body's defense mechanisms. Promoters may also alter body tissues, predisposing them to cancer growth. A diet that is high in fat can make toxic chemicals much more efficient promoters. This is because chemicals can accumulate in fatty tissues, from where they can leach back into the body, causing continual damage and, eventually, the development of disease.

Because cancer can lie dormant for many years before it begins to grow and spread, it can be difficult to link it conclusively with toxic exposures. Nevertheless, when cancer clusters (large numbers of people in one area with the same type of cancer) appear, environmental factors, such as toxic exposure, are always the leading suspects. It is estimated that between 10 and 30 percent of cancers are the result of regular exposure to toxic chemicals.

Asthma and Allergies

An allergy is a response to something the body identifies as foreign or toxic. Around 15 to 20 percent of the population experience significant allergic reactions to consumer products.

Asthma is an extreme allergic response. It can be triggered by a variety of stimuli, the nature of which varies from individual to individual. Upper-respiratory-tract infections, either viral or bacterial, can often trigger an asthmatic attack. Changes in weather or temperature, exposure to molds, animal dander, grass, or tree pollens may all be triggers for asthmatics, and so are the preservatives, fragrances, and colorings used in prepackaged foods, cosmetics, toiletries, and household cleaners.

Fragrances in particular are major triggers for asthma attacks, with around 70 percent of asthmatics reporting that exposure to perfumes can worsen their condition. Other chemical triggers include the formaldehyde used in such products as medicated shampoos, germicidal soaps, mouthwashes, and toothpastes. The solvents commonly found in toiletries and household cleaners can also cause respiratory problems.

Often, the triggers for such reactions can remain undetected for years, only revealing themselves as toxins when they are taken out of the diet or environment and the body is given a chance to recover and repair itself.

Skin Disorders

Rashes and other disorders of the skin now constitute a frequent complaint in the GP's office. Commonly reported problems range from simple hives to more complicated conditions, such as eczema and psoriasis.

The skin is the largest organ in the body and performs many life-sustaining functions. It is a physical barrier that protects us from harmful organisms in our environment, but it is also a major organ of excretion. Skin reactions are commonly localized reactions to something that has come into contact with the skin. But they can also be the result of the body trying to rid itself of circulating toxins deep within the body.

The fragrance portion of toiletries and cleaning products is responsible for a large percentage of skin reactions. Other chemicals are also implicated, however. These include preservatives, detergents, and antibacterial agents.

While the skin does act as a barrier, it can be easily breached by harsh chemicals that dissolve the protective oils lying on the surface of the skin, thereby allowing toxins to be more easily absorbed into the bloodstream. Many substances, such as solvents, perfumes, preservatives, fatty acids, and other emollients and nanoparticles, actually aid the absorption of other, more harmful chemicals into the body. These agents are known as penetration enhancers (see chapter 6). Skin permeability is also increased by heat, such as when taking a hot bath or shower.

Headaches

If you get headaches regularly, it is likely because your body is under some kind of stress. In fact, the most common type of headache is the tension headache. While we often dismiss such headaches as the result of emotional stress, they are also likely to be the result of biological stress—due to food allergies or exposure to pollutants and toxins. Migraines are more complex, but also respond remarkably well to the removal of allergens and synthetic chemicals from the environment.

Research into migraines shows that fragrances are a common trigger. This is because scents can breach the blood-brain barrier and gain direct access to the central nervous system. Many other chemicals, such as solvents and propellants, which are so prevalent in toiletries and household products, also affect the central nervous and vascular systems, and are implicated in chronic headaches.

Research shows that pregnant women who frequently use aerosol products, such as air fresheners, deodorants, furniture polishes, and hairsprays, have significantly higher rates of headaches and postnatal depression compared with those who use these products less than once a week.

Depression

There is some evidence that environmental pollutants can both cause and exacerbate depression and other emotional problems. The chemicals known to trigger depression include solvents, VOCs, and endocrine-disrupting chemicals. The fragrances used in perfumes, toiletries, and household cleaners contain many of these substances and, not surprisingly, are often implicated in mood swings and emotional problems.

Many environmental practitioners have had good results in relieving depression by putting mild to moderately depressed patients on chemical-free regimes. Once patients begin to limit their exposure to compounds like fragrances, they often then find it easier to recognize when a particular chemical ingredient or fragrance has triggered a depressive episode.

Depression also has a circular link with immunity. Depressed immune function—often a result of toxic overload—can affect mood. Likewise, a depressed mood can lead to impaired immune function, resulting in a vicious circle of poor mental and emotional health. Similarly, hormone disruption can also be a factor in depression.

Infertility and Reproductive Problems

Many of the chemicals in everyday products are hormone-disrupting. Often, they mimic the effects of estrogen in the body. While women (and men) need estrogen to remain healthy, too much of this hormone has profound effects on our well-being, and on our sexual and reproductive health, as well as being a known risk factor for estrogen-dependent cancers of the breast, ovary, endometrium, and prostate.

Much of what we know about the influence of everyday toxins on fertility comes from research into those who work with these chemicals every day. A Canadian study, published in the *Journal of the American Medical Association*, showed that women who work with organic solvents—such as artists, graphic designers, laboratory technicians, veterinary technicians, cleaners, factory workers, office workers, and chemists—have a greatly increased risk of both miscarriage and of giving birth to premature, low-birth-weight, or damaged babies compared with women who aren't so exposed.

Hairdressers and others who work in the beauty industry are also exposed to these kinds of organic solvents. And again, they have much higher rates of infertility, miscarriage, and babies with birth defects than women who are not exposed to these chemicals every day.

These kinds of solvents are not restricted to the workplace. They are also commonly used in cleaning products, toiletries, and paints. Pregnant women who live near petrochemical factories also experience more threatened abortions, toxemia (toxic spread of an infection via the bloodstream), anemia, nausea, and vomiting.

A man's fertility can also be affected by chemical exposures. Men who work in jobs that bring them into regular contact with pesticides and toxic chemicals are more likely to father children with birth defects. Such men often bring residues from their work home with them on their clothes and hair, and in their semen, increasing their partners' exposure to these toxins as well.

Hormone-disrupting chemicals that find their way into the food chain are now believed to be responsible for the global decline in sperm counts. Some twenty different toxic chemicals with the potential to harm sperm quality and production have been found in studies of sperm quality. In contrast, there is evidence suggesting that men who eat organic foods have sperm counts that are twice as high as those who don't.

Finally, studies show that more than 350 man-made toxic chemicals are being passed on to babies in increasing amounts through such pathways as the placenta. Unlike adults, a developing baby is very sensitive to changes in the supply of nutrients and the presence of poisons.

Eating Disorders

Both obesity and weight-loss disorders have been linked to toxins in the body. Continual ingestion of toxins can, for instance, produce nutritional deficiencies, particularly in zinc. Several studies show that zinc deficiency is a contributing factor to weight-loss disorders, such as anorexia. Hormone disruption may also cause weight-loss disorders.

One German review concluded that distorted hormonal patterns are often found in young women before the onset of anorexia. Other researchers have found that one reason why bulimics report feeling uncomfortably full after eating may be irregularities in the hormonal process that regulates fluid volume in the body. Where this hormonal disruption comes from, and whether it begins at a young age with exposure to everyday toxins, may be useful avenues of research in coming years.

Similarly, some experts believe that obesity can be a response to accumulated toxins in the body. This may be due to the way toxins can alter thyroid function, making it more sluggish and unable to respond to the energy intake of the body.

It may also be because some of the most harmful toxins are absorbed by the body and stored in fat, however. As a rule, the body doesn't like to allow the concentration of potentially harmful substances to rise too high, and will excrete them if it can. If for some reason the body cannot excrete them, however, or cannot excrete them quickly enough, the body's other option is to "dilute" the toxins by storing them in fat cells. Under these circumstances, fat becomes the body's way of controlling and preventing high levels of toxins from circulating around the body.

During weight loss, as we lose fat we release toxins into the body. This may be why some dieters feel so unwell when they begin a weight-loss regime. To protect your body from the release of toxins while dieting, you need to ensure a greater intake of water and fiber, and of the antioxidant nutrients, such as vitamins C and E, beta-carotene, selenium, and zinc.

Another way in which the body attempts to dilute toxins is through the accumulation of water. Those who feel that their extra weight is the result of water retention may also benefit from a sensible detoxification program.

Making Changes

Few of us have the choice of living in an unpolluted environment. City dwellers are often obliged to travel and live in places where pollution from cars and factories is a fact of life. In fact, many of us work and live in buildings so full of chemicals that they have come to be known as sick buildings. Good evidence shows that many of the substances that we come into contact with each day are causing a health crisis in our bodies, and it behooves us to do what we can to reduce our exposure whenever and wherever we can.

Because they tend to bypass our conscious awareness, environmental and other stressors that are not emotional or psychological in nature are arguably the most harmful to our health. But, in a body overwhelmed by environmental poisons, the usual recommendations, such as relaxation and exercise, may no longer be enough to completely counteract the effects of stress.

To cope with environmental stress, you need to be aware of the environment and to understand how it affects you even when you are not immediately aware of these effects. Once you know the particular sources of your environmental stress, you can begin to make positive changes in your home and in your regular routines. The first step is to remove as many chemical pollutants as you can from your everyday activities.

Other supportive steps include:

Improve your diet. Little changes can make a big difference. Switch to organic foods when you can, and make sure your diet includes lots of fresh fruit and vegetables. Fresh produce contains those important nutrients called antioxidants, which help to correct the damage caused by pollutants. In addition, the water-soluble fiber in these foods can help eliminate accumulated toxins. A diet that is low in saturated fat will also keep toxins from accumulating in the body. Try to choose oily fish over red meat whenever possible, as the essential fatty acids in mackerel, trout, salmon, herring, and sardines can also help fight the effects of chemical exposure in the body.

Exercise regularly. Our bodies are designed to be used. When we don't use them to their optimal extent, muscles deteriorate, metabolism becomes sluggish, and breathing becomes shallow. For these reasons, it is desirable to develop good, sensible habits of exercise—whether they are aerobic routines, an active lifestyle, or weight training—that you can easily incorporate into your life for the rest of your life.

Studies also show that regular aerobic exercise can help detoxify the body, so choose two or three activities that you really enjoy and work these into your schedule each week. Aerobic exercise—or anything that makes you sweat (such as a regular sauna)—is particularly useful for boosting metabolism and aiding the release of toxins through the skin.

Investigate stress relief. The state of your body often reflects the state of your mind. Too much stress depletes the body of nutrients needed to fight the effects of pollution. Any activity that absorbs you completely and allows you to switch off can be useful in lowering stress levels. Activities that involve deep breathing, however, such as yoga or meditation, can be very relaxing as well as promote the release of toxins via the lungs. Any activity that relaxes you will also have a positive effect on your immune system, helping it to function more efficiently.

Have regular massage. Consider booking an appointment for regular massage. It's relaxing and can improve the movement of blood and lymph through the body, encouraging the removal of toxins, cell regeneration, and better all-round circulation.

Try hydrotherapy. Water in all its states helps to purify the body. Try a relaxing bath with cider vinegar; add Epsom or sea salts to stimulate the skin to release toxins. Invest in a home whirlpool for your bath. Or, if you belong to a health club with a steam sauna, make regular use of it.

Use plant power. A two-year study by NASA scientists suggests that the most sophisticated pollution-absorbing device in your home is a potted plant. Living, green, and flowering plants have an amazing ability to remove several toxic chemicals, including formaldehyde, *benzene*, and carbon monoxide from the air. You can use plants in your home or office to improve the quality of the air as well as to make it a more pleasant place to live and work, where people feel better, perform better, and enjoy life more.

The fifteen most effective houseplants for this job are: English ivy, spider plant, golden pothos, peace lily, Chinese evergreen, bamboo or reed palm, snake plant, heartleaf philodendron, selloum or elephant-ear philodendron, red-edged *Dracaena*, cornstalk *Dracaena*, Janet Craig *Dracaena*, Warneck *Dracaena*, and weeping fig.

Use food therapy. There are some simple kitchen cupboard solutions to help you combat everyday toxins. For instance, all leafy, dark-green vegetables, but especially cruciferous vegetables (belonging to the cabbage family), can inhibit the carcinogenic effects of chemicals. So, include plenty of kale, spinach, broccoli, and brussels sprouts in your diet. (See page 363 for an extended list of foods that fight toxic damage.) Other foods are helpful, too:

- The pectin found in apple and pear seeds can protect your body from damage by toxic metals. These work by blocking the absorption of toxins while aiding detoxification. Try making apples or pears, stewed with their seeds, a regular part of your diet.

- Garlic and onions contain powerful antioxidants that aid the body's natural day-to-day efforts to detox. Use these liberally in cooking.

- Peas, beans, and lentils also contain special antioxidants. They are also high in fiber that can bind to toxins and aid their excretion from the body. Legumes are a good alternative source of protein, so why not substitute a couple of meat meals each week for one based on (organic) legumes.

- Bananas have been shown to have antioxidant qualities.

- Eggs protect against lead and mercury contamination.

- A high-fiber diet in general is useful for trapping toxins and assisting in the elimination of heavy metals. Consider adding water-soluble, mucilaginous fibers, such as psyllium seeds and flaxseeds, to your diet. These can be ground up and added to cereals, soups, and baked foods.

- Seaweeds and alginates can also bind to heavy metals. There is evidence, for instance, that the freshwater green algae chlorella can draw persistent chemicals, such as PCBs, out of the system.

Learn to breathe properly (and preferably in a clean environment). Most of us breathe in a shallow, inefficient way high into the chest. This reduces oxygen consumption and denies the benefits of breathing. When the breath is shallow, we not only don't take in enough oxygen, but we also don't get rid of enough carbon dioxide. As a result, our bodies become oxygen-starved, allowing toxins to build up. In addition, shallow breathing fails to exercise the lungs and so reduces their ability to function optimally, creating a vicious circle of lost vitality.

The kind of deep-breathing practices found in yoga, for example, draw air into the very bottom of the lungs, helping to clear the lungs and bloodstream of toxic buildup. Studies also show that breathing deeply is more relaxing, and so lowers levels of stress hormones and encourages the immune system to work more efficiently. Getting more oxygen into the lungs is reputed to have the added effect of improving the function of your eliminatory organs, such as the liver and kidneys, as well as your digestive tract. Oxygen-rich blood also feeds the nervous system, in particular the brain, which requires three times more oxygen to work properly than other organs in the body.

Kick the habit. Excess use of tobacco products, alcohol, and caffeine wreak havoc on your body. They also encourage toxic damage. Smoking exposes you to cadmium and carcinogenic *polycyclic aromatic hydrocarbons* (PAHs). Alcohol can alter immune and endocrine functions, and is poisonous to your internal organs—specifically your liver. In this day and age, no one needs to justify advice to cut down. Too much caffeine dehydrates the body, and a dehydrated body is less able to function properly to fight off infection and the effects of toxic exposures.

4. ESPECIALLY FOR PARENTS

Most parents know that the greatest gift they can give their children is good health. Once upon a time, this may have seemed like a simple matter of putting a roof over their heads, making sure they had a good winter coat, and giving them decent food. The rest, parents may have reasoned, was up to chance, genetics, or Divine intervention.

Today, life is more complex. We live in a polluted world surrounded daily by hundreds of man-made toxins that we can't see, taste, or even smell, but that nevertheless have the potential to damage human health. When we go to the supermarket, we buy "fresh" foods that are covered with pesticides and not really fresh at all. Instead, they have been stored for long periods of time, during which time they have been sprayed with even more chemicals to maintain the appearance of freshness. As our schedules get busier, we rely more and more on convenience foods laced with additives, flavorings, colors, and aromas, all of which can cause a variety of health problems.

While it may appear that, in spite of all this, our children are being born alive and well, a closer look at infant health trends says otherwise.

Children Are More Vulnerable

Children are uniquely vulnerable to environmental pollution, in part because their response to toxic exposure is often very different from that of adults. Good examples of this are the paradoxical responses to phenobarbital and methylphenidate (Ritalin) in children compared with adults. Phenobarbital acts like a sedative in adults, but produces hyperactivity in children; Ritalin, a cocainelike drug, is used as an anti-hyperactivity drug in children, but has a stimulant effect in grown-ups.

There are many reasons for this paradoxical response, but perhaps the most influential is that in the womb and during the first two years after birth, children undergo extraordinary cell growth in every part of their bodies, from brain neurons to immune cells, so there are more disruptive opportunities for toxic compounds. During childhood, different systems and organs develop at different rates and in different phases. Growing tissue is also much more sensitive to toxic exposure than other tissues, and remains sensitive right through to the teen years. Indeed, studies of exposure to cigarette smoke have shown that the risk of dying of breast cancer is greater for those who started smoking before the age of sixteen than for those who started smoking after the age of twenty.

In addition to growing and developing, children differ from adults in a number of other ways that can increase their susceptibility to toxins. For example:

• Their systems have a less-developed ability to break down toxic substances and their bodies may also have less capacity to repair any damage as well.

• They eat, drink, and breathe in more for their weight than adults, which means they take in more toxins per pound than grown-ups—in fact, even at rest, an infant breathes in twice the volume of air as an adult does.

• They crawl around on the floor near dust and other potentially toxic particles.

• They are more likely to put things in their mouths and eat things that they shouldn't.

The developing fetus reacts strongly to toxic chemicals. This is because the developing body is extremely sensitive to the signals and complex interactions of hormones. Disruption of these signals and interactions can permanently skew the body's development.

Many studies show that hypertension, coronary heart disease, thyroid dysfunction, cancer, diabetes, asthma, arthritis, and even Alzheimer's disease—things that can't be picked up on a prenatal scan—are all programmed into a baby while still in the womb. What determines the programming is maternal nutrition and exposure to environmental toxins.

More Cancer

The worst effects of environmental poisons on children can clearly be seen in the increasing rate of childhood cancers.

According to medical scientists, the reason for the rise in childhood cancers is something of a mystery. Indeed, some experts continue to promote the idea that childhood cancer is rare. Yet, statistics show that, after accidents, childhood cancer is the second biggest killer of children.

Just like adults, children can develop cancer at any site in the body, but two—the bones and the brain—are now particularly common sites for cancer. Figures from the National Cancer Institute show that most childhood cancers are on the rise. Rates for acute lymphocytic leukemia (ALL) have risen 10 percent in the last fifteen years, and the incidence of central-nervous-system tumors are up by more than 30 percent.

Cancer is, of course, a multifactorial disease—many things can trigger it. But while scientists continue to focus their research on the genetic links to childhood cancer, important environmental triggers—in the form of mercury-containing vaccines, pesticides, food additives, and electromagnetic radiation—are being ignored.

In addition to obvious birth defects and cancer, more subtle trends have emerged. Population studies tell us that the rate of birth defects has actually gone up in recent years. In the United States, one report showed that eighteen of the twenty most common birth defects were on the rise—some by as much as 1,700 percent. Reports from the U.K. show a similar trend. But this fact has been successfully obscured by an increase in medical terminations—as long as the baby is not born at term, the fact that it had an abnormality does not count in the official records. Also, in the West, some problems, such as undescended testicles, have become so commonplace that they are no longer recorded as malformations.

Furthermore, rates of asthma and other respiratory problems among children are on the rise, as are skin conditions, learning and behavioral difficulties, and such serious conditions as attention deficit/hyperactivity disorder (ADHD).

Life in the Womb

Many parents-to-be believe that as long as the baby is inside its mother, it is safe from environmental toxins. This belief stems from a long-standing view that the placenta—the baby's life-support system—acts like a filter, letting only the nutrients and immune-protective agents like antibodies into the baby's system. In reality, the placenta acts more like a sponge.

The placenta consists of a complex mass of blood vessels (if laid out flat, there would be enough to completely cover more than half a tennis court) that carry nutrients and oxygen to the baby, and remove waste products and carbon dioxide. While the placenta can protect your baby to some degree, it is not a total barrier; studies show that, nowadays, more than 350 man-made toxic chemicals are being passed on to babies in increasing amounts through such pathways as the placenta.

Absolutely *everything* that enters the mother's system also enters the baby's system via the placenta. So, along with all those vitamins, minerals, amino acids, and antibodies, there are also heavy metals, car fumes, pesticides, cigarette smoke, drugs, and the chemicals from household cleaners and cosmetics.

The World Wildlife Fund (WWF) in the U.K. has stated, in its report *Chemical Trespass: A Toxic Legacy*, that: "It is now recognized that the fetus can be damaged by relatively low levels of contaminants which do not affect the adult. . . . Exposure in the womb can cause birth defects and can affect our children's future ability to reproduce and their susceptibility to diseases such as cancer. Functional deficits may also be caused, such that some children may not reach their full potential. Put simply, the integrity of the next generation is at stake."

There is a huge body of evidence to show that a combination of inadequate nutrition and exposure to environmental toxins can have a profound effect on the developing child. Consider the following:

Cutting Down on Toxic Toiletries

Certain everyday toiletries may also pose a threat to your unborn child's health. There is a substantial body of evidence to show that hairdressers are at greater risk of having babies with malformations than other women, and that they are more prone to miscarriages as well. This is because hairdressers are exposed daily to the poisonous chemicals in hair preparations, such as shampoo, conditioners, hairsprays, gels, mousses, and hair dyes. The average woman is not exposed to these chemicals in the same concentrations, but a quick look through your bathroom cupboard may give you pause for thought. If it is filled with lots of different types of hair-care products, you may wish to consider cutting down.

Similarly, a University of Bristol study of fourteen thousand women revealed that pregnant women who constantly use aerosol products, such as air fresheners, deodorants, furniture polishes, and hairsprays, have significantly higher rates of headaches and postnatal depression than those who use these products less than once a week. The high users' babies had higher rates of ear infections and diarrhea (see "Air Fresheners," page 157).

Cutting down on unnecessary toiletries is a good habit to get into now, as it may help you to resist the temptation to smother your baby with the unnecessary and harsh chemicals contained in many baby products.

• According to the National Birth Defects Prevention Network in the United States, a 50 percent reduction in birth defects could be achieved if parents simply improved their diets and limited their exposure to toxic substances.

• The U.K.'s preconceptual care group Foresight has published figures showing that a prepregnancy health program that includes dietary correction and reduction of toxins can lead to an overall birth-defect rate of less than 1 percent—compared with the 5–7 percent that is the national average.

• Everyday toxins, such as food additives and those in unfiltered, contaminated tap water, raise the risk of your baby having a birth defect. Pesticide exposure during pregnancy has also been linked to an increase in birth defects, along with a greater risk of cancer later in life.

• Hormone disrupters, which can be found in large amounts in pesticide residues, but also in everyday household detergents and toiletries, and even in disposable diapers, may alter a child's thyroid function and sexual characteristics. These types of chemicals have already been implicated as responsible for low sperm counts in young men, and there is fear that exposure to too many of these synthetic estrogens may predispose young girls to estrogen-dependent cancers of the breast, ovary, and endometrium later in life.

The Toxic Baby

Human babies are unlike any other young animals in that they are born completely helpless and with many of their bodily functions, such as their digestive and immune systems, still not fully functioning. This is why extra consideration is worthwhile when making choices about feeding, and when looking around for potential sources of exposure to toxic chemicals and fumes in the home.

Babies also indulge in lots of hand-to-mouth activity, making it easy to transfer more foreign substances into their bodies. Young children are also more likely to have close encounters with the pesticides on lawns or in pet collars, and toxins in carpets, as they spend a lot of time playing or crawling on the ground.

There are other, less obvious threats to their health as well. The average newborn, with his faster metabolism and immature immune and detoxification systems, may:

• Spend his first year of life in a new crib with a mattress that's been treated with pesticides and fire-retardant chemicals. The foam inside the mattress can give off toxic formaldehyde gas, and the dyes used in the sheets and covers are usually carcinogenic. The typical crib headboard or bed frame is constructed from particleboard—wood shavings pressed and glued together with a urea-formaldehyde resin that also gives off toxic gases.

- Wear disposable diapers made of bleached paper that emits a slow, steady dose of cancer-causing dioxins. These diapers also contain a "chemical sponge" that emits hormone-disrupting chemicals.

- Obtain some or all of his nourishment from plastic bottles that give off phthalates (plasticizers) in amounts that can be measured in the bloodstream.

- Travel in brand-new, molded, plastic baby carriers and car seats that have been treated with toxic flame retardants and that off-gas *toluene* and more plasticizers.

The average parent may simply shrug and reason that none of these things on their own could possibly expose their child to enough toxins to cause illness. In a sense, that is correct. None of these things individually is likely to cause harm. But collectively, they create a powerful combination of harmful chemicals from which a baby has no escape.

Household Cleaners Raise Asthma Risk

Household chemicals, such as bleach, disinfectant, and cleaning fluid, have been blamed for the huge surge in childhood asthma, and the data suggest that the chemical formaldehyde present in many household products could be the reason. A 2004 British study of more than seven thousand children found that those born into households that are high users of such products are twice as likely to suffer persistent wheezing, often a precursor to asthma. The results, published in the journal *Thorax*, came from an ongoing study at Bristol University dubbed "Children of the '90s," as it has been following children born in the Avon, England, area in the early 1990s and tracking their health in relation to chemical exposure in the home.

Their findings echoed those of an Australian study published earlier in 2004 that linked volatile chemicals in household products with asthma.

According to these two studies, the following household products were the ones most likely to trigger an asthma attack:

- aerosols
- air freshener
- bleach
- carpet cleaner
- disinfectant
- dry-cleaning fluid
- paint or varnish
- paint stripper
- pesticide
- white spirit
- window cleaner

Toddler to Child

Children grow quickly and, watching their remarkable progress from help-less babies to walking and talking individuals, it is easy to believe that they are no longer as vulnerable as they were as newborns. To some extent, this is true. Your child's immune system has matured—but not fully.

As a child grows, so does the potential for greater exposure to environmental toxins. Playgroups or nursery schools can expose a child to more bacteria, viruses, and allergens than are normally encountered at home. To combat this, parents may start giving their children conventional medicines. Time constraints and faddy eating habits may mean resorting more and more to convenience foods. More time out of the house also means more exposure to pollutants and, if it is sunny, more chemicals in the form of sunscreens.

Scientists are only just beginning to make the connection between toxic ex-posure in childhood and developmental disorders. For instance, researchers at Johns Hopkins University School of Hygiene and Public Health recently went on record saying that childhood exposure to lead, mercury, pesticides, and poly-chlorinated biphenyls (PCBs) can affect brain development, and may be linked to eventual ADHD, autism, Parkinson's disease, and other developmental disorders.

Children's brain development and behavior are vitally important to their health and to their ability to contribute to society throughout life. Yet, there is currently no system for testing pesticides and other chemicals to see what impact their ingestion has on the brain and neurological system of growing children. This research is desperately needed, but in the meantime, some parents may feel it's prudent to live by the axiom "Look before you leap."

What You Can Do

Overexposure to chemical toxins is not inevitable for your children at any stage, nor is it out of your control. There are many simple ways to protect your developing baby and your child, and to keep everyday chemical exposures to a minimum.

If You Are Pregnant or Trying for a Baby

Change your lifestyle before you become pregnant. As little as six months of ef-fort can make all the difference, and many parents might reason that this effort is nothing compared to the emotional, physical, mental, and financial drain it may be to look after a handicapped child.

Don't forget Dad. While the mother's health plays a major role in the state of her child, fathers do have some influence as well. Men who smoke are more likely to father children of low birth weights. Those who work in jobs that bring them into contact with pesticides and toxic chemicals are more likely to have children with birth defects. Such men often bring residues from their work home with them, raising their partners' exposure to toxins through contact with clothing and semen.

As mentioned earlier, some twenty different toxic chemicals with the potential to harm sperm quality and production have been found in random male samples. Contrast this with evidence suggesting that men who eat organic foods have sperm counts that are twice as high as those who don't.

Eat organic foods. Organic foods are free from pesticide residues, food additives, and GM (genetically modified) additives. Organic foods are also significantly higher in nutrients. One U.S. study found that organic tomatoes had 500 percent more calcium than the conventionally grown variety. You'll also get more iron, potassium, magnesium, manganese, and copper in every bite as well, which is good for you and your baby.

If you're thinking of making the switch to organic but budgeting is an issue, then consider buying organic for those foods you eat the most of. Even a small switch to organic teas and coffee (preferably decaffeinated) can substantially reduce your intake of pesticides. Or you may wish to replace the most contaminated types of conventional foods with organic alternatives. This means dairy products and meats (especially beef). Watch out also for orchard fruits, such as strawberries, cherries, apricots, and apples. Research into pesticide residues on such produce shows that these types of fruits are among the most heavily contaminated.

Cut out caffeine. You probably don't think of caffeine as a toxin, but in large quantities and especially when you're pregnant, it is. Caffeine, which is found in coffee, tea, sodas, and chocolate, leaches essential nutrients out of your system, leaving little for your baby to grow on.

The most recent medical evidence also suggests that consuming large amounts of coffee daily—five to six cups—can encourage miscarriage. What isn't known is whether this risk is higher in some women than in others. Caffeine also dehydrates the body. This means that the relative concentration of toxins in your blood will be higher than in a woman who limits caffeine. Instead of caffeinated beverages, try drinking herbal teas, or grain coffees, such as dandelion and chicory.

Limit or avoid cured meats, such as hot dogs, salami, bacon, and smoked fish. These are treated with known carcinogens called *nitrites*. Prenatal exposure to nitrites raises the risk of your child developing cancer. For example, it has been found that men who regularly consume hot dogs run the risk of fathering children with an increased risk of leukemia. Women who eat cured meats during pregnancy appear to increase their child's chances of developing brain cancer. Read the labels on organic cured meats carefully, because organic standards in most countries allow the use of nitrites in cured meats.

Use non-fluoride toothpaste. Also check with your local water authority to see if your water is fluoridated. If it is, switch to filtered water. Fluoride is a toxic substance that arrives at the toothpaste manufacturer in a barrel marked with a skull and crossbones. Pregnant women who consume large amounts of fluoride increase their children's risk of birth defects and cancer.

Limit alcohol. This is especially important in the crucial preconceptual stage and during the first few months of life in the womb. Binge drinking and chronic alcoholism can deplete your body of nutrients, such as vitamin B_6, iron, and zinc, and interfere with normal hormonal function. It also interferes with the proper formation of organs, such as the kidneys, and raises the risk of congenital malformations.

There is also evidence to show that consuming alcohol can interfere with a woman's ability to conceive. Once you are pregnant, it can stop your baby from developing properly. There are no official rules for preconceptual and prenatal drinking, but government guidelines suggest that pregnant women should not drink more than one or two units of alcohol (one unit equals one small glass of wine) once or twice a week. Nevertheless, many women still prefer to avoid alcohol while trying to conceive and during the first trimester, when the fetus is developing.

Rethink soft drinks. Fizzy drinks like colas and lemonade provide empty calories and have the potential to cause harm. They contain caffeine as well as sugar, which can significantly depress immune function and leach nutrients from the body. They can also contain artificial sweeteners, such as *aspartame*, and other harmful ingredients, such as *phosphoric acid*.

Artificial sweeteners have been shown to harm the developing brain of young animals, and scientists now believe they are likely to do the same in developing human babies (see chapter 5). They have also been shown to increase your sweet tooth, so, ultimately, these calorie-sparing drinks may defeat their purpose.

Recently, American researchers made the connection between soft drink consumption and brittle bones in teenagers. They are now turning their attention to what happens when mothers consume large quantities of phosphoric acid during the developmentally sensitive time in the womb. Phosphoric acid blocks the absorption of calcium and magnesium by the intestines, which means less is available for your developing baby's bones.

Quit smoking. Smoking can poison your body with carcinogenic nicotine and the toxic metal cadmium. Once you are pregnant, smoking decreases the flow of blood and oxygen to the placenta and reduces the availability of essential amino acids necessary for proper growth. Smokers are also twice as likely as nonsmokers to miscarry or have an ectopic pregnancy (when the egg gets implanted outside of the womb). According to recent data, women who smoke also have a 78 percent higher risk of giving birth to a baby with a cleft palate or lip. In addition, babies of smokers are also more likely to have chronic breathing problems. Studies have shown that the lungs of babies whose parents smoke are 10 percent smaller than those of nonsmoking parents, and their risk of cancer is 50 percent greater. Babies of smokers are born with fewer natural reserves to fight off infection, and have a 43 percent higher risk of blood disorders, neurological and sensory disorders, bladder and kidney problems, and skin disorders than children of nonsmokers.

Follow a stress-relief program. Stress depletes the body of essential nutrients—especially the B vitamins. Mothers who are under lots of stress tend to have babies that are smaller and less active in the womb. Stress also depresses the immune system—making you less able to fight off the effects of any toxins that are ingested and inhaled.

In a recent U.S. study, women who had strenuous jobs, such as those that require repetitive tasks, had a higher rate of problems during pregnancy, including preeclampsia, premature delivery, and low-birth-weight babies. Not all stresses can be dealt with easily, but try to do what you can. A large study in Sweden has recently found that the kinds of stress most likely to affect a baby's growth are a lack of emotional and practical support, social isolation, and an unstable home life.

Anything that relaxes you—whether it is yoga, swimming, or just vegging out in front of the TV—should become a regular part of your routine.

After Your Child Is Born

Serve organic foods. It may be the most important step you take. In spite of what appears to be a junk-food culture, children still eat fruit and vegetables at a much higher rate than adults do, thus consuming up to twelve times as much pesticide residues. In the United States, it is estimated that 3 to 4 million children now have toxic lead levels in their bodies. So-called safe levels of lead and pesticides as defined by government agencies are only applicable to adults. No safe levels have been established for children, and, indeed, many argue that there is no such thing as a safe level of these toxins.

In addition, make sure that your children get plenty of variety in their diets. Many children's day-to-day diets are made up of the same types of foods over and over again. This can lead to food allergies and nutritional deficiencies, which can alter appetite and weaken the immune system (see page 60).

Use a non-fluoride toothpaste. Fluoride is only slightly less toxic than lead and more toxic than *arsenic*, yet we continue to add it to toothpaste and to our water supplies. As we can take in fluoride from other sources—such as produce grown in soil with a high fluoride content or sprayed with fluoride as a pesticide, Teflon cooking utensils, and car exhausts and other industrial pollution—our children may be getting between four and twelve times the "safe" limit of 1 milligram per day. Mounting evidence shows that fluoride overdose can cause such health problems as fatigue, skin rashes, visual disturbances, stomach problems, headaches, and dizziness. In the long term, it is also considered to be a carcinogen.

Breast or Bottle?

Your baby is born with an immature immune system. Just as she relied upon you for protection in the womb, she will rely upon you for some time to come for protection outside the womb. The first and most important step in providing this protection is by breast-feeding your baby for as long as possible.

No matter what formula manufacturers claim, no matter how healthy the baby in the magazine ad looks and no matter how much some would like to believe it, artificial milk cannot provide anywhere near the full range of short- and long-term advantages that breast milk does.

Breast milk is economical, always the right temperature, and always "on tap." While you are breast-feeding your baby, you are providing, among other things:

- Good bacteria that guard against intestinal infection and aid digestion.
- Essential fatty acids, necessary for brain function and to help kill off parasites, such as *Giardia lamblia*, a common cause of diarrhea in infants.
- Antioxidants, to help your baby fight off infection and the effects of pollution.
- Immune boosters, such as antibodies, immunoglobulins, and interferon.
- Active protection from disease, as mothers pass on their own immunity to several diseases against which babies are routinely vaccinated.

Toxic Breast Milk?

There has been a great deal of attention in the press recently regarding toxins in breast milk. Women who are considering breast-feeding their children have expressed concerns that the benefits of breast milk may be negated by the pres-

Avoid exposure to passive smoke. There is nothing passive about passive smoke. It actively destroys health. Children breathing in secondhand smoke have higher rates of respiratory illness than those who do not. Remember: healthy lungs are necessary to excrete accumulated toxins. Passive smoke depletes levels of the antioxidant vitamin C by as much as 20 percent and increases the risk of cancer over the short and long term, and the risk of heart disease by 25 percent.

Rethink storage. Brightly colored plastics in a child's room, such as storage crates, plastic toys, or vinyl wallpaper, give off poisonous gases, such as formaldehyde. We may not always be able to smell these gases, but they are entering our bodies and have the potential to cause harm. Consider untreated wood boxes or traditional wooden toy chests for toy storage.

ence of harmful chemicals, such as dioxins and PCBs (polychlorinated biphenyls).

According to a World Health Organization (WHO) survey, published in the *British Medical Journal*, the daily estimated intake of dioxins and PCBs by breast-fed infants is around 170 pg/kg of body weight at two months and 39 pg/kg at ten months. The tolerated daily intake is around 10 pg/kg of body weight.

So, how can we know whether or not breast milk is safe? This is an area that has been extensively studied, and the overwhelming conclusion is that while prenatal exposure to these levels of toxins has a definite negative effect on neurological development, exposure via breast milk did not have the same dramatic effect.

This does not mean that the issue of contaminated breast milk is not serious. It is. But along with any contaminants, breast milk also has constituents that fight against toxic overload. The overwhelming opinion among pediatricians and child-health experts is that the benefits of breast-feeding still far outweigh the potential risk of ingesting chemicals. What's more, according to the child-health expert Dr. Michel Odent, of the Primal Research Centre in London, if a woman is following an organic regime, the longer a woman breast-feeds, the less contaminated her milk can become. Breast-feeding uses up calories (it burns up fat), and as toxic fat is burned up, this is replaced by nontoxic fat.

Remember also that a baby formula made with conventional tap water is likely to contain many harmful chemicals and heavy metals, without conferring even a whisper of the benefits that breast milk has.

Go fragrance-free. Fragrances, used in room fresheners, soaps, deodorants, baby wipes and lotions, and cleaning agents, all contain highly volatile fragrance compounds that have been shown to be both carcinogenic and allergenic. If that's not bad enough, fragrance also alters central-nervous-system function and lowers immunity. Using fragrance-free products goes part of the way toward reducing your child's risk of such toxic exposure.

Consider supplements. It would be nice to think that our children could get all the nutrients they need from their diets, but this is just not possible. As our world becomes more and more polluted, it is even more important to give your child a daily multivitamin and mineral supplement, as a well-nourished body is better able to cope with environmental insults. Many popular brands of children's vitamins only contain a few essentials, such as vitamins A, B, C, D, and E. These are not enough. You may need to make a trip to the health-food store to find a supplement designed for children with a full range of nutrients.

Teach your children to drink water. Sodas, fruit juices, and milk top the list of favorite drinks for many children. Equally, some parents feel that they are somehow depriving their children of a "good" drink if they only offer water. But water is necessary for life and is more thirst-quenching than any other drink. An adequate amount of water can also help the body to flush out toxins, and is necessary to maintain the efficiency of many other bodily functions.

5. FOOD AND DRINK

The food we eat is inexorably linked with our well-being. It is the bedrock on which a healthy life is based. It is the body's ready store of nutrients and energy—the thing that holds us up, bolsters our immunity, fights free-radical damage, and maintains our energy cycles in the face of an increasingly polluted world.

We have to eat and drink to live, and yet, increasingly, eating and drinking has become an act of faith, as most of what we consume today does not resemble food in any reasonable sense of the word.

Indeed, much of what we call food today would only have existed in the realms of science fiction a hundred years ago: exotic items grown without soil, flown in daily from far away, made from ingredients synthesized in test tubes, and preserved long beyond their natural shelf life using a variety of industrial chemicals derived from petroleum by-products.

We eat meat by-products enhanced with artificial meat flavors to make them palatable. We eat processed, quick-cook microwave and oven meals. Even the so-called healthy cereals we eat for breakfast are so highly processed and nutritionally poor that the manufacturers have to add vitamins to them simply so that they can be classified as foods.

These foods also contain a myriad of additives—occasionally at higher levels than any actual nutrients in them—and contaminants, such as pesticides. These days, it is estimated that every one of us ingests a gallon of pesticides and herbicides a year from our daily diet.

Every day, we put this nutritionally poor, adulterated, unbalanced stuff into our bodies, and when our bodies eventually stop functioning properly, we wonder why. The fact is, our daily diets are the most influential aspect of our day-to-day health. What we eat is reflected in the strength of our immune and hormonal systems, the way our minds function, our muscle coordination, the health of our bones, the quality of our skin and hair, and the short- and long-term health of the children we produce. The health problems associated with a poor diet—heart disease, obesity, cancer, arthritis, and diabetes—are real and tangible.

Eat, Drink, and Be Worried

Food can be bad for you in lots of ways. You can eat too much of it and become obese (a major risk factor for heart disease, stroke, and diabetes, among other things). It can contain pesticides, contaminants, and "anti-nutrients" (substances, such as soy flour, that prevent the body from absorbing essential nutrients). Or it can contain so few nutrients that you "starve" even when you appear to be eating plenty.

Each of these problems is linked. For instance, when you eat nutrient-poor food, your body doesn't get all it needs to stay healthy. The body instinctively knows this, and craves more and more food to get what it needs. When you give in to these cravings and continue to eat calorie-rich but nutritionally poor foods, you gain weight. The more excess weight you carry, the more capacity you have for storing compounds, such as pesticides and other synthetic chemicals, in your body. And the more chemicals in your body, the greater the risk of declining health.

Food fads have also drastically altered the way we eat. Most of us have a list of "good" and "bad" foods compiled by the cult of food "experts" who offer advice in newspapers, books, and magazines and subtly inform our food choices. Much of the constantly changing advice of dietitians and government bodies—reduce fat, eat raw foods, follow a "Mediterranean diet"—has never been researched in detail, with the result that some of it can be downright damaging to our health. In fact, it has been said that you have a better chance of winning the lottery than you have of hitting on clear and accurate advice as to what you should be eating.

Humans thrive on variety, yet diet faddists encourage us to cut out specific types of foods, even entire food groups, from our daily diet for the sake of being healthy. At the same time, market forces encourage us to consume a whole range of new and novel convenience foods—often in great quantity—that may not be good for us.

Anyone interested in long-term good health would certainly benefit from a healthy daily dose of skepticism about food fads and question whom all this ever-changing dietary advice really serves. Chances are, you will find that, ultimately, it benefits multinational food manufacturers.

These companies have massive influence worldwide and have no interest in our eating fresh, unprocessed food. A steak is a steak is a steak, for instance. But a prepared meat product, seasoned and formed from "select cuts of beef" is a patented recipe, and patented recipes (which, with a bit of clever marketing, can be sold to the public as healthy, nutritious, quick, and easy) are where the profits are. Fresh food is not high on the priority lists because there is considerably less profit in it.

It is the lack of variety, toxic additives, long storage times, and highly processed foods that have led us to where, nutritionally, we are today—a place where the food we eat detracts from, rather than adds to, our ongoing sense of well-being.

Synthetic Additives

There are thousands of food additives approved for use in our foods. If your diet is high in processed or convenience foods, you will be consuming a staggering amount of these additives and artificial ingredients each year.

Sugar, corn sweeteners, salt, *citric acid*, pepper, vegetable colors, mustard, yeast, and baking soda account for the vast majority—some 98 percent—of the total amount of food additives we consume. But, even though the rest are used in very small amounts, it has been estimated that the average American, for example, consumes five pounds of additives per year. If you include refined sugar—the food-processing industry's most used and abused additive—the total skyrockets to 135 pounds a year.

Additives are placed in foods for a number of reasons. They facilitate the preparation of processed foods or lengthen shelf life. They can make food more appealing. With the use of chemical additives, food technicians are able to mimic natural flavors and to color foods that are well past their nutritional best to make them look more "natural" or "fresh." They are used to preserve foods for increasingly longer periods of time and allow the creation of highly manipulated forms of bread, biscuits, fruits, vegetables, meats, and dairy products.

Chemicals can also be used to make the product more marketable in some way—for example, by adding a sugar substitute, a manufacturer can advertise its product as sugar-free. Some "foods," such as coffee creamers, chewing gum, and sweets, consist almost entirely of artificial ingredients derived from synthetic chemicals.

Are All Additives Harmful?

Although we eat them every day, food additives are not subject to the same scrutiny by the regulatory authorities as drugs are, and the history of food additives includes a number of products that were once deemed safe but were later banned or allowed to be used only if accompanied by warnings. Certain food colorings, the artificial sweeteners *cyclamate* and *saccharin*, and the flavor enhancer *monosodium glutamate (MSG)* are examples of such products.

At their best, additives add little or no nutritional value to a food product. At their worst, they can detract from your health and your day-to-day well-being. Moreover, some food additives provoke powerful adverse effects in some people while appearing to cause no problems for others. For instance, *sulphites*, a group of preservatives/antioxidants used in dried fruits and wines, are known to cause sensitive individuals (such as those suffering from asthma) to experience severe reactions. People with the genetic disorder phenylketonuria (PKU) are unable to fully metabolize the artificial sweetener aspartame, which can lead to a buildup of its breakdown products in their body that can potentially result in serious brain damage. The flavor enhancer MSG, a relative of aspartame and also a neurotoxin, can cause sensitive individuals to have headaches, nausea, weakness, and breathing difficulties.

While food additives and preservatives undergo a required series of premarketing tests, often involving laboratory animals being given huge doses of individual additives, no one can ever test for what really happens when all the different additives in a food break down and interact with each other in your body.

The Problem of Mixtures

When we eat processed foods, we ingest a mixture of different chemicals, and yet until recently very few studies had been conducted to enlighten us as to what risks might be attached to this.

Recent reports have shown that we should be paying more attention to the problem of mixtures. In 2005, British researchers at the University of Liverpool examined the toxic effects on nerve cells in the laboratory using a combination of four common food additives: aspartame, MSG, and the artificial colorings Brilliant Blue and Quinoline Yellow. The findings, published in the journal *Toxicological Sciences*, revealed that when nerve cells were exposed to MSG and Brilliant Blue or to aspartame and Quinoline Yellow, in concentrations that are easily found in the bloodstream after a typical children's snack and drink, the paired additives stopped the nerve cells from growing and interfered with proper signaling processes. Mixing the additives had a much more potent effect on the nerve cells than each additive had on its own.

Not long after this report was published, in the United States, the Environmental Working Group (EWG) sampled a range of popular juices and sodas and presented evidence showing that two ingredients—ascorbic acid (vitamin C) and either *sodium benzoate* or potassium benzoate—found in many popular children's drinks, when mixed together can form the potent cancer-causing chemical benzene. After this was revealed, consumer groups elsewhere in the world began testing for and finding benzene in a range of popular soft drinks.

The EWG found that the Food and Drug Administration (FDA) had known about this interaction since 1990, but instead of notifying the public and acting to ban the use of the combination, the FDA left it to the beverage industry to voluntarily reformulate its products, while keeping quiet about the problem.

As more data like these emerge, it becomes clear that our ability to formulate foods from chemical mixtures has far outstripped our ability to ensure that these mixtures are safe. The next time you buy yourself a chemical meal, ask yourself a simple question: Just because it is on sale, does it mean that it is safe to eat?

Food for Thought

We tend to think of food as being fuel for the body. Government campaigns on health often focus on the importance of a good diet to combat conditions like heart disease, diabetes, and cancer, and most of us accept that poor-quality food can produce poor physical health. Less often publicized is the role that good-quality food plays in shaping our minds.

Your brain is the most metabolically active organ in your body. It uses up 20 percent of the body's energy stores. It is extremely sensitive to changes in its chemical environment. In fact, one of the first reactions to a poor diet, or to ingesting toxins, will be mental and behavioral rather than physical.

In the last hundred years or so, we have drastically altered the number and kinds of chemicals we take into our bodies—and at a rate much faster than any human organ could evolve to cope with. When people complain about the dumbing-down of society, or about the seeming rise in senseless violence, aggression, and crime, few make the connection between not feeding the brain with necessary nutrients and a brain-dead society.

Yet consider studies done among prison populations, where prisoners were given food and supplements that met all the body's and brain's requirements. In these populations, aggressive behavior and recidivism were cut by an average of 40 percent. Furthermore, these individuals were not given megadoses of expensive supplements, but just basic, recommended daily allowance (RDA) levels of what each of us needs to not fall ill. In addition, there are now over five hundred studies linking diet to a range of mental-health conditions, including depression, schizophrenia, Alzheimer's and other types of dementia, as well as attention deficit/hyperactivity disorder (ADHD).

No one is suggesting that a poor diet is the only cause of these problems, but it can make a substantial contribution. In many cases, making some simple dietary adjustments can significantly improve symptoms and modify problem behavior. Ensuring that both children and adults get adequate nutrition each day, then, seems a simple, safe, inexpensive, effective, and humane step in the direction of turning the world into a more peaceful and more thoughtful place.

A Lesson in Labels

Food labels are the inevitable result of our reliance on prepackaged, highly processed convenience foods. Most of us have become so accustomed to buying food with labels that we can hardly imagine purchasing a food that doesn't come with an ingredients list, and cooking, heating, and storage instructions. Totally natural foods need no cooking instructions, no statements about nutritional content (or lack of it), no cautions about containing traces of nuts or other allergens, no disclaimers about how this information affects your statutory rights, and no hype about how much better this product is for you than a dozen other similar products on the supermarket shelves.

Given how ubiquitous processed food is in our diets, some label information is useful. Statements about fat, protein, carbohydrate, sodium, and calorie content can be helpful. But the truth is, most labels are designed for a less worthy purpose. Food companies use packaging and labels as mini-advertisements for their products. Sometimes, the two functions of a label—to provide accurate information and to entice someone to buy the product—are in conflict. When this happens, the manufacturer will do everything possible to distract you from the truth about their product. For this reason, food labels can be misleading, especially if you don't learn how to read between the lines and examine the fine print. Knowing what the words on the label really mean is a big step in learning to make better choices at the supermarket.

Getting Beyond the Hype

Smart shoppers ignore the hype on the front of the package. This part of the label is designed by the company's marketing and advertising departments and contains whatever pleasing images and fashionable words will best help sell the product.

While there are laws regulating the meanings of many of the terms found on food packages, it's still easy to be deceived by them. In spite of reassuring claims made by the manufacturers on the front of the package, the product inside may not always be what it seems. While manufacturers cannot legally lie on a food label, they are allowed, within reason, to stretch the truth. Be wary of these tricky terms:

Pure. Everyone wants to eat food that's pure. No one would want to eat contaminated food or serve it up to their family. Unfortunately, the word "pure" has no regulated meaning in food labeling. A product can claim to be pure and still contain ingredients that should not be there, such as unwanted processing aids and contaminants. The packaging of most ready-made foods can leach chemicals, such as adhesives, polyvinyls, and hormone-disrupting bisphenol A and phthalates, into food. This is especially true of canned goods and foods that go from the freezer to the oven.

Natural. This is probably one of the most abused label terms. Once again, there is no universal or legal definition of "natural" in the food business. While it sounds appealing, "natural" says little about the nutritional quality of the food, or even its safety. "Natural," for example, doesn't necessarily mean nutritious. The vast majority of "natural flavors" you find in many processed foods are synthesized in the lab to be "natural identical." They contain nothing that the average person would equate with a product that is truly natural. Instead, they're derived from a range of neurotoxic and carcinogenic chemicals that are best avoided in any diet.

Made from . . . This simply refers to a starting material. For example, the claim "made from 100 percent vegetable oil" may be technically correct. But it can also be misleading. Many simple vegetable oils are processed and changed beyond recognition before they end up in our food or as a tub of margarine or spread. Along the way they may have been diluted or hydrogenated, changing them from a generally healthy fat to an artery-damaging trans fat. Another common label claim—"made from natural . . ."—doesn't necessarily mean the end product is natural. It only means that the manufacturer started with a natural source. But by the time the food reaches your table it may bear little resemblance to anything natural or healthy. Think chicken nuggets and ask yourself: Which part of the chicken? In many cheap products every bit of the animal, including organs, feet, beaks, and other nonnutritious parts, is included to support the "made from natural . . ." claim.

Made with real fruit. This claim is particularly prevalent in snacks for children. Unfortunately, there is no law requiring labels to say how much real fruit is in the product. A quick scan of the label will reveal that many "real fruit" snacks contain more sugar, preservatives, and colors than fruit.

Made with whole grains. This is a common claim on cereals and breads. It should indicate to the consumer that they are buying and eating a healthy food full of whole grains. But the label rarely says, and is not legally required to say, how much whole grain is in the product. This means that the main ingredient could be highly refined white flour with a minimal amount of whole wheat (and brown coloring) added. If this is the case, your bread or cereal won't contain all the fiber and other nutrients associated with whole grains.

Fat-free. Fat content provides the pleasing "mouth feel" in natural foods, and removing it deeply alters the consistency of food as well as the way it tastes. As a result, fat-free foods are often full of emulsifiers, modified starches, sugar (or worse, poisonous sweeteners), salt, and artificial flavorings. Sugary foods may not contain fat, but when you eat more sugar than your body can effectively process, not only will it increase your risk of diabetes, it will eventually result in your body storing this extra sugar as fat.

Some intake of fat is necessary for health and we need a mixture of saturated and unsaturated fats in our diet each day. A good example of why can be seen in salads. The dominant nutrients in fresh vegetables are mostly fat-soluble nutrients known as carotenes. Carotenes are powerful antioxidant and disease-fighting substances. Adding a drizzle of oily dressing to your salad aids your absorption of these nutrients, whereas studies show that a fat-free dressing or no dressing at all effectively stops your body from absorbing any of these beneficial nutrients from fresh vegetables.

Enriched. This word is often a clue that the product you are buying has been rendered so nutritionally poor through processing and a potentially long shelf life that the manufacturers needed to put some of the good stuff back in, usually in the form of added vitamins and minerals, in order to call it food. Enriched flour, enriched white bread, and enriched cereals are all good examples of foods that have been processed in such a way that all the beneficial nutrients have been removed. Enriched foods are not as healthy as their whole-food counterparts because they are often missing important cofactors found in natural foods.

Smoked. Legally, this term describes the flavor of the food, not how it was smoked. You might think that such foods are smoked in an old-fashioned smokehouse. In truth, they are likely to have been artificially or chemically smoked and/or just contain smoked flavoring. In spite of this they can still, legally, be labeled "smoked."

Fruit drink. When the word "drink" appears on the label, it tells you the product is not 100 percent juice. In fact, a fruit drink may contain little or no real fruit juice. You will need to scan the ingredients to know what's really in the bottle. More often than not it is mostly sugar and water, with added vitamin C. Enriching the drink in this way enables the manufacturer to add another buyer incentive—"high in vitamin C"—even if the product is a long way from being real orange juice.

Experienced label readers have learned to look right past the bold banners and colorful claims on the front of the package and instead look for the important facts in small print on the back.

What to Avoid

While many of us are now used to checking labels for salt and sugar content, and even for artificial colorings or artificial flavorings, it can be difficult to get into the habit of searching for other undesirable ingredients, too. Of course, the way to get out of reading labels altogether is to buy fresh food and prepare your own meals. If you are not willing to give up the convenience food habit, however, then there are a number of additives you and your family could do without.

To find them, you have to get into the habit of reading food labels as you shop. Don't be fooled into thinking that a high price tag guarantees quality. Some very high-priced name-brand convenience foods are full of the worst kinds of additives, while some of the more moderately priced, non-name brands may be perfectly acceptable. Equally, some organic foods, especially cakes and biscuits, can contain more sugar and fat than conventional brands.

With more than ten thousand chemicals added to our foods nowadays, it can be a daunting task to decipher labels and decide which products you should and should not be buying. The best way to avoid synthetic chemicals in your food is to buy fresh ingredients and make it yourself. But on those occasions when you do resort to second best, consider avoiding foods that use certain ingredients (see table, below). In Europe, these additives will usually be listed by their "E number." In Australia, they tend to use the same numbers, but without the E prefix. This system is due to be adopted internationally in the next few years, so while it isn't used in the United States at the moment, you can still scan the labels for specific additive names you would like to avoid until the more convenient E numbers are put into practice.

When shopping for food, try to avoid products that contain the following additives. (See chapter 10 for further health information on additives.)

ADDITIVE	E NUMBER	FOUND IN
Allura Red AC	E129	Food coloring in snacks, sauces, preserves, soups, wine, cider, etc.
Amaranth	E123	Food coloring in wine, spirits, fish roe
aspartame	E951	Sweetener in snacks, sweets, alcohol, desserts, "diet" foods
benzoic acid	E210	Preservative in many foods, including drinks, low-sugar products, cereals, meat products
Brilliant Black BN	E151	Coloring in drinks, sauces, snacks, wines, cheese, etc.

continues on following page . . .

ADDITIVE	E NUMBER	FOUND IN
butylated hydroxyanisole (BHA)	E320	Preservative, particularly in fat-containing foods, confectionery, meats
calcium benzoate	E213	Preservative in many foods, including drinks, low-sugar products, cereals, meat products
calcium sulphite	E226	Preservative in a vast array of foods—from burgers to cookies, frozen mushrooms to horseradish; used to make old produce look fresh
carboxymethyl cellulose sodium salt	E466	Bulking agent found in ice creams, beverages, and other foods
carrageenan (seaweed extract)	E407	Thickener used in a wide variety of foods, including dressings, ice cream, jams, and custards
monosodium glutamate (MSG)	E621	Ubiquitous flavor enhancer found in almost every preprepared food
nitrite chemicals	E249–252	Curing agents commonly found in cured or preserved meats
polyoxyethylene sorbitan chemicals	E432–E436	Emulsifiers found in spreads, cake mixes, dressings, desserts, and beverages
Ponceau 4R, Cochineal Red A	E124	Food coloring found in sweets, desserts, and beverages
potassium benzoate	E212	See calcium benzoate
potassium nitrite	E249	Preservative in cured meats and canned meat products
propyl p-hydroxybenzoate, propylparaben, parabens	E216	Preservative in cereals, snacks, paté, meat products, confectionery
saccharin and its sodium, potassium, and calcium salts	E954	Sweetener in diet and no-sugar products
sodium metabisulphite	E223	Preservative and antioxidant used in dried and frozen fruits and fruit fillings
sodium sulphite	E221	Preservative used in wine making and other processed foods
soy protein isolates	—	Protein source widely used in ready-made meals and breads
stannous chloride (tin)	E512	Antioxidant and color-retention agent in canned and bottled foods, fruit juices
sulphur dioxide	E220	Preservative found in dried fruits and condiments

ADDITIVE	E NUMBER	FOUND IN
Sunset Yellow FCF, Orange Yellow S	E110	Food coloring found in sweets, desserts, and beverages
tartrazine	E102	Yellow food coloring found in sweets, desserts, and beverages
tri- and polyphosphate chemicals	E450(b)	Added to meat to make it take up water to increase weight (and so the price) at no extra cost to the manufacturer

Hidden Additives

Apart from the known additives that are listed on the labels, modern processed foods also contain a number of unintentional contaminants, such as pesticides, genetically modified (GM) ingredients, chemicals that have leached from the packaging, and, most recently, nanoparticles. Many of these hidden additives can have a profound effect on health, and, what's more, as they are generally industrial chemicals, food will not be your only source of exposure to them. That's why choosing to cut your exposure to them whenever and wherever you can makes good sense.

Pesticides

Health professionals recommend that you eat at least five servings of fruit and vegetables every day as part of a varied diet. Unfortunately, if you eat conventionally grown produce, you may also unknowingly be ingesting a mixture of harmful pesticides, including:

• insecticides to control insects

• rodenticides to control rodents

• herbicides to control weeds

• fungicides to control mold and fungus

• antimicrobials to control bacteria

Just because you can't see or taste them doesn't mean they aren't there. The most comprehensive testing for the presence of unwanted chemicals in food is the ongoing U.S. Total Diet Study (TDS), conducted by the FDA and updated yearly. The TDS looks for the presence of many different chemicals in food, but its findings on levels of chlorinated pesticides have been particularly distressing. In its 1988 report, *DDE* (dichlorodiphenyldichloroethylene), a close relative of DDT (dichlorodiphenyltrichloroethane), was found in every single sample of raisins, spinach (fresh and frozen), chili con carne (beef and beans), and beef.

DDE was also present in 93 percent of processed cheeses, mince, hot dogs, collards (spring greens), chicken, turkey, and ice-cream sandwiches sampled. It was also present in 87 percent of lamb chops, salami, canned spinach, meat loaf, and butter, and in 81 percent of sauces and creamed spinach.

Since DDT and DDE have been banned in the United States since 1972, it is likely that some of this contamination is from produce imported from other countries that still use these chemicals. But some of it is also due to the persistence of these chemicals in the soil. Growing crops or rearing animals on land contaminated with DDT and DDE means that we recycle these toxins back into the food chain.

In the intervening years, things didn't get much better. The 1999 TDS report showed that, among the foods sampled, seventeen different pesticides were found in butter, thirty-two different ones in cherries, twenty-nine in strawberries, and twenty-seven in apples. The baked potato samples contained twenty-three pesticides, and hamburger, twenty-two. Milk chocolate samples contained eighteen different pesticides. Once again, DDE/DDT was the residue most often found, with *chlorpyrifos-methyl*, *malathion*, *endosulfan*, *dieldrin*, and *chlorpyrifos* also being very common. (See also chapter 8, page 207, on pesticides.)

In the U.K., the 1999 Annual Report by the Working Party on Pesticide Residues (WPPR) found that 27 percent of the full range of foods tested showed pesticide residues. Among them, DDT (which is banned in the U.K.) was found in beef slices, corned beef, and lamb's kidney, and 2,4-D (also banned in the U.K.) was found in over half the oranges tested. Oranges, pears, lettuces, chocolate, and apples contained the highest numbers and levels of residues. Three-quarters of the chocolate samples contained *lindane* (a relative of DDT), and one in eight jars of baby food were also contaminated. Surveys in Australia and New Zealand have found similarly high levels of pesticides in foods.

Government surveys around the world continue to show that many everyday foods can increase our exposure to this cocktail of chemicals exponentially. For instance, in the U.K.:

• **Apples.** In 2003, 71 percent contained residues and 39 percent had residues of more than one chemical.

- **Beer.** In 1999, 35 percent contained pesticide residues. Growing nonorganic hops involves twelve to fourteen annual sprays using an average of around fifteen chemical products.

- **Bread.** In 2003, residues were found in 61 percent of the ordinary bread sampled, and 12 percent contained multiple residues.

- **Cereal bars.** Two surveys were carried out in 2001. The first found that 64 percent contained detectable residues, with 22 percent of these containing multiple residues; the second found that 71 percent had detectable residues, with 14 percent containing more than one chemical. There is currently no maximum residue limit for cereal bars.

- **Feta cheese.** In 1999, 67 percent of samples contained residues of DDT.

- **Cucumber.** In 2003, 24 percent contained residues, and 4 percent had multiple residues.

- **Grapes.** In 2003, 63 percent contained residues and 32 percent had multiple residues.

- **Lemons.** In two surveys carried out in 2001, one found that 100 percent contained detectable residues, with 90 percent of them containing multiple residues, while the other found 93 percent with detectable residues, 81 percent containing multiple residues.

- **Pears.** In 2003, 58 percent of those tested contained residues, and 22 percent had multiple residues.

- **Potatoes.** In 2003, 35 percent contained residues, with 9 percent containing multiple residues.

- **Raspberries.** In 2003, 57 percent contained residues, 31 percent with multiple residues.

- **Rice.** In 2003, 54 percent of samples contained residues, with 10 percent containing multiple residues.

- **Spinach.** In 2003, 24 percent of samples contained residues.

- **Wine.** In 2003, 10 percent contained residues.

Pesticides are harmful to people—no one would dispute that. We can't always detect the immediate health effects from eating pesticide-laden food, but that doesn't mean that they are safe. The World Health Organization (WHO) estimates that between 3.5 and 5 million people globally suffer acute pesticide poisoning every year.

Studies of people regularly exposed to pesticides show that these poisons can cause nerve damage, cancer, diabetes, and other effects that can take a long time to manifest. These ill effects depend on how toxic the pesticide is and how much of it is taken in. Also, when researchers test the amount of pesticide in a single carrot or apple and declare that it is too low to be harmful, they are missing an important point. In the real world, we do not eat foods singly. We eat them in quantity and in combination, day in and day out.

As with food additives, little is known of the effects of multiple residues— the cocktail effect (see chapter 2, page 28). Very little research has been done, but the current knowledge points to the distinct possibility that these chemicals would react with each other to form even more potent toxins.

Officials continue to argue that levels of pesticide residues in food are within legal limits, but until those limits are proven safe beyond all reasonable doubt, we should not allow ourselves to be lulled into a false sense of security—legal does not necessarily mean safe.

How to Avoid Pesticides in Your Food

Once they are on or in food, pesticides are very difficult to avoid. Some authorities recommend that we wash and scrub all fresh fruit and vegetables thoroughly under running water. Running water has an abrasive effect that soaking doesn't have, so this may help to remove traces of chemicals from the surface of these foods as well as dirt from crevices. But not all pesticide residues can be removed just by washing, because many are designed to be water-resistant so they won't wash off crops when it rains.

Peeling the skin off fruit and vegetables whenever possible and discarding the outer leaves of leafy vegetables can reduce your exposure. Trimming the fat from meat and the skin from poultry and fish will also help, as most pesticide residues collect in fat.

Eating a variety of foods is sometimes recommended to help reduce your exposure to any one pesticide. It is uncertain how effective this is, however, as most pesticides work in similar ways, whatever the produce. Also, on the journey from farm to table, many foods are coated with multiple pesticides and fungicides. From a nutritional health standpoint, however, eating food from a variety of sources will give you a more comprehensive mix of nutrients, which may have a protective effect.

In fact, the best, and probably the only, way to avoid pesticides in your food is to include as much organic food in your diet as possible (see page 84).

You Are What They Eat

In recent decades, our consumption of meat products has grown dramatically. In the West, the average person eats around 137 pounds of beef, chicken, fish, and shellfish per year. But, if you're a meat eater, then you are also eating whatever the animal ate before it was slaughtered.

There was a time when animals reared for food ate what grew naturally—cows and chickens ate grass and grain, and big fish ate small fish or other sea creatures. In industrialized meat production—often a thirty-thousand-cow feedlot or a sixty-thousand-chicken coop—things are very different. The artificial conditions the animals are kept in—often without light or regular exercise—and the requirement for the animals to grow quickly to a saleable weight means that the animals require special "scientific" diets.

Such facilities thus require huge quantities of high-protein rations, and this has coincided with the need for slaughterhouses to find a cheap, safe way to dispose of more and more waste. Both industries have now entered into a marriage of convenience, which means that a number of animal by-products are now included in animal feeds—even for those animals that are not normally carnivores.

Cattle and chickens are still given plant-based feed: corn (for carbohydrates) and soybean meal (for amino acids) make up 70 to 90 percent of most commercial animal feeds. But the remaining 10 to 30 percent of feeds can differ radically from what cows and poultry would normally eat in their natural habitats.

Processed feathers, for instance, are an acceptable source of protein in cattle feed, as is chicken feces. Plastic pellets are permitted as roughage. Chickens can be fed meat and bonemeal. And, in addition to their main diet of fishmeal and fish oil, farmed fish may be given rendered meat, bone, and feather meal. These animal by-products can be contaminated with bacteria, such as salmonella, and the recycling of animal by-products into animal feed is an acknowledged risk for mad cow disease.

Other animal-feed additives contain worrisome industrial toxins. Every year in the United States, 11 billion pounds of animal fat are recycled into animal feed—a serious cause for concern, as many toxins and pesticides, such as dioxins and PCBs, concentrate naturally in animal fat. Dioxins are also found in the clays that occasionally get mixed into animal feeds.

Also included in the food of intensively reared animals are medications, such as growth promoters and antibiotics, given routinely even to healthy cattle and chickens to hasten growth and keep infections at bay. There is growing concern over the high use of antibiotics and its possible effects on human health. Antimicrobial drug residues in food (including antibiotics) are suspected to cause allergies, cancer, paralysis, respiratory failure, anaphylactic shock, and aplastic anemia in both humans and animals. In particular, every time we ingest antibiotics via our meat, we are contributing to the worldwide problem of antibiotic resistance. Nevertheless, the default position of many official government committees is that these residues pose no risk to consumers.

Stress Affects Meat Quality

Animals are, of course, subject to the same stresses that we humans are. Like us, extremes in temperature, humidity, light, sound, and confinement, as well as excitement, fatigue, pain, hunger, and thirst, can stress animals out—and so can environmental toxins, such as sheep dip and pesticides, in their food. Dairy cows and sheep living near sources of electromagnetic radiation, such as power lines, also exhibit signs of greater stress and lowered immunity.

When an animal is under severe stress due to fear or pain, increased levels of stress-related hormones, such as epinephrine (adrenaline) and cortisone, are found not only in the blood but also in body tissues. The stress experienced before slaughter is not only cruel but can cause undesirable effects on the quality of the meat, resulting in PSE (pale, soft, exudative) meat, which, as the name suggests, is colorless and overly liquid, or DFD (dark, firm, dry) meat, which lies at the other end of the scale.

The quality of the meat may also be compromised in other, more important ways. As stress levels in animals go up, immunity goes down, making them more prone to bacterial and viral infections (and more likely to be given antibiotics and other medicines as prevention and treatment). These microbes and chemicals as well as all the other toxins, such as pesticides, remain in the fat and muscle of the animal and are passed on to humans when we consume conventionally reared meats. The health effects of this have not yet been properly evaluated; however, it may be an early and persuasive argument against eating commercially reared meats, reducing your overall meat intake, or, for some, switching to a vegetarian diet.

Genetically Modified Ingredients

Increasingly, news headlines about genetic modification leave many of us anxious and confused about the food we eat. We now have the technology to alter the most basic building blocks of life. Sadly, we have not conducted the studies necessary to prove or disprove the safety of GM foods over either the long or short term. It is still not clear whether GM foods can, for instance, cause damage to a vulnerable fetus at certain stages of its development.

GM foods don't taste better and are not cheaper to buy; they have, however, been implicated in increased resistance to antibiotics and the creation of superbugs. They have also been linked to an increased incidence of allergies, unpredictable rises of toxins in the body, increased cancer rates, and a decline in the nutritional quality of foods. Ironically, studies show that, contrary to most industry reports, U.S. farmers growing GM crops are using just as many toxic pesticides and herbicides as conventional farmers—and, in some cases, more.

For farmers, these pesticide-resistant crops have certain benefits. For example, they can spray large quantities of herbicides on and around them to kill weeds without damaging their crop. Because of this widespread practice, scientists estimate that herbicide-resistant crops planted around the globe will triple the amount of toxic, broad-spectrum herbicides used in agriculture.

Although it is claimed by the biotechnology companies that there have been no ill effects seen in people consuming GM food in the United States, there have been no large or in-depth studies to support this statement. Observations in the medical press, however, suggest that negative effects are becoming more apparent. For instance, according to a report by the U.K.'s Soil Association, "Genetic Engineering and Human Health":

- **In the U.K.** A 50 percent rise in soy allergies has been reported since imports of GM food started.

- **In Ireland.** Doctors have reported an increase in child soy allergies since the start of GM soy imports.

- **In the United States.** Coinciding with the introduction of GM ingredients, food-derived illnesses are believed to have doubled over the last seven years.

Food can either be genetically modified itself or contain genetically modified ingredients. The issues are complex, but, if you are concerned, you might want to consider avoiding or limiting:

- **Tomatoes (and tomato purée).** The first GM foods to be sold. In the United States, you can buy fresh tomatoes that have been genetically modified; in the U.K., you can only buy puree made from these tomatoes. Watch out for ready-made foods, such as pizza, that may use GM tomato purée.

- **Soy.** Modified to resist weed killer. In the United States, the supplier of most of the world's soy, GM and unmodified soy are not kept separate, and processed foods may contain both. Soy is present in most baked and prepackaged foods in several forms: oil (often just labeled as "vegetable oil"), vegetable fat, flour, lecithin, and vegetable protein.

- **Corn.** Modified to contain bacteria toxic to a common crop pest. Corn is used as a grain, as cornmeal, cornstarch, corn syrup, dextrose, glucose, fructose,

xanthan gum, and maltodextrin, and as corn oil. Be aware of things like chocolate bars and sweet drinks that contain sugars derived from corn.

- **Cheese.** Can be made with a GM enzyme called chymosin instead of traditional rennet. Chymosin is used in many vegetarian cheeses and increasingly in
hard cheeses for general consumption.

- *Enzymes.* Used in a large number of products, including drinks, bakery goods,
and dairy products. Manufacturers are not obliged to include these on the
product information.

- **Canola, or rapeseed.** Mainly used as oil. Some crops now contain human
genes.

- **Yeast.** Has been genetically modified and approved for making bread; it is difficult to know the extent to which it is used in bakery products.

- **Vitamin B$_2$.** Known as riboflavin, and now widely produced from genetically
modified microorganisms. It is generally added to breakfast cereals, soft drinks,
baby foods, and diet foods.

To spot GM foods, you will have to read the labels. But even this will not guarantee that your diet will be GM-free. Labeling laws can be very confusing, and
seem to exist mostly to protect the manufacturer rather than the consumer. Certain GM ingredients, such as flavorings and additives, do not need to be listed on
the label, and very few manufacturers volunteer this information. For the moment, the best way to avoid GM foods is to eat as much organic and freshly prepared (by you in your home) food as possible, and to avoid prepackaged foods
when you can.

In addition to GM organisms in our food, concerns have recently been expressed that some excipients (inert ingredients) in nutritional supplements may
also include genetically modified ingredients. Most health supplements that are
not licensed medicines are classed as foods and, as such, are obliged to carry
warnings to the consumer on the label if they are known to contain GM ingredients. Supplements that are licensed medicines (for instance, some folic acid and
cod liver oil supplements) are not required to carry alerts to consumers to the
presence of GM ingredients or derivatives, and so could contain these ingredients without any indication on the label.

According to Genetic Food Alert (GFA) in the U.K., unless expressly denied
by the manufacturer, the following excipients may be genetically modified:

- Derivatives of soy, corn, cotton, or rapeseed, including oils that are used as carriers for vitamins (A, D, and E) in supplements; lecithin and vitamin E, which

are used as antioxidants; and sweeteners, such as dextrose, glucose, dextrins, maltodextrins, and sorbitol.

- GM microorganisms or their products, including some bacteria, brewer's yeast, and baker's yeast. Products of GM bacteria can include aspartame and enzymes used as processing aids (which may not be listed on the label), such as alpha-acetolactate decarboxylase, alpha-amylase, catalase, chymosin a, chymosin b, cyclodextrin-glucosyltransferase, beta-glucanase, glucose isomerase, glucose oxidase, hemicellulase (xylanase), lipase, triacylglycerol, maltogenic amylase, pectinesterase, protease, and pullulanase.

- Products of GM-fed or -treated animals, including gelatin, bonemeal, and albumen from animals raised on GM ingredients or injected with GM growth hormones, such as BST (bovine somatotropin).

Packaging

A wide range of materials come into contact with food during its production, processing, packaging, storage, and preparation. All of these have the potential to leach chemicals into the product.

If your intake of packaged foods is high, then your potential exposure to the chemicals that migrate from packaging into the foodstuffs is also high. In the EU, the "safe" exposure of migrants from food-contact materials (FCMs) is an estimated intake of 2.2 pounds of packaged food per 130-pound person per day. But this figure applies only to adults. Children tend to consume more food than adults per pound of body weight. Worse, food products that are targeted specifically at children are often packaged in small single portions, so the potential for greater migration into the food is higher. There is no reliable safe limit of food-contact materials for children.

Following are examples of the kinds of chemicals that can migrate from package to food.

- **Toxins leaching from plastic or foam packaging** can be absorbed by foods, and are associated with such health problems as cancer. The chemical of concern is *1,3-butadiene*, but, because of the varying amounts of this chemical that are used in plastics and foam packaging, it is impossible to make an accurate estimate of how much gets into your food from any one container.

- **Aseptic or Tetra Paks** have recently been shown to leach *isopropylthioxanthone* (ITX). ITX can get into any fatty product like milk when it is exposed to sunlight's ultraviolet rays. Little information is available as to the safety of ITX, which is a chemical produced in relatively small quantities globally. The U.S. Environmental Protection Agency (EPA) considers it a potentially high hazard in the environment based on studies showing that it is toxic to aquatic species. Manufacturers have yet to provide clear, verifiable information on the health effects of ITX, especially if it is consumed as a contaminant in foodstuffs. But some evidence suggests that people exposed occupationally to ITX can develop skin rashes when exposure to the chemical is followed by exposure to the sun.

• **Teflon** is widely used in the paper wrapping of fast and microwaveable foods, such as french fries, popcorn, and pizza, as well as candy wrappers and other products. It helps to prevent grease stains from coming through the wrappers. You don't see it, you don't feel it, and you can't taste it, but when you open that bag and start removing your french fries from it, you are extracting and eating a fluorochemical called Zonyl, which can further break down into perfluorooctanoic acid (PFOA). According to the EPA, PFOA stays in the bloodstream and is a suspected carcinogen. The U.S. government says this chemical is now believed to be in the blood of nearly every American.

• **Aluminum** is found in the packaging of freezer-to-oven ready-made meals and in soda cans, and is implicated in a range of neurological disorders. The more acidic the food product is, the greater the chances that aluminum will migrate into it.

• **Plastics** are used for microwaveable packaging and as liners in trash cans. They contain several chemicals that mimic the action of estrogen, including phthalates and bisphenol A. The latter has recently been found to provoke insulin resistance, a prediabetic condition in which tissues lose their normal sensitivity to insulin. Plastic wrapping on microwaveable foods can also transmit the chemicals during heating.

Less obvious packaging materials that can pose health risks include *isocyanates*, adhesive components in laminates and can coatings; *semicarbazide*, used in the plastic sealing gaskets on jars of food, especially baby food; volatile substances, such as those present in adhesives and in the printing inks used for packaging; and microwave susceptors, usually a mixture of metals and minerals incorporated into a plastic film to ensure that microwaved foods crisp during cooking.

Even if your food isn't in something that you recognize as packaging, it may have been "packaged" in some way to make it more appealing on the supermarket shelf. Fresh fruit is a good example. Many fresh foods are coated in petroleum-derived waxes to help maintain freshness. The waxes on fruit and vegetables are based on petrochemicals and may trigger allergies. They may also contain *morpho-*

line, which, according to World Health Organization reports, turns into the carcinogen *N*-nitrosomorpholine.

Foods that are regularly waxed include thin-skinned produce, such as cucumbers, peppers, and apples. In addition, all fruit and vegetables are repeatedly sprayed with a multitude of pesticides and fungicides while in storage. Unwanted additives can also seep in from packaging. For example, if the plastic packaging is derived from vinyl chloride—a known carcinogen and endocrine disrupter—this can easily migrate into foods, especially those that are acidic or fatty.

Nano Additives

Nanotechnology deals with particles so small—a million of them would fit on a pinhead—that the laws of classical physics no longer apply. After experiencing widespread rejection of genetically modified foods, the food industry is somewhat skittish about owning up to its research into "atomically modified" food products. But this research is ongoing and nanofood products are already on the shelves.

According to a 2004 study entitled "Nanotechnology in Food and Food Processing Industry Worldwide," around two hundred food-manufacturing companies are already working on ways to insert nanotechnology into foods. These companies are already celebrating the future profits of their endeavors. The food industry calculates that the nanofood market was already worth around $7 billion in 2006 and that this figure will grow to $20 billion by 2010.

But no research at all has been done to investigate how these particles might affect human health (in this, there is a disturbing parallel with GM). Worse, no one knows how to regulate these technologies, as they span the regulatory boundaries between pharmaceuticals, medical devices, and biological agents. The U.S. Food and Drug Administration considers that particle size is not the issue in regulation; but this is clearly not the case, since the defining characteristic of nanoparticles is that, because of their size, they behave in ways that defy classical physics and, thus, may interact with the body in entirely unpredictable ways. None of the current crop of safety tests is designed to investigate the effects of nanoparticles, and none can prove them to be entirely safe for human consumption.

Where Does Your Food Come From?

One of the inevitable consequences of advanced preservation systems for food is our newfound ability to ship food over long distances and store it for long periods of time without provoking spoilage. Thus, people in the middle of a dark winter morning by the North Sea can have papayas or lychees for breakfast, if they so desire.

There is a price to pay, however, for the luxury of eating long-haul foods. A recent survey in the U.K. showed that an alarming number of children have no real understanding of how, where, or why their food is produced. Indeed, many didn't know that eggs came from chickens or hamburgers from cows.

Some of the one hundred youngsters—aged between ten and fourteen and living in England and Wales—who took part in the survey for the Country Landowners Association thought that a ewe was a bird, that mutton came from rabbits, that "free range" means "not genetic" and that cows produce milk because they eat grass. If this survey had been carried out twenty or thirty years ago, it would have produced a very different set of answers.

Nevertheless, grown-ups shouldn't feel too superior either. Many know little more than the basics as to the origins of their food or the consequences of the overuse of certain ingredients. Few can claim to understand, for instance, how the overuse of palm oil in junk foods is killing off orangutans in far-flung corners of the world, such as Borneo and Sumatra, by destroying their natural habitats. And few know just how significantly our love of long-haul food contributes to the destruction of our natural environment.

Yet, according to the Soil Association, which is the U.K.'s main organic-certification board, the number of food miles accumulated by many of the foods we take for granted every day is staggering. Indeed, the carbon-dioxide emissions from moving food around the planet is a direct contributor to the catastrophic problem of global warming. For instance:

- Through the food consumed, the average person is responsible for 9.63 tons of carbon-dioxide emissions.

- A weekly basket of imported food for a family of four could add 1.1 tons to per capita emissions.

- A typical Sunday meal could travel forty-nine thousand miles—equivalent to two journeys around the world and releasing eighty-two pounds of carbon dioxide.

- Distributing products by plane results in fifty times more carbon dioxide than sea freight.

- For every thousand fruit products bought in the U.K., only six will be grown there.

- The food system accounts for up to 40 percent of all U.K. road freight.

What Is Missing from Your Food?

Apart from the things that are added intentionally or otherwise to our food supply, there is a whole host of things that we have lost due to modern intensive agricultural practices. These also have important implications for our long-term health.

While fruit, vegetables, and whole grains are commonly thought to be high in essential nutrients, the majority of today's produce and grains are grown in depleted soil, doused with pesticides, and stored for long periods of time (all the while being sprayed with more insecticides and fungicides) before being sold. They may be stored for an even longer time after purchase, before being eaten or used in cooking.

Because of this, some modern nutritionists believe that, in the midst of all this plenty, many people in the West are starving—for the basic nutrients that were once in our everyday food.

Conventional farmers are caught in a vicious circle of production. They add chemical fertilizers to the soil in the hope of increasing crop yields, but doing this ultimately increases many plants' susceptibility to pests. So more pesticides are used. But the pesticides they use can also affect the soil's capacity to sustain and generate fertility.

Using synthetic fertilizers to make plants grow in otherwise depleted soils has other disturbing consequences. For instance, while the fertilizer will stimulate the plant to grow in the absence of any of the usual protective nutrients they should contain, the plants will also take up more of the heavy metals in the soil, such as aluminum, mercury, and lead, and these, in turn, are passed on up through the food chain.

All the while, the nutritional value of our food is plummeting.

Nutrient Deficits

In 1940, the British chemists Robert McCance and Elsie Widdowson published the first of what would be their periodical examinations of the nutrient content of food. When the fifth edition of this tome—which has over the years become a standard reference work on the subject—was published in 1991, the British geologist-turned-nutritionist David Thomas undertook the work of comparing the values as published in the first and latest editions of the book.

He examined the data for twenty-eight raw vegetables and forty-four cooked vegetables, seventeen fruits, and ten types of meat, poultry, and game. His findings make frightening reading. What he found was that, among today's foods:

- **All fruits** contain 27 percent less zinc.

- **All meats** contain 41 percent less calcium and 54 percent less iron.

- **Apples and oranges** have 67 percent less iron.

- **Broccoli** (boiled) has 75 percent less calcium.

- **Carrots** have 75 percent less magnesium, 48 percent less calcium, 46 percent less iron, and 75 percent less copper.

- **Potatoes** have 30 percent less magnesium, 35 percent less calcium, 45 percent less iron, and 47 percent less copper.

- **Rutabaga** has 71 percent less iron.

- **Scallions** have 74 percent less calcium.

- **Spinach** (boiled) has 60 percent less iron and 96 percent less copper.

- **Watercress** has 93 percent less copper.

Among the other worrisome findings was that the practice of seeding the soil with only certain minerals (sodium, phosphorus, and potassium) has greatly altered the natural mineral profile of our foods. Thus, rutabaga now contains 110 percent of the phosphorus it once did. Humans who eat this nutritionally altered food cannot help but experience an alteration in the natural mineral profiles of their own body tissues and bones as well, which can affect their health.

A similar exercise was carried out in the United States in 1999, when the nutritionist Alex Jack compared nutrient values in that year's U.S. Department of Agriculture (USDA) handbook with those published in 1975. He discovered a number of mineral deficits, as well as the fact that cauliflower had 40 percent less vitamin C than it did in 1975.

Many classes of herbicide can alter plant metabolism and, thus, nutrient composition. For example, herbicides that inhibit photosynthesis (such as triazine or phenoyacetics) produce effects similar to growing a plant in low-light conditions. Under such conditions, the carbohydrate, alpha-tocopherol (vitamin E), and beta-carotene (a precursor of vitamin A) content of a plant is reduced, and protein, free amino acid, and *nitrate* levels are increased. Equally, bleaching herbicides can reduce beta-carotene levels, and sulphonylurea herbicides are known to reduce levels of branched-chain amino acids (which people need to maintain muscle tissue).

Making Changes

When you begin to realize the health risks associated with processed foods and food additives, it makes good sense to start eating less of them or, better yet, cutting them out altogether. The problem is that the widespread use of additives has greatly changed our perception of what food is and should be. Food riddled with additives is convenient. It can be bought in bulk and stored for long periods of time. It's always on tap. It is highly flavored and brightly colored, appealing to our senses.

If giving up all the foods you like seems too big a task, then start slowly. If there are special treats that you just can't imagine living without, have them on occasion. But be aware of what those special treats contain. Where possible, look for wholesome alternatives that taste just as good and that don't put your health at risk.

Also, consider changing your buying habits. Are there farmers' markets in the area where you could shop frequently? If you don't know, use the Internet or the local paper to find out. Is there a natural-foods market with organic produce nearby that you've never bothered to patronize? If so, now is the time to investigate it.

Eating Locally

When it comes to eating good food, most of us would automatically think organic. Organic food has undoubted advantages but, in the big picture of food production, locally produced food has a much more important role to play in keeping our bodies and communities healthy.

Consider the conclusions of a British study, "Farm Costs and Food Miles: An Assessment of the Full Cost of the UK Weekly Food Basket," published in 2005 in the journal *Food Policy*. It calculated a shopping cart's hidden costs, which grow as produce is transported over large distances. The study found that road miles account for proportionately more environmental damage than air miles. While organic farming is valuable, the distance that organic food often travels to reach our plates creates environmental damage that outweighs the benefit of buying organic.

Instead, these scientists argued that people can help the environment even more by buying food from within a twelve-mile radius. By their calculations, if all foods originated within twelve miles of where they were consumed, environmental and congestion costs would fall from more than $4.4 billion to under $450 million—an "environmental saving" of $4 billion annually.

Buying locally produced food might seem impossible if you live in a big city. But by patronizing farmers' markets, you can drastically cut your contribution to food miles and put fresher, better food on your table.

Locally produced food has other benefits as well:

- **Fresher, riper, better-tasting.** Produce that is purchased in the supermarket or a big-box store has been in transit or cold-stored for days or weeks, whereas produce that you purchase at your local farmers' market has often been picked within twenty-four hours of your buying it. This freshness not only affects the taste of your food but also the nutritional value, which inevitably declines during long storage times. In addition, because local produce doesn't have to stand up to the rigors of shipping, it can be allowed to ripen naturally on the tree or vine and sold ripe and ready to eat.

- **Seasonal.** By eating with the seasons, we are eating foods when they are at their peak taste, are the most abundant, and are the least expensive.

- **Full of variety.** Supermarkets are only interested in selling name-brand fruit and vegetables, such as romaine lettuce, Red Delicious apples, and russet potatoes. Local producers have more freedom to try growing new varieties that might have a shorter shelf life or don't produce high yields, and so don't make it to a large supermarket.

- **More personal.** Buying direct from the farm or at a farmers' market means that you get to know the people who grow and sell your food. Knowing some of the story of your food can be an important part of enjoying a meal, but equally important is the fact that knowing the person who grew your food provides you with a fail-safe and actual person to speak to should you find the produce (or bread, or fish, or meat) below standard. This kind of immediate person-to-person contact is good for you and good for the food producer.

- **The key to responsible land development.** When you buy locally, you give those with local open spaces—farms and pastures—an economic reason to remain open and undeveloped.

Eating Organic

The increased demand for organic food has been the result of many shifts in consumer consciousness. Food scares, such as bovine spongiform encephalopathy (BSE, or mad cow disease) and other food-borne diseases have affected consumer confidence in conventional farming. Greater awareness of environmental issues has made many people make the ethical choice of eating organic foods. Also, the increasing use of alternative therapies that rely on organically grown foods has helped to renew interest in the quality of the food we eat.

Interestingly, there have been few human studies into the benefits of organic foods. So, we can only guess at how beneficial they may be, and whether consumers of organic foods are truly healthier than those who consume conventionally produced foods. Even if there were research to prove the superior health of organic consumers, however, the nutrient content of the food would be only one element in their total health picture. Consumers of organic foods may also, for instance, be more active. They may walk or cycle instead of taking the car. They may restrict their use of hazardous chemicals in the home. They may be better able to manage stress.

Nevertheless, one review of what research there is found that when all the data are taken together, there is a clear trend supporting the notion that organic foods are indeed more nutritious. For instance, according to a report by the U.K.'s Soil Association, "Organic Food: Facts and Figures 2005":

- Organic food contains, on average, higher levels of vitamin C and essential minerals, such as calcium, magnesium, iron, and chromium.

- In a review of forty-one studies from around the world, organic crops were shown to have statistically significantly higher levels of vitamin C, magnesium, iron, and phosphorus. Spinach, lettuce, cabbage, and potatoes showed particularly high levels of minerals.

- Nitrate levels in organic foods are, on average, 15 percent lower than in conventionally grown foods. Scientists at Glasgow University found a link between the levels of nitrates in vegetables and throat cancer, the numbers of which have tripled over the last twenty years and claim more than three thousand lives a year. They believe that an increase in the use of nitrate fertilizers since World War II may be one of the major reasons for the rise in this cancer.

- Organic vegetables have higher levels (between 10 and 50 percent) of secondary nutrients. These include antioxidants that help to mop up harmful free radicals implicated in cancer.

- Deficiencies in certain vitamins and minerals can lead to a variety of symptoms, including muscle cramps and depression.

- Between 1940 and 1991, trace minerals in conventional U.K. fruit and vegetables fell by up to 76 percent; U.S. figures showed a similar trend.

- In a survey of organic vegetable soups, researchers found that they contained almost six times as much salicylic acid as nonorganic vegetable soups. This acid helps combat arteriosclerosis (hardening of the arteries) and bowel cancer, and is responsible for the anti-inflammatory action of aspirin. It is naturally used by plants as a defense against disease.

Supporters of organic food also point out that organically grown foods contain more secondary metabolites than conventionally grown plants. Secondary metabolites are substances that form part of plants' immune systems and also help to fight cancer in humans.

But the claim for the superiority of organic foods is not based on nutrient content alone. In some ways, the nutrient-content argument may even be misleading, as it's not what is in organic foods but what is not in them that is more important—pesticides and, according to the prevailing regulatory standards for organic processed foods, the full range of worrisome additives. But this brings us to the thorny question of whether organic convenience food is in keeping with either the spirit or letter of organic principles.

Slow Food

In his bestselling book *Fast Food Nation*, author Eric Schlosser writes of the growing costs of our love affair with fast foods. "Fast food," he argues, "has triggered the homogenization of our society . . . has hastened the malling of our landscape, a widening of the chasm between rich and poor, fueled an epidemic of obesity, and propelled the juggernaut of American cultural imperialism abroad." This must-read book documents how fast food has lured us into choosing diets that are deficient in nearly everything except calories, and into supporting practices that are deceptive in every aspect—from advertising to flavoring—as well as systems that degrade nearly everyone and everything involved.

As a result, for many of us, the shopping, preparation, and eating of food have become just one more rushed chore in an already packed day. Yet, according to the Slow Food movement, it doesn't need to be that way.

The Slow Food movement began in Italy in 1986 as an act of resistance against fast food. Since then, it has expanded globally to one hundred countries and now has eighty-three thousand members in the United States, Europe, Japan, and elsewhere. Its view is that processed fast food is not only changing the physical landscape through intensive farming, but is also eroding the way of life that revolved around the producing and eating of great food in a relaxed, sociable way.

As an antidote to this loss of the pleasures of sharing good food, its members are keen to "protect the pleasures of the table from the homogenization of modern fast food and life." They want to know where their food comes from and how it is produced. They want local foods produced by someone they know and trust, and they want to help motivate other ordinary people into taking control of how they live, work, and eat.

By promoting "gastronomic culture," Slow Food is committed to promoting the diversity of local and regional quality food that is produced and marketed in a way that protects traditional foods at risk of extinction, and guarantees farmers a fair price while protecting the environment and the natural landscape.

Even if you are not a committed food campaigner, you can embrace the principles of slow food in your everyday life by considering some of the suggestions at the end of this chapter.

Organic Junk Food

A significant proportion of the organic market is now made up of convenience foods. As the market booms, there is a genuine risk that the kind of commercial success demonstrated in recent years by organic foods will attract people with the wrong motives and wrong values to take up organic farming.

A quick look at the supermarket shelves will also confirm that the majority of organic items stocked in any supermarket are convenience foods. Preprepared

What Is Good Food?

What is it that makes food good? Since food is central to so much of our social experiences as well as the foundation for continuing good health, this question is worth pondering.

For some, quality is defined by what you pay for food; for others, it is defined by how fresh it is or whether it's organic. In fact, good food is defined by a number of factors, some of which may seem like a utopian ideal in the food desert we now occupy. And while every meal you eat may not meet these high criteria, it's still worth aiming high. For food to be good, it must be:

- **Authentic.** In other words, it should not have been synthesized or adulterated during its production, processing, or storage. It must be what it promises to be and what consumers expect it to be—for example, the brown color of brown bread is real, not just a synthetic color added to white bread.
- **Sensual.** Food should feel good to eat. It should combine taste, smell, texture, look, and feel. Think of the incomparable blend of sensations when you bite into a genuinely ripe peach or eat a freshly caught fish. If you can't recall these sensations, you've been away from genuinely good food for too long.
- **Functional.** How appropriate is a specific food to its purpose? For example, different varieties of potatoes are more or less suitable for boiling, baking, roasting, or frying. When we are denied variety in our diet, the functional quality of food in making a dish special disappears.
- **Nutritious.** How does what you eat benefit your body? Good fresh food has enormous value for its protein, fat, and carbohydrate contents as well as its levels of vitamins, minerals, trace elements, beneficial enzymes, and live organisms (as found in live yogurt).
- **Ethical.** Everything you eat has social and political implications. Food should be produced in such a way as to protect and honor the planet and the people on it. Instead, the industrialization of food has had negative impacts on human rights, animal rights, and the environment. How much rain forest was destroyed for the hamburger you're eating? Did a farmer in Ghana go bankrupt producing your favorite chocolate bar? Pondering these questions makes it increasingly hard to justify eating according to the fast-food habit.

sauces, burgers, chips, pizza, ice cream, peanut butter, jam, sausages, and chocolate are all big sellers. It is highly unlikely that any of these foods are substantially better for you (or more nutritious) than their conventional counterparts.

Unfortunately, there's no basic difference in the processing of some organic foods and nonorganic foods. Many organic foods are not really produced in the traditional way at all. They're still produced using conventional industrial methods. For instance, organic bread can still use highly refined flours. Manufacturers of organic products are also using preservatives, such as sugar. In fact, some organic cookies have more sugar and fat in them than a conventional cookie.

Focusing on nutrient counts and a lack of pesticide residues is important, but it also narrows our vision. The boom in organic food has come about largely because of clever marketing on the part of the big supermarkets. They have sold us the idea that buying organic is something healthy that you don't have to change your lifestyle to do. In reality, buying better food, be it local or organic, will require a shift in your mind-set and your scheduling. As these giant retailers fall over themselves to package and shift more and more organic convenience foods, another issue has emerged. Many countries already have a strict definition of "organic," but what we really need is a better definition of "food."

Return to Real Food

The more we learn about the toxic potential of modern foods, the greater the need for a new food culture that values wholesomeness, nutrition, freshness, and flavor. Raising our expectations of food and embracing these values has the added effect of protecting the natural environment, treating animals humanely, protecting our soil, and respecting the farmers and food-industry workers who are involved in the food-production process. It also leads to a stronger preference for foods that are produced locally.

Getting back to good food is much easier than you think. Consider these tips:

• **Eat the best quality you can afford.** Avoid junk foods (such as cookies, sweets, and sodas), which are not only chock-full of artificial colors and other additives but are also of little nutritional value—high in calories, sugar, fats, and/or sodium. This is especially good advice for children, who are the main consumers of junk food and at increased risk of health problems involving additives. In addition, while frozen foods may be convenient, freezing destroys vital nutrients, and there is even some indication that refrigeration causes similar effects.

- **Eat freshly prepared.** Consider removing the microwave from your kitchen. If you only use it to heat coffee, or cook potatoes or prepackaged meals, you probably don't need it. Getting rid of your microwave will also vastly improve the quality of the food you eat, as food that has been microwaved has fewer nutrients in it. In addition, proteins, such as those found in meats, are significantly altered during the microwave process. Eating food directly from the microwave may also mean ingesting food that is still giving off radiation; this is why users are advised to let food sit for a few minutes afterward—to let all this radiation disperse.

- **Eat natural.** If it comes in a box or container, or tray or jar—or if it's a color you don't normally see in nature—think twice before putting it in your mouth.

- **Eat variety.** This may limit your exposure to any one additive—safer in the event that it turns out to have long-term health risks.

- **Eat seasonally.** It is less expensive, provides greater variety in the diet, and will reduce your exposure to the antifungal and antibacterial chemicals commonly used to extend the shelf life of products grown out of season or shipped halfway across the globe.

- **Eat slowly.** If it's a choice between a burger shack or the local café or restaurant, ditch the burger shack. If it's a choice between wolfing down a sandwich at your desk or sitting on a park bench, go to the park. Wherever possible, try to sit down and enjoy your meal, and teach your children to do the same.

- **Eat what you like.** Be guided by your taste buds, and be aware that the more you change your eating habits, the more your taste will start to return to normal. Cravings for salty, sugary, highly processed foods will disappear and, with them, the tendency to overeat foods that are not good for your health.

6. TOILETRIES AND COSMETICS

We use them to make us feel good, smell good, and look good. We spend vast amounts of money on them—globally more than $200 billion a year—and with that investment comes a lot of blind faith that the hair products and skin products, toothpastes and makeup will somehow improve us. Whatever your head may know, your heart still wants to believe that there is some instant magic in the toiletries and cosmetics you buy that will—at least for a little while—make you younger, sexier, more beautiful, and more vibrant than before.

The magic of all the toiletries and cosmetics we buy is strong and the promises on the fronts of the packages are so seductive that most of us never bother to look on the back to find out what's actually in all these products we buy. Even if you do check the label of your favorite cosmetics, the chances are that all you will see is an incomprehensible alphabet soup of words.

It's easier, and certainly more comforting, to believe in magic than it is to learn to makes sense of the often impenetrable labels on personal-care products. But the effort might just be worth making, since, whatever the front-of-the-package come-on is, the truth is that achieving a cosmetic quick fix requires a cocktail of largely synthetic ingredients, which are known to cause, among other things, cancer, central-nervous-system disruption, birth defects, and immune damage.

The chemicals in personal-care products are a particularly insidious form of pollution because they enter the body through multiple routes. We can swallow them, inhale them, and absorb them through the skin, as well as through the mucous membranes in the eyes, mouth, and nose. In addition, cosmetics commonly contain emollients (oils and fats), solvents (for instance, *propylene glycol*), and humectants (such as *glycerin*), which, while relatively harmless in their own right, increase the skin's permeability, which, in turn, increases the amount of other, more toxic ingredients in the mix that is absorbed into the bloodstream.

While many people assume that the government oversees the safety and efficacy of cosmetics and toiletries, most regulatory agencies do not require manufacturers to demonstrate that their products are either safe or effective.

Such regulations as there are do little to protect consumers. While regulators have approved more than three thousand ingredients for cosmetic use in Europe, many more substances find their way into cosmetics and toiletries through loopholes in the law—for instance, those that allow products to contain traces of contaminants and other banned substances that are difficult to remove during or after manufacture.

In an ideal world, we would all be able to judge the safety of a product by its labeling. Sadly, manufacturers are inconsistent in their labeling practices and many actively resist full disclosure of ingredients on their labels because of the fear of customer backlash. What this means is that, on any supermarket shelf, you will find some products where the labels are printed on the container, and others where they are listed on peel-away labels stuck on the underside of the product. Others print them on the packaging (which is often thrown away without as much as a glance), and some use vague wording or, worse, don't list all of their ingredients, or only make the ingredients list available on request at the point of sale. What this means is that it's currently difficult for all but the most motivated among us to make good decisions about what products are safe.

Where the Problem Starts

When it comes to cosmetics and toiletries, certain types of ingredients, such as preservatives, perfumes, and colors, are known to be a significant cause of skin reactions. In fact, skin reactions are the most frequently reported adverse effect of using cosmetics, with between 10 and 30 percent of adults experiencing skin problems from exposure to preservatives and fragrances in cosmetic products.

There is evidence to suggest that the number of people experiencing skin reactions to cosmetics is increasing. At this time, more than 80 percent of those who develop reactions to cosmetics are healthy individuals without any prior skin problems.

It can be fairly easy to pinpoint the cosmetic causes of skin reactions, such as dermatitis. But tracking the causes of more significant or longer-term problems like depression and migraines, and even cancer, is a much more difficult task. And yet, as research into cosmetic ingredients advances, scientists are finding that many of the same substances that can cause short-term problems are also long-term poisons. Skin reactions, then, could be seen as the body's early-warning system kicking in and telling you to stop using particular products or to avoid certain ingredients.

Preservatives

Preservatives by their very nature are designed to kill things. Specifically, they work by killing cells and preventing their dissemination, and are intended to prevent the growth of bacteria and fungi—mainly, *Candida albicans*, *Pseudomonas aeruginosa*, *Escherichia coli*, *Aspergillus niger*, and *Staphylococcus aureus*—which can potentially cause serious infections on the skin and in the body.

The problem is that human skin also comprises living cells, so preservatives, even if used in small quantities, present a risk to the integrity of the skin and, should they be absorbed into the bloodstream, to the rest of the body, too. For this reason, most cosmetic preservatives have restrictions on their use—usually limiting them to a small percentage of the total formula.

For cosmetic formulators, finding new preservatives is complicated, because to be considered effective a preservative has to fulfill several criteria. It must be:

- effective across a wide range of microbes
- long-lasting, in that it continues to keep the product free from contaminants for the life of the product
- rapid-acting, at the first sign of contamination
- nonsensitizing (it won't cause an allergic response)
- nontoxic and nonirritating
- compatible with the other ingredients in the mix
- stable (it won't break down during storage and stays active across a wide pH range)
- inactive, except as an antimicrobial (it won't interact with other ingredients)
- soluble, so that it mixes well with whatever base (water or oil) it's in
- acceptable in odor and color
- cost-effective

No single preservative, synthetic or natural, fulfills all of these criteria, which is one reason why manufacturers often use several different preservatives in a single product. Another reason is solubility: some preservatives are water-soluble and some are oil-soluble; in a water-oil emulsion, such as a hand lotion, formulators need to use both types.

The most commonly used cosmetic preservatives belong to a family of chemicals known as alkyl hydroxy benzoates, or *parabens*. Look on any cosmetic ingredients label and it's likely you will find *methylparaben, ethylparaben, butylparaben*, and propylparaben listed, either singly or, more often, in combination.

All the most commonly used preservatives can cause dermatitis and other skin reactions—some more so than others. Parabens are universally recognized as skin sensitizers. But, in late 1998, researchers at Brunel University in the U.K. published a study that identified parabens as estrogen mimics as well, each with a different estrogenic potency. Methylparaben was the least potent, followed by ethylparaben, propylparaben, and, finally, butylparaben. In studies of breast tumors, traces of parabens were also found in every single sample, suggesting that this estrogenic effect is not just an artifact of the lab.

After parabens, *Kathon CG*—the main constituents of which are *methylisothiazolinone* and *methylchloroisothiazolinone*—is the most common preservative ingredient used in cosmetics. Like parabens, it too is a common allergen.

But not so long ago, a study from the University of Texas Health Science Center found that Kathon CG was also mutagenic—in other words, capable of causing genes to mutate. This study was the first to test commercially available products containing this preservative. The researchers noted that when a product is both a sensitizer and a mutagen, then it also has the potential to cause cancer and that "more adequate testing for its cancer-causing potential is needed." Since then, laboratory studies have found that methylchloroisothiazolinone is also a neurotoxin.

Fragrances

The addition of "fragrance" is a particularly thorny issue for consumers because most of us will never know which fragrance chemicals are in the products we use. Manufacturers are allowed to list them under simple, shorthand names that belie the often hundreds of different ingredients that are involved in producing a single scent. (Even the simplest fragrances can contain between thirty and fifty ingredients.)

The fragrance portion of a product is thought to account for as much as 15 percent of all allergic reactions in eczema patients, and this trend is increasing. And while synthetic fragrances are the most commonly used and, thus, the most commonly implicated, emerging evidence suggests that natural fragrances may also cause allergic reactions.

But most fragrance chemicals are potentially more damaging, as they are composed of neurotoxic solvents associated with central-nervous-system (CNS) disorders, such as multiple sclerosis, Parkinson's disease, Alzheimer's disease, and sudden infant death syndrome, and many of these solvents have been labeled as toxic waste by the U.S. Food and Drug Administration. It's not just adult cosmetics that are a problem. Play makeup and perfumes aimed at children often contain unacceptably high levels of these substances.

According to the 1991 U.S. Environmental Protection Agency (EPA) report "Health Hazard Information," the twenty most common fragrance ingredients make up a toxic soup that no thinking person would volunteer to be exposed to. Among these chemicals, seven—1,8-cineole, beta-citronellol, beta-myrcene, nerol, ocimene, beta-phenethyl alcohol, and alpha-terpinolene—are completely lacking in safety data. Among the rest:

- *Acetone* is on the hazardous waste lists of several government agencies. It is primarily a CNS depressant that can cause dryness of the mouth and throat, dizziness, nausea, lack of coordination, slurred speech, drowsiness, and, in severe exposures, coma.

- *Benzaldehyde* acts as a local anesthetic and CNS depressant. It can cause irritation to the mouth, throat, eyes, skin, lungs, and gastrointestinal (GI) tract, causing nausea and abdominal pain. It can also cause kidney damage.

- *Benzyl acetate* is an environmental pollutant and potential carcinogen linked to pancreatic cancer. Its vapors are irritating to the eyes and respiratory passages, and it can also be absorbed through the skin, causing system-wide effects.

- *Benzyl alcohol* is irritating to the upper respiratory tract. It can cause headache, nausea, vomiting, dizziness, a fall in blood pressure, CNS depression, and, in severe cases, death due to respiratory failure.

- *Camphor* is a local irritant and CNS stimulant that is readily absorbed through body tissues. Inhalation can irritate the eyes, nose, and throat, and cause dizziness, confusion, nausea, muscle twitches, and convulsions.

- Ethanol is on the EPA's hazardous waste list. It causes CNS disorders and is irritating to the eyes and upper respiratory tract even in low concentrations. Inhalation of its vapors has the same effects as ingestion, including an initial stimulatory effect followed by drowsiness, impaired vision, loss of muscle coordination, and stupor.

- *Ethyl acetate* is also on the EPA's hazardous waste list. It's a narcotic, is irritating to the eyes and respiratory tract, and can cause headache and stupor. Its defatting effects may cause drying and cracking of the skin. In extreme cases, it may cause anemia with leucocytosis and liver or kidney damage.

- *Limonene* is a carcinogen as well as a skin and eye irritant and allergen.

- *Linalool* is a narcotic and cause of CNS disorders. It can produce sometimes fatal respiratory disturbances, poor muscular coordination, reduced spontaneous motor activity, and depression. Animal tests indicate that it may also affect the heart.

- *Methylene chloride* was banned in the United States by the FDA in 1988, but no enforcement is possible due to trade-secret laws that protect the chemical-fragrance industry. It is on the hazardous waste lists of several government agencies. It is a carcinogen and CNS disrupter; it's absorbed and stored in body fat; and it metabolizes to carbon monoxide, thereby reducing the oxygen-carrying capacity of the blood. Other adverse effects include headache, giddiness, stupor, irritability, fatigue, and tingling in the limbs.

- Alpha-Pinene is a sensitizer, and can damage the immune system.

- *Gamma-Terpinene (g-Terpinene)* causes asthma and CNS disorders.

- *Alpha-Terpineol (a-Terpineol)* is highly irritating to mucus membranes; aspiration into the lungs can produce a pneumonitis or even fatal edema; it can also cause nervous excitement, loss of muscle coordination, hypothermia, CNS and respiratory depression, and headache. Scientific data warn against repeated or prolonged skin contact.

In the EU, certain fragrance ingredients with a high potential to cause allergic reactions must now be listed separately on the product label. These are:

- amyl cinnamal
- amylcinnamyl alcohol
- anisyl alcohol
- benzyl alcohol
- benzyl benzoate
- *benzyl cinnamate*
- *benzyl salicylate*
- cinnamal
- *cinnamyl alcohol*
- *citral*
- *citronellol*

- *coumarin*

- *d-limonene*

- *eugenol*

- *farnesol*

- *-gamma-Methylionone* [3-methyl-4-(2,6,6-trimethyl-2-cyclohexen-1-yl)-3-buten-2-one]

- *geraniol*

- *hexylcinnamaldehyde*

- *hydroxycitronellal*

- hydroxymethylpentylcyclohexenecarboxaldehyde

- *isoeugenol*

- *lilial* [2-(4-tert-butylbenzyl)propionaldehyde]

- linalool

- *methyl heptine carbonate*

- oak moss

- tree moss

Penetration Enhancers

Your skin absorbs up to 60 percent of the chemicals in products that come into contact with the skin, and sends them directly into the bloodstream. Scientists estimate that it takes as little as twenty-six seconds for some substances to go from the skin to every major organ of the body. This is why nicotine or birth-control patches are so effective.

But the job of estimating how little or how much of a particular product actually enters the body is complicated. It is made more so by the fact that certain ingredients, while considered inert or generally recognized as safe (GRAS), may enhance the skin penetration of other, more toxic chemicals.

These ingredients are known as penetration enhancers. Emollient or moisturizing ingredients that are easily absorbed into the skin act as penetration enhancers. And so, too, do things like microscopic liposomes and nanosomes, which are forms of nanotechnology designed specifically to drive ingredients deeper into the skin. Others, such as solvents used in perfumes, and detergents used in shampoos and shower gels, can alter the structure of the skin in some way, usually by dissolving its protective oily barrier—in this way, allowing other chemicals in the mix to penetrate deeper into the skin. Because the skin is laced with tiny blood vessels, these chemicals will also eventually find their way into the bloodstream and internal organs.

The list of ingredients that can act as penetration enhancers is incredibly long, but often includes:

- **Ionic compounds**, such as ionic surfactants, *sodium lauryl sulphate*, sodium carboxylate, sodium hyaluronate, and sodium ascorbate.

- **Solvents** such as acetone, ethanol, limonene, *polyethylene glycol (PEG)*, propylene glycol (PPG), *xylene*, *acetamide*, and trichloroethanol.

- **Fatty-acid esters**, such as butyl acetate, diethyl succinate, ethyl acetate, and some isopropyl, methyl, and sorbitan compounds.

- **Fatty acids**, such as capric acid, *lactic acid*, linoleic acid, *oleic acid*, and *palmitic acid*.

- **Complexing agents**, such as liposomes, *naphthalene*, classical and nonionic surfactants, and nonoxynol.

Carcinogens

Most of us are aware of the allergenic potential of cosmetics and toiletries, and manufacturers work hard to reduce the irritation factor of most of their products. But what may come as a shock is that there are longer-term risks associated with the continual use of cosmetics and toiletries. Many, for instance, contain known carcinogens.

Manufacturers argue that these ingredients are only present in small amounts and so could not possibly be harmful, and without the long-term research that manufacturers are unwilling to fund, the possibility that cosmetic use could lead to cancer is difficult to prove. Nevertheless, some types of cosmetics, such as hair dyes, are already being linked to higher rates of specific cancers among users (see page 128).

According to Dr. Samuel Epstein, the chairman of the Cancer Prevention Coalition, there are two classes of major cancer-causing ingredients in our cosmetics and toiletries.

The first class includes those ingredients that are carcinogenic in themselves—these are known as frank carcinogens. The second group are called hidden or cocarcinogens. These chemicals, while not carcinogenic in themselves, may under certain conditions—for instance, when mixed together—develop cancer-causing properties or increase the carcinogenic potential of other chemicals.

Over forty frank carcinogens and more than thirty hidden carcinogens are commonly used in everyday beauty products and toiletries—even those intended for children.

Frank Carcinogens

This list comprises mostly the synthetic coal-tar dyes commonly used to color cosmetics and hair dyes, as well as solvents and preservatives that appear on almost every cosmetic label. As an eye-opening exercise, check for yourself if any of your favorite products contain any of the following ingredients:

- benzyl acetate
- *butyl benzyl phthalate*
- *butylated hydroxyanisole (BHA)*
- *butylated hyroxytoluene (BHT)*
- *crystalline silica*
- D&C Green 5 (CI61570)
- D&C Orange 17 (CI12075)
- D&C Red 2, 3, 4, 10, 17*
- D&C Red 8, 9, 19, 33 (CI15585, CI45170, CI17200)
- *diaminophenol*
- *diethanolamine (DEA)*
- *dioctyl adipate*
- Disperse Blue 1 (CI64500)
- Disperse Yellow 3 (CI11855)
- *ethyl alcohol*
- FD&C Blue 1, 2 (CI42090, CI73015)
- FD&C Blue 4*

- FD&C Green 3 (CI42053)
- FD&C Red 4, 40 (CI14700, CI16035)
- FD&C Red 10*
- FD&C Yellow 5, 6 (CI19140, CI15985)
- fluoride
- formaldehyde
- *glutaral*
- *hydroquinone*
- methylene chloride
- *nitrophenylenediamine*
- *phenyl-p-phenylenediamine*
- polyvinylpyrrolidone
- *p-phenylenediamine*
- pyrocatechol
- saccharin
- *talc*
- *titanium dioxide*

*Now banned from cosmetics in the United States and Europe.

Hidden Carcinogens

In general, these can be broken down into three main categories: formaldehyde releasers, nitrosamine precursors, and contaminants. Formaldehyde releasers and nitrosamine precursors are generally preservatives, solvents, carriers, and detergents/surfactants. These are always listed on the label.

Formaldehyde is a skin irritant and known carcinogen, so products with formaldehyde ingredients on their own carry a certain amount of risk. But when formaldehyde releasers and nitrosamine precursors are mixed in the same formula, they can produce potent cancer-causing agents called nitrosamines. Studies show that between 42 and 93 percent of toiletries and cosmetics on the shelf contain these compounds, which are quickly and easily absorbed into the skin from both leave-on and wash-off products. Check the labels of your favorite cosmetics for these formaldehyde-releasing substances:

- *2-bromo-2-nitropropane-1,3-diol (bronopol)*
- *diazolidinyl urea*
- *DMDM hydantoin*
- *imidazolidinyl urea*
- metheneamine
- quaternium-15
- *sodium hydroxymethylglycinate*

Nitrosamine precursors are among the most dangerous chemicals that we put in and on our bodies in the name of beauty each day. They belong to a family of hormone-disrupting chemicals, and are almost always found in products that foam, including bubble bath, body washes and shower gels, shampoos, liquid soaps, and facial cleansers. Some of the most common of these ingredients are:

- *bromonitrodioxane*
- *bronopol (2-bromo-2-nitropropane-1,3-diol)*
- *cocamide DEA*
- *cocamide MEA*
- *DEA-cetyl phosphate*
- *DEA-oleth-3 phosphate*
- diethanolamine (DEA)
- *lauramide DEA*
- linoleamide MEA
- metheneamine
- *monethanolamine (MEA)*

- morpholine
- *Myristamide DEA*
- *oleamide DEA*
- *padimate-O (octyldimethyl para-amino benzoic acid)*
- pyroglutamic acid

- *stearalkonium chloride*
- *stearamide MEA*
- *TEA lauryl sulphate*
- *TEA-sodium lauryl sulphate*
- *triethanolamine (TEA)*

Once added to the product, these chemicals readily react with any nitrites present to form the carcinogenic nitrosamine NDELA (*N*-nitrosodiethanolamine). Nitrosamines are also one of the major carcinogens in cigarettes, and are also found in cured meats. In the 1970s, nitrosamine contamination of bacon and other cured meats became a worldwide public-health issue. As a result, the nitrosamine content of cured meats has dropped drastically in recent years; however, the nitrosamine content of toiletries remains alarmingly high. In a single shampoo, you could absorb 50 to 100 micrograms of nitrosamine through the skin. A typical portion of bacon would supply only 1 microgram of the chemical.

Nitrites get into personal-care products in several ways. They can be added as anticorrosive agents or be present as contaminants in the raw materials. They can also result from the presence of formaldehyde-releasing chemicals in the mix.

The long shelf life of most toiletries increases the risk of this carcinogenic chemical reaction. Stored for extended periods at raised temperatures, nitrates will continue to form in a product, accelerated by the presence of certain other chemicals, such as formaldehyde, paraformaldehyde, thiocyanate, nitrophenols, and certain metal salts.

Inadequate and confusing labeling means that consumers may never know which products are most likely to be contaminated. According to a 1980 FDA report, however, approximately 42 percent of all cosmetics were contaminated with NDELA, with shampoos having the highest concentrations. In two reports released in 1991, twenty-seven out of twenty-nine products tested were contaminated with NDELA.

While manufacturers plead that DEA and its relatives are safe in products that are designed for brief or discontinuous use, or are washed off, there is evidence from both human and animal studies that DEA is quickly absorbed through the skin. Also, this argument does not explain why these chemicals crop up regularly in body lotions and facial moisturizers, which are not washed off.

As far back as 1978, the International Agency for Research on Cancer (IARC) concluded that N-nitrosodiethanolamine should be regarded for practical purposes as if it were carcinogenic to humans. The IARC maintains this position on NDELA even today.

In 1994, the U.S. National Toxicology Program similarly concluded in its "7th Annual Report on Carcinogens" that: "There is sufficient evidence for the carcinogenicity of N-nitrosodiethanolamine in experimental animals." They noted that, of over forty-four different animal species in which NDELA compounds have been tested, all were susceptible, and that humans were most unlikely to be an exception to this trend.

But the response of the cosmetic industry to the problem of nitrosamine formation in their products has been to put even more chemicals, such as preservatives and antioxidants, into the products we use in an attempt to slow or inhibit the formation of NDELA. Yet, none has been proved adequate against the possible nitrosating agents found in everyday cosmetics.

Contaminants

Carcinogens can get into your toiletries in other ways as well. Contaminants end up in cosmetics due to careless processing of the starting materials and, as such, are not listed on the label. These include:

- aflatoxin, in peanut oil and flour

- arsenic, in *coal-tar* dyes, polyvinyl acetate, PEG (polyethylene glycol) compounds

- chloroaniline, in *chlorhexidine*

- crystalline silica, in amorphous (powdered) *silicates* used in toothpastes and makeup

- DDT, dieldrin, endrin, and other organochlorine pesticides, in lanolin, hydrogenated cottonseed oil, and quaternium-26

- DEA (diethanolamine), in DEA-cocamide/lauramide condensates and quaternium-26

- 1,4-*dioxane*, in ethoxylated alcohols, including PEGs, *polysorbate* 60 and 80, nonoxynol, and chemicals with "eth" in their names (such as choleth-24, ceteareth-3, and laureths)

- ethylhexylacrylate, in *acrylate* and methacrylate polymers

- *ethylene oxide*, in PEGs, *oleths*, ceteareth-3, *laureths*, polysorbate 60 and 80, and nonoxynol

- formaldehyde, in polyoxymethylene urea

- lead, in coal-tar dyes, polyvinyl acetate, PEG (polyethylene glycol) compounds.

In addition to these, many of today's toiletries are based on compounds called ethoxylated alcohols. Ethoxylates can be contaminated with the carcinogen 1,4-dioxane. Commonly used ethoxylates include polyethylene, polyethylene glycol (PEG), polyoxyethylene, and "eth" compounds, such as sodium laureth sulphate and those with "oxynol" ingredients. Polysorbate 60 and 80 may also contain these contaminants.

In one 1991 study of a range of products including shampoos, liquid soaps, sun creams, bath foams, moisturizing lotions, aftershave lotions, cleansing milks, baby lotions, facial creams, and hair lotions, more than half the products contained dioxanes at levels potentially harmful to human health.

Bath Soaps and Body Washes

These days, most of us don't use soap at all—for anything. Instead, we use body washes, bath foams, baby wash and shower gels, facial washes and scrubs, all of which rely on complex modern detergents—often the same ones used in heavy industry—to wash away simple dirt.

The difference between soap and detergent is rather like the difference between cotton and nylon. Soap and cotton are produced from natural products by a relatively small modification. Detergents and nylon are produced entirely in a chemical factory. Detergents have a greater impact on the environment than soaps, both from the waste stream they generate during their manufacture and in their lesser biodegradability.

The detergents we use every day are part of a larger group of chemicals called surfactants (short for "surface-active agents"). Surfactants work by changing the properties of water. For instance, they can lower the surface tension of water, making it "wetter" and better able to interact with other cleaning agents in the mixture. Detergents have similar properties to surfactants and may also add foaming ability. Both detergents and surfactants can be synthesized from either plants or petrochemicals. There is no difference between the detergents that are in your household cleaning products and those you use in your bath. It is simply a matter of concentration.

Detergents, which replaced simple soap in our hygiene routine soon after World War II and which form a major part of most bath products, were originally developed for industrial use in hard-water areas, where they were thought to clean more efficiently. Since then, research has shown that simple soap and detergent perform equally well in most types of waters, although hard water appears to increase the potential of both types of cleaners to irritate the skin.

Manufacturers also boast that, unlike soap, detergents do not produce precipitate—the scummy substance that floats on the water or sticks to the side of the bath or shower. This is not strictly true: all washing products produce some degree of precipitate, and claims about precipitate simply serve to illustrate how much manufacturers rely on aesthetics rather than effectiveness to sell their products.

The problem can arise during the rinse. In hard-water areas, both types of cleaners can be difficult to wash off, and old-fashioned soaps even more so. Genuine castile soap, however, made with a high percentage of coconut oil, appears to rinse equally well in both types of water.

Having said this, even among detergents there is a wide variation in both effectiveness and ecological impact. Those based on plant materials are somewhat kinder to the body and environment than those based on petroleum. And while for some industrial applications detergent is an appropriate choice, it is totally unnecessary, and potentially toxic, when used to clean the body.

Milder Detergents

Detergents can only be produced synthetically, and the damage they can do to skin, hair, eyes, and mucous membranes varies according to how harsh and denaturing they are. If you are determined to buy detergent-based body-care products, you can make safer choices by choosing those with ingredients that have a milder action on the skin and/or don't contain potential carcinogens. Avoid shampoos, body washes, and foam baths with ingredients that contain the acronyms DEA, TEA, or MEA, and look instead for those that are based on the following milder detergents:

- amphoteric-2
- amphoteric-20
- amphoteric-6
- cocamidopropyl hydroxysultaine
- cocoa betaine
- cocoa glucoside
- decyl glucose
- decyl polyglucose
- lauryl betaine
- lauryl glucoside
- polysorbate-20
- polysorbate-40
- sodium cocoyl isethionate
- sodium lauraminopropionate
- sorbitan laurate
- sorbitan palmate
- sorbitan stearate

Soap is a simple, effective, and largely natural cleanser. It is a simple substance that is made in a one-step process that creates little waste in its manufacture, and little waste in its use. To make soap, all you need is fat or oil and a strong alkali solution.

Bath Bars

That good old bar in the bath or shower is the mainstay of most people's personal-care regime. While they may all look the same, manufacturers claim significant differences in terms of effectiveness and mildness among their products. There is a genuine basis for such claims. For example, glycerin-based soaps are among the mildest on the market, while deodorant and antibacterial soaps are among the harshest and most irritating to skin.

Most bath bars are made from synthetic and semisynthetic detergents, including *sodium tallowate*—made from animal fats—and *sodium palmate*, *sodium palm kernelate*, and *sodium cocoate*, which, although of vegetable origin, can be highly processed and retain none of their original vegetable characteristics. They can also contain glycerin (a humectant), water softeners, such as *pentasodium* and *disodium EDTA*, and *tetrasodium EDTA*, skin conditioners, such as *stearic acid*, and rinse aids, such as *sodium chloride*, as well as fragrances and synthetic colors.

Bubble Baths and Body Washes

Of all the available bath products, bubble baths, which are highly fragranced, have the greatest potential to cause skin irritation, allergic skin reactions, and headaches.

A bigger problem with using bubble baths is that they can irritate more than just your skin. Regular bubble bath use is associated with a high rate of urogenital infections. The harsh detergents in these products can strip away protective oils from sensitive areas of skin as well as strip away the mucus that lines the genitourinary tract. Removing this natural protection allows bacteria to take hold and cause infection. Children are particularly vulnerable, and bubble baths are a major cause of urogenital infections in babies.

In the United States, bubble baths are now obliged to carry a health warning, advising users to follow directions carefully and warning that prolonged use can cause skin irritation and raise the risk of urinary tract infections.

Body washes come in liquids, gels, and foams, but, essentially, they are the same product containing the same basic ingredients as a bubble bath. Soaking in any bath product will prolong its contact with your skin, increasing the risk that chemicals will be absorbed. Hot water also increases your skin's permeability and helps to vaporize some of the chemicals in the product, making them more easily inhaled. So both bubble baths and shower gels have the potential to penetrate into the skin and lungs.

Your bubble bath or shower foam is likely to contain detergents like *sodium laureth sulphate* and *cocamidopropyl betaine*, preservatives such as tetrasodium EDTA, methylchloroisothiazolinone and methylisothiazolinone, and humectants, such as propylene glycol or *butylene glycol*. If your bubble bath contains cocamide DEA (or similar compounds ending with DEA, TEA, or MEA) along with formaldehyde-forming substances, such as 2-bromo-2-nitropropane-1,3-diol (bronopol or BNP), DMDM hydantoin, diazolidinyl urea, imidazolidinyl urea, and quaternium-15, you shouldn't be using it because it is likely to contain cancer-causing nitrosamines. (See page 99 for more information.)

Try This Instead . . .

Most bath products are frankly unnecessary. Anything that produces a lot of foam has been made to appeal to your emotions and senses rather than to your desire to be clean, as foam adds no cleaning ability; however, manufacturers constantly add more detergent and additional foam boosters to produce the foam that they believe consumers can't possibly live without. The increased concentration of detergent creates the need for conditioners and other additives, generating an even more complex cocktail of ingredients in the attempt to limit any skin reaction to the detergents.

The best alternative is to stick to bath bars, avoid bubble baths altogether, and limit your use of bath foams and shower gels. If you are looking for the mildest way to clean your skin, then:

Always opt for vegetable- and glycerin-based soaps over harsher petrochemical-based varieties.

Buy real soap made from at least 70 percent vegetable oil. Many health-food stores stock such soaps, or they can be ordered from specialty suppliers.

Choose a liquid castile soap instead of a body wash. Liquid castile soaps (such as those made by Dr. Bronner) foam beautifully and are made from enriching oils, such as coconut, hemp, and olive. They are usually fragranced with essential oils (but check the label), and even come unscented so you can add your own fragrance.

If you must have bubble baths, have them less often and make sure the room is well ventilated to avoid inhaling too many chemicals.

For the more ambitious, making your own bath products means you can have exactly the right scent to suit your mood on any given day. It also ensures that you are not soaking in or inhaling a bathtub full of potentially harmful chemicals.

Use essential oils to fragrance your bath. To help them disperse in the water, mix 4–10 drops of essential oil in 1 tablespoon of milk (semi-skimmed or whole). The fat in the milk will distribute the oils evenly around the bath. Alternatively, mix in a carrier oil, such as almond or grapeseed. Choose oils that match your skin type: for greasy skin: lavender, orange, lemon, clary sage, neroli, cypress, ylang-ylang, bergamot; for normal skin: palma rosa, geranium, lavender, Roman chamomile, jasmine, neroli, ylang-ylang, frankincense, sandalwood, patchouli; for sensitive skin: geranium, lavender, German chamomile; for dry or damaged skin: geranium, lavender, German chamomile, Roman chamomile, clary sage, nisouli, thyme linalol, myrrh, or a blend of eucalyptus and lemon or peppermint.

A fragrant mineral bath will eliminate the need for you to buy expensive brands. Add a generous handful of Epsom salts and a few drops of your favorite essential oil (mixed in a carrier oil, as noted above). Epsom salts can be purchased at any pharmacy in large bags for a fraction of the cost of name brands that are essentially the same thing. For a bit of fizz in the bath, add a handful of baking soda as well. Epsom salts are a good way to encourage the skin to release accumulated toxins, so, in addition to being pleasant and safe to soak in, they are therapeutic as well.

Make your own bath bomb, because commercially made bath bombs often have dubious chemicals and colors in them. Instead, if you want your bath to fizz nicely, mix 3 tablespoons of baking soda with 1½ tablespoons of citric acid in a bowl together with 8–10 drops of your favorite essential oil. Drizzle a scant teaspoon of water over the dry ingredients and mix well. This is enough for one large bath bomb. You can press it into a mold (an old film cartridge or an ice-cube tray will do) and store in a plastic bag for later. Or you can use it right away by sprinkling the mixture in the bath just as you are getting in.

Have an herbal bath by brewing up a strong infusion of your favorite herbal tea and mixing this into your bathwater. Good choices include peppermint, chamomile, lavender, and lime flower.

For dry, irritated skin, try making your own herbal wash bag. Cut the foot off of an old pair of tights, about six inches from the end. Fill the pouch with a handful of oatmeal, some soothing herbs, such as chamomile or lavender, and 2 tablespoons of finely ground almonds. Tie a knot in the open end of the pouch. You can now use this in the bath or shower. One wash bag will last one day at most—keep it in the fridge in a plastic bag if you intend to use it morning and night, but don't try to store it for longer than this, as it can accumulate bacteria. When wet, it will produce a lovely creamy liquid that will clean and nourish your skin without drying it. This is great for adults, but it's also good for babies and children who have dry skin.

Dental Care

Brushing your teeth several times daily will keep them clean, clear the mouth of plaque-forming bacteria, and freshen the breath. There is now a staggering variety of toothpaste products, including family toothpastes, whitening toothpastes, children's toothpastes, tartar-control toothpastes, toothpastes plus mouthwash, gels, creams, and stripes, and mild mint, fresh mint, baking soda, and herbal toothpastes, each one claiming to do something specific and/or unique.

But while there is such a wide variety of dentifrices on the market, most are basically the same—there is no advantage to gel toothpaste, for example, over cream formulas. And while many toothpastes appear to make grand claims about what they can do for your teeth, look closely at the wording on the label the next time you buy. It won't actually say it will prevent plaque or tartar buildup; instead, it says it "fights" it or "can help prevent" it. This is a convenient way for manufacturers to sound like they are making a medicinal claim (and thus encouraging the trust of the purchaser) when they really aren't.

While it may make your mouth feel fresh, toothpaste is not actually necessary for cleaning your teeth. Dry brushing can do the job just as effectively.

Tartar-control toothpastes cannot remove existing tartar. Likewise, those pastes that claim to prevent gum disease cannot treat existing gum disease. In both cases, a trip to the dentist is necessary. Smoker's toothpaste, which claims to remove stains, can be highly abrasive. Excessive abrasion on the teeth can damage tooth enamel and cause the gums to recede.

The problems of dental decay and gum disease are very real and impact more than just the mouth. A vast amount of scientific research links periodontal disease to other conditions, such as heart disease. Indeed, your risk of developing heart disease is much higher if you have poor oral health than if you smoke or have high cholesterol. One theory for why this is suggests that oral bacteria can enter the bloodstream, attach to fatty plaques in the coronary (heart) arteries, and contribute to clot formation.

Another possibility is that the inflammation caused by periodontal disease increases plaque buildup, which may contribute to swelling of the arteries. Researchers have found that people with periodontal disease are almost twice as likely to suffer from coronary artery disease as those without periodontal disease. Poor oral health also raises your risk of stroke, peripheral vascular disease, osteoporosis, respiratory diseases, diabetes, and preterm pregnancy.

But brushing, like so many daily tasks, can sometimes be boring, so major manufacturers have begun to advertise toothpaste in a way that suggests it is a beauty or luxury product rather than simply an aid to personal hygiene. One major brand even promises to provide noticeable improvement for all five signs of healthy teeth—fewer cavities, less tartar, healthy gums, naturally white teeth, and fresh breath—in much the same way that antiwrinkle creams fight the "seven signs of aging."

By turning basic daily necessities into more attractive, premium purchases, manufacturers are encouraging consumers to buy more—and buy them at a higher price. This has the added effect of drawing attention away from the product ingredients.

Looking at the label on a typical toothpaste tube, you might wonder why you would want to put this product in your mouth at all. In a market crowded with alternatives, each brand has to make bigger claims about what it can do. And to back up these claims, manufacturers add more and more chemicals. Should you be worried? Probably.

Hard to Swallow

Several of the active ingredients in toothpaste are worrisome. The industrial-strength detergent sodium lauryl sulphate (SLS) is a suspected gastrointestinal or liver toxicant. There is also concern that by irritating and stripping away the protective mucous membrane of the mouth, SLS could increase the incidence of mouth ulcers and may also be involved in an increased risk of oral cancer.

Triclosan is one of the most common antibacterial agents used in toothpaste. It is often found in antibacterial and antiplaque formulas, and there is evidence that it can help reduce plaque buildup. Although tartar-control formulas may prevent 40–50 percent of new tartar buildup, they can do nothing for plaque that is already present.

Triclosan, like SLS, is an irritant, and there is some evidence that the two substances can combine synergistically to become an even more powerful irritant. Triclosan is also associated with a rise in superbugs, bacteria that are resistant to many kinds of antiseptics and antibiotics. (See "Antibacterial Cleaners," page 173.)

Sensitive-teeth formulas contain nerve-deadening chemicals, such as *strontium chloride* or potassium nitrite. But don't expect these toothpastes to work immediately, like they do on TV—most people won't notice any improvement for four to six weeks. If your teeth are very sensitive, you'll need to make a trip to the dentist to rule out an underlying problem, such as a cracked tooth or gum disease.

Certain abrasives, such as *silica*, are also potentially harmful. Recent studies have shown that fine granules of this mineral can build up under the surface of the gums, causing granulomas—small nodules of inflamed tissue. Other fine-grained abrasives can have a similar effect, leading to symptoms that can mimic gingivitis, but which may also leave the gums more vulnerable to infection.

Many toothpastes also contain gluelike substances, such as PVM/MA copolymer, that keep the active ingredients in contact with the teeth even after rinsing.

Fluoride Myths

Without doubt, the most controversial ingredient in toothpaste is fluoride. Many of us still buy fluoride-containing toothpastes, believing that the chemical protects teeth. There is, however, little convincing scientific evidence to support this. In fact, fluoride is a systemic poison, and there is enough in the average-sized tube of family toothpaste to kill a small child if it is ingested. For this reason, both the American Food and Drug Administration (FDA) and the Swedish National Food Administration now require that toothpaste containing fluoride should be labeled with a special "poison" warning.

Studies have shown a clear relationship between mouth cancer and fluoride intake in both animals and humans. For instance, benign squamous papilloma, which appears as a white patch on the inside of the mouth and is the precursor of squamous cell carcinoma, can also be triggered by fluoride exposure.

Fluoride can cause sensitivity or allergic-type reactions and is now a suspect in a host of illnesses, including gastroesophageal reflux disease (GERD), bone problems, diabetes, thyroid malfunction, and mental impairment. Fluoride exposure from toothpaste, supplements, and water before the age of six is also an important risk factor for dental fluorosis, which leads to mottled and discolored teeth.

Young children have a tendency to swallow toothpaste and, with it, the toxic fluoride. This may be because they are too young to control the swallowing reflex, or it may simply be that the sweet flavors and pretty colors make toothpaste as appealing as candy to swallow.

For both these reasons, it is now widely accepted that family toothpastes, which generally contain the highest amounts of fluoride (around 1,500 ppm, or parts per million) are unsuitable for children under the age of eight.

More recently, fluoride has been found to activate and interfere with substances known as G-proteins—chemical messengers that play a vital role in the activities of hormones and neurotransmitters. By activating G-proteins, fluoride may actually be promoting gingivitis (gum disease), thus contributing to the range of diseases associated with that problem.

Whitening Toothpastes

These toothpastes work in two ways—either by bleaching the teeth with chemicals, such as *hydrogen peroxide* (which can be a slow process), or by using gritty particles to scrape away stains. Such toothpastes are popular among smokers and among those with low self-esteem; however, the abrasive action is harmful to your teeth. Although the jury is still out on chemical bleaching, problems have been observed.

At best, whitening toothpastes may produce a mild cleaning or bleaching action that only lasts as long as you keep using the product. At worst, they can make your teeth painfully sensitive to heat and cold, or they may irritate your gums and permanently destroy tooth enamel. Concern has also been expressed that the new chemical whiteners are still something of an unknown quantity. Peroxide, for instance, is highly reactive and may interact with other chemicals in the paste to form new, harmful chemicals.

Mouthwash and Breath Fresheners

The traditional purpose of a mouthwash is as an antiseptic gargle to help remove germs that can lead to bad breath. Today, mouthwashes come in many more complex forms that purport to fight plaque, strengthen teeth, fight tooth

---

The Low-down on Dental Floss

Although we think of flossing as a recent development in dental care, evidence gleaned from the skulls of prehistoric humans suggests that we have been flossing in one way or another for a very long time. In the 1800s, floss was made of fine unwaxed silk thread. Now it is made of thin nylon string.

Some holistic dentists have expressed concerns that modern dental floss can be contaminated with mercury-containing antiseptics. Certainly, some flosses are impregnated with unnecessary flavorings derived from petrochemicals, and some are even colored. Often, they are coated with waxes of petrochemical origin as well.

The American naturopath Dr. Hulda Clark has gone so far as to recommend that flossing is best done with a two- or four-pound monofilament fishing line (doubled and twisted for strength). She also suggests that the thin plastic used for most shopping bags is also serviceable. Tear off a thin strip and roll it slightly to make a quick, effective floss.

If you don't fancy that or don't have a fisherman in the family, you might just try to be a little more aware of the types of dental floss you use. Choose one without flavor or color, and don't overfloss. It can wear a groove in your teeth and tear up your gums, making them more susceptible to infection.

decay, and freshen breath—in addition to killing germs. The result is a complex mixture of chemicals that, in the long run, may do more harm than good.

Although they are mostly made of water, there are several problems with the current crop of mouthwashes. First, most contain alcohol. Using an alcohol-containing mouthwash is associated with an increased risk of throat and mouth cancers. This is because alcohol is drying, changes the pH of the mouth, and strips away the protective mucous membrane in the mouth and throat. Although in a low concentration, most mouthwashes also contain fluoride. Drinking alcohol- and fluoride-containing mouthwash is a major source of poisoning among young children.

Breath fresheners—often sprays—are concentrated forms of mouthwash. Typically, they contain more alcohol than water, as well as *isobutane*, glycerin, sweeteners, such as saccharin or *sorbitol*, flavorings, and even colors. Because these products are so high in alcohol and are not rinsed out of the mouth, regular users are at an increased risk of throat cancer. And incidentally, using a spray will not stop you from having bad breath.

With good oral hygiene, mouthwashes and breath sprays are never necessary. A healthy mouth simply has no odor. If you are experiencing a problem with persistent bad breath, it could be because of gum disease or some other underlying infection. This problem is most effectively addressed by a trip to the dentist.

Try This Instead . . .

Remember that it's not the paste but the brush that cleans your teeth. Equally, it's not how hard you brush but how long and how thoroughly. Brushing hard and fast won't clean your teeth better, and it may damage your gums. So, instead of just running the brush quickly over your teeth and hoping the toothpaste (or mouthwash) will catch what you don't, consider spending at least a minute (if not two) in gently but thoroughly brushing your teeth every morning and night.

The type of brush you use is also important, so, for optimal dental health, invest in a good one with lots of filaments packed tightly together. A soft-to-medium brush is fine for most people (very few really need a firm brush), and the angle of the head is mostly immaterial. Many a weird-shaped brush has been developed in recent years—largely to try to make up for the lazy way in which most people brush their teeth; however, there is little evidence that they are substantially better than a standard straight-handled brush. Replace your toothbrush regularly at the first signs of wear.

If you still want to use commercial brands of toothpaste, consider these options:

Use less. In spite of what you see on TV, you only need a pea-sized amount of toothpaste (about a quarter of the advertised amount) to clean your teeth. And while children are advised to use a pea-sized amount, they can clean their teeth adequately with half this amount—in other words, just a smear.

Dilute it. Turn toothpaste into a cream by diluting it with cooled boiled water. Store it in a small squeeze-top bottle. It will still foam and clean well.

Use a low-fluoride toothpaste. Among the brands aimed at adults, a low-fluoride content is around 500 ppm. Several children's brands contain even less, and there is nothing (apart from aesthetics) stopping the whole family from using a children's paste to clean their teeth.

Buy a fluoride-free brand and, if you can, one that is SLS-free. In most large supermarkets and pharmacies, it will be almost impossible to find a toothpaste that is fluoride-free and SLS-free. Health-food stores will stock a wider range; but check the labels of "natural" alternatives for detergents and other dubious chemicals.

Alternatives to conventional toothpastes are not hard to find; they are plentiful in health-food stores, by mail order, and on the Internet, and they are beginning to be sold in supermarkets, too. A quick scan of many ingredient labels, however, will show that many of the so-called alternatives are not very alternative. Many contain SLS and may also contain fluoride. Some also contain contentious preservatives, such as parabens, a potential hormone disrupter.

While chalk or baking soda (*sodium bicarbonate*) can be substituted for silica, essential oils for triclosan, and glycerin for more harmful humectants, such as propylene glycol, the basic mixture is the same. The trick with toothpaste alternatives is to read the labels and find one with a basic mix that is as natural as possible while still providing the degree of effectiveness, the feel in the mouth, and the taste that you are used to.

Very few toothpastes are free from worrisome chemicals of one sort or another. If you feel strongly that you shouldn't put anything in your mouth that you aren't prepared to swallow, then brushing regularly with a tiny amount of baking soda or food-grade hydrogen peroxide will clean your teeth adequately. Hydrogen peroxide provides the bonus of gently whitening your teeth.

Baking soda is a useful mild abrasive and comes with antibacterial properties. Undiluted, straight baking soda can be hard on tooth enamel (particularly as you get older and enamel begins to soften), so try dissolving a teaspoonful in a little water first, and then dipping your toothbrush into the liquid frequently during brushing. (Do the same when using hydrogen peroxide.)

Since baking soda doesn't taste great, you can try making it more palatable by mixing the dry powder in a small, airtight container with a few drops of peppermint oil. Mix together well and then store for use as and when you need it.

It's also rather easy to make your own toothpaste and mouthwash.

Simple toothpaste can be made from baking soda, vegetable glycerin, and essential oil of peppermint, lemon, or fennel.

As a general rule, use one part liquid to two parts baking soda—for example, 4 heaping tablespoons of glycerine to 8 heaping tablespoons of baking soda. You may have to play with the proportions until you get just the consistency you like. Add five drops of the essential oil of your choice to pep up the flavor. Shake well before use.

This mixture can be stored in a small squeezable or pump dispenser (such as those used for travel). Use it sparingly. Don't be tempted to make more than about 2 ounces at a time. Although the essential oils will act as preservatives, when making your own toiletries it is always safest to make small amounts as needed rather than risk the product going stale.

Another way of making this mixture is to substitute a natural mouthwash—one without alcohol, fluoride, chemical preservatives, flavors, or colors—for the glycerin. Mix this with baking soda in approximately the same ratio as above.

Simple mouthwash. The simplest mouthwash is a couple of drops of peppermint oil or sage tincture in a cup of water. To make around 1/2 cup of a more complex blend, you need:

1 Tbsp lavender tincture
1 Tbsp calendula tincture
2 tsp aloe juice
2 Tbsp cooled boiled water
2 Tbsp vegetable glycerin
5 drops peppermint essential oil

Mix the ingredients together and pour them into a bottle. This mixture will keep for up to six months. If you have an infection in the mouth or gums, substitute echinacea, myrrh, or goldenseal tinctures for the lavender.

Deodorants and Antiperspirants

Deodorants were the first products to be developed to help combat the problem of body odor. They are basically strong perfumes that mask the odor produced by bacteria in your armpits. Antiperspirants, which prevent sweat from leaking out of the armpits, were developed later. Nowadays, there is a huge range of antiperspirants, deodorants, and antiperspirant deodorants on the market in a variety of formulations, including creams, roll-ons, solids, and sprays. A quick look at the labels will tell you that there isn't much of a difference among the ingredients in any of them.

Antiperspirants and deodorants typically contain a range of moisturizers, solvents, preservatives (such as parabens), synthetic perfumes, and antibacterial agents, such as triclosan (which can be absorbed through the skin, and which has been shown to cause liver damage in animal experiments).

While nobody wants to go around smelling like a compost heap (and nobody enjoys being around someone who does), it's worth asking what price we are paying for trying to stay shower-fresh all day long.

Finding an answer to this question became more urgent in 2002, when U.K. researchers highlighted the potential risks associated with parabens (or para-hydroxybenzoic acids) in deodorants. The researchers at the University of Reading found traces of parabens in every single tumor sample taken from a small group of women with breast cancer.

Parabens are used in a wide variety of cosmetics, and the scientists suggested that the chemicals had seeped into body tissues after being applied to the skin, probably via deodorants. These findings are worrisome because parabens are estrogen mimics, and this makes them potential triggers for the growth of human breast tumors.

Aluminum Worries

But before bad news about parabens came out, it was the *aluminum* content of antiperspirants that was a major cause of concern.

Most antiperspirants contain some form of aluminum, most commonly *aluminum chlorohydrate, aluminum zirconium tetrachlorohydrex GLY, aluminum chloride, aluminum sulphate*, and *aluminum phenosulphate*.

No one knows exactly how aluminum compounds work to reduce underarm wetness. They may prevent sweat by clogging the sweat ducts, which, in turn, increases the pressure inside of the ducts due to the sweat building up. It is thought that this pressure buildup then causes the sweat glands to stop secreting.

Alternatively, they may cause perforations in the glands so that the sweat seeps out into the surrounding tissues rather than coming out through the surface of the skin. Or they may block the transmission of the nervous impulses that activate sweat glands.

Whatever the mechanism, aluminum is absorbed through the skin, however superficially. The recently acknowledged link between Alzheimer's disease and aluminum has raised a furious debate as to whether it is safe to put aluminum compounds into deodorants. Unfortunately, this is not a question that has benefited from much scientific evaluation. Only one study reports an association between Alzheimer's and a lifetime's use of deodorant. No other studies have been conducted that refute or confirm these findings.

Nevertheless, other evidence from looking at the incidence of breast cancer among four hundred American women suggests that it may be the combination of underarm shaving and deodorant use that allows chemicals to seep into breast tissue. In this study, women who shaved three times a week and applied deodorant at least twice a week were almost fifteen years younger when diagnosed with cancer than women who did neither. The researchers suggested that aluminum compounds could act as a breast-cancer trigger.

Certainly, aluminum-based deodorants are a major cause of skin irritation and, for this reason alone, should be approached with caution by users. Aluminum zirconium products have been shown to cause granulomas (small nodules of chronically inflamed tissue) under the arms with prolonged use.

Alum versus Aluminum

Rock crystals are the newest alternative to aluminum-containing antiperspirants. Some of these are made from magnesium sulphate, while others are made from *alum*. These products often claim to be aluminum-free or free of aluminum chlorohydrate, yet alum by its other name is aluminum sulphate. Manufacturers suggest that aluminum sulphate has a much higher molecular weight than aluminum chlorohydrate—which is true—and so cannot be absorbed through the skin; however, this may be too simplistic. While aluminum chlorohydrate has a lower molecular weight, it is also less soluble in water (or sweat).

Sulphates, on the other hand, are highly soluble in water, and alum may break down into its component parts more readily in a sweaty armpit. Does this mean that the aluminum will be absorbed into the skin? Without the emollient ingredients found in most conventional formulations, it is unlikely, but it would be reassuring if there were more conclusive research evidence to enlighten us.

Try This Instead . . .

Body odor can be caused by bacteria in your armpits, but it can also be caused by what's inside your body—for instance, what you eat, and how polluted your body is by toxins and allergens.

If you can, try to avoid aluminum-based antiperspirants. Aluminum is highly toxic, and there is too little evidence of safety with aluminum-containing products applied to the skin. The presence of such ingredients as *magnesium oxide* and *zinc oxide* will buffer the irritant properties of aluminum- and zirconium-based compounds, but they, too, can cause skin irritation.

In addition, when selecting conventional antiperspirants and deodorants:

Avoid aerosols, which surround you and those in your immediate area with a cloud of easily inhaled and toxic chemicals. Aerosols can contain planet-poisoning *hydrochlorofluorocarbons* (HCFCs), as well as the neurotoxic and reproductive toxins propane, butane, and isopropane.

Switch to a solid or stick variety, because these are less emollient, and are therefore less likely to aid the absorption of ingredients into the skin. Sticks also tend to produce less irritation.

Never apply antiperspirants or deodorants to broken or newly shaved skin, because the chemicals in them will be much more easily absorbed into your system if your skin is broken in any way.

Avoid colored products, which won't help you stay drier, and the coal-tar- and petrochemical-derived colors used in these products are easily absorbed into the skin and can be carcinogenic.

Avoid products containing quaternium-18, which can cause rashes even beyond the area of application.

Your health-food store may sell deodorants based on plant extracts and essential oils (but remember to read the label to find out what is really in them). Some also sell crystal deodorants (made from mineral salts). These can be very effective, but always check what they're made of—some are aluminum-based (see box, page 115). Don't buy crystal deodorants with labels that are in any way unclear about the mineral used.

If you are feeling more ambitious, you can make your own antiperspirants and deodorants from a few simple ingredients.

Dust under your arms with plain cornstarch. If you don't sweat heavily, this may be all you need.

Try a simple astringent, such as witch hazel. This helps to temporarily contract the tissues around the sweat glands, and may be all some people need (but do not apply to broken skin, as it may sting).

Use a mixture of unflavored vitamin C powder or citric acid and water. This works well for some people. Mix ¼ teaspoon of powdered vitamin C or citric acid to 16 ounces of water. Dab this sparingly under your arms after a bath, or spritz a little on from a spray bottle. If you can't wait around for it to dry, dust with cornstarch afterward.

For a more ambitious spray, the owners of Neal's Yard, one of the U.K.'s most respected natural toiletry manufacturers, recommend the following:

6 Tbsp witch hazel
2 tsp vegetable glycerin
2 drops each of clove, coriander, and lavender essential oils
5 drops each of grapefruit, lime, and palma rosa essential oils
10 drops of lemon essential oil

Mix the witch hazel and vegetable glycerin together, then add the essential oils. Shake well. Store in a dark glass or plastic bottle with a spray top. The mixture will last for up to six months.

To make an effective foot deodorant, all you need is 2 tablespoons of witch hazel and 5 drops each of lavender and grapefruit essential oils. Blend the ingredients together, store in a spray bottle (preferably made of dark-colored glass or plastic). Spray regularly onto clean feet. Shake before applying. This mixture will keep for up to two months.

For a simple foot powder, use cornstarch. If you want a powder that perfumes and deodorizes, mix 5 drops each of lemon and coriander essential oils with the cornstarch. Store the perfumed mixture in an old talcum-powder dispenser or similar type of container.

Body Sprays

Body sprays serve no useful function. They are not deodorants, they are not quite strong enough to be perfumes, and they can't stop you from sweating.

Nevertheless, the market for body sprays, for men and women, has expanded exponentially in recent years.

Advertising for such products suggests that using them will make you more attractive to the opposite sex, or give you the courage to do wild and outrageous things. In reality, they are likely to give you a headache (which may stop you from doing wild and outrageous things), cause you to become forgetful, tired, and listless, and may even make the people around you feel sick as well.

Body sprays are mostly solvents, propellants, and fragrances. The perfumes can cause allergic reactions, headaches, dizziness, fatigue, and a range of mental symptoms; the solvents and propellants are neurotoxic and have been implicated in reproductive problems, such as miscarriage and birth defects.

Try This Instead . . .

The best alternative of all is to toss these unnecessary and expensive items. If you must add yet another fragrance to your body, try to keep it as natural as possible.

Use food-grade flower waters. Rose and orange flower waters can be purchased in any supermarket or pharmacy. While not chemical-free, these have somewhat fewer nasties in them than conventional body sprays. Either splash them on or transfer them to a spray bottle and spritz on.

You can make a pleasant body spray from water and essential oils. Try mixing 5 drops each of lavender, sage, lemon, rosemary, and grapefruit essential oils with 3 drops of peppermint oil into 2 teaspoons of vodka. Shake to mix, then add 7 tablespoons of white vinegar. Leave this mixture to sit for an hour or so to fix the scent. Next, add the scented mixture to 2 cups of spring or filtered water and shake again.

You can also substitute natural vanilla essence for the essential oils. By learning more about essential oils, you can make an infinite number of light splashes and sprays to suit your every mood.

Talc

Talcum powder is a traditional mainstay of freshness. We use it liberally on babies' bottoms and to absorb perspiration on hot summer days and nights. A few of us are old enough to remember our mothers having special dishes of talc in the bathroom that had big, inviting powder puffs to help you dust your body—and most of the bathroom floor—with the stuff.

But time marches on, and the romantic illusion of talc has taken a huge blow.

Talc, or magnesium silicate, is made up of finely ground particles of stone. As it originates in the ground and is a mined product, it can be contaminated with other substances. Asbestos is a good example, and recent reports of the talc used in crayon manufacture being contaminated with this poisonous substance have caused alarm to every parent whose child has ever chewed on a crayon.

The harmful effects of talc on human tissue were first recorded in the 1930s. More recently, a report from the U.S. National Toxicology Program concluded that talc is carcinogenic.

An ominous series of studies has linked talc to ovarian cancer; in these cases, talc was found in a number of ovarian and uterine tumors as well as in ovarian tissue. It has since been confirmed that talc, either placed on the perineum (or on the surface of underwear or sanitary towels), can reach the ovaries by ascending the fallopian tubes. It is now estimated that women who frequently use talc have three times the risk of developing ovarian cancer compared to nonusers.

The talc used in the manufacture of condoms carries a similar risk. In the 1960s, the medical journal *Lancet* reported the first case of a woman who had a significant amount of talc in her peritoneal (abdominal) cavity. Laboratory tests confirmed that the talc in her body matched that found on her husband's condoms. The authors concluded that talc had traveled up through the fallopian tubes and become implanted in her abdomen. Talc sprinkled on diaphragms may also be implicated in such problems.

Talc use is also associated with respiratory problems. Because it comprises finely ground stone, it can lodge in the lungs and never leave. Babies whose mothers smother them in talc have more breathing difficulties and/or urogenital problems than other infants. Women are also at risk since, even if they don't use talcum powder on their bodies, they are likely to be using cosmetics (face powders, eyeshadows, blushers) that are talc-based.

Try This Instead . . .

Don't use products containing talc. Giving up body powders is relatively easy. Giving up your eyeshadow may be less so (try applying it with a damp sponge to minimize fallout). Whatever you can do to cut your exposure to talc will benefit your health.

Make your own. You can quickly and easily make a very efficient and inexpensive body powder based on cornstarch. Combine one part baking soda to eight parts cornstarch. Mix these up in a blender and add 10–15 drops of your favorite essential oil (optional). Store in an airtight container (either a jar or an old talc container, or you could recycle one of those Parmesan cheese shakers).

Babies' bottoms do not need talc or any other powder to stay fresh. Instead, let your baby go without diapers as often as possible, or investigate cotton diapers, which allow the skin to breathe and have been shown to cause less diaper rash than disposables.

Use talc-free condoms, but be aware that many talc-free condoms contain other particles, such as vegetable starches, silica (another carcinogen), mica, diatomaceous earth, and lycopodium (club moss) spores. Lycopodium can be contaminated with talc, sulphur, and/or gypsum, and is linked with inflammation of the soft tissues. It is not known how many chronic "women's problems" may be the result of an overuse of talc or, indeed, allergy to the latex used in condoms, or other contraceptives, such as the diaphragm, and all the paraphernalia that go with them (spermicidal jellies, foams, creams, and lubricants).

Feminine Deodorants

Feminine deodorants and douches are totally unnecessary. The majority are bought and used simply out of a media-fueled paranoia, which makes women worry that the people around them can detect any faint odors coming from their genitals.

If you really have a problem with strong and unpleasant vaginal odors, go to your doctor to sort out the underlying cause of the problem. You may have a low-grade vaginal infection that can easily be cleared up.

Ironically, the use of feminine deodorants—which are no different from most body sprays—can cause the very vaginal infections that may be the cause of unpleasant odors. More worrisome, in one study involving nearly seven hundred women over three years, researchers found that those who used vaginal douches more than once a week experienced a fourfold risk for cervical cancer. It did not matter which preparation was used, since all douches alter the chemical balance of the vagina, making the cervix more susceptible to bacterial infection and tissue changes.

Feminine deodorants are almost always aerosols, which means that you inhale harmful chemicals when you use them, and they are always highly perfumed. Douches contain harsh detergents, perfumes, and colors, none of which should be coming into contact with this delicate part of your body.

Try This Instead . . .

Have a little confidence in yourself and toss these toxic products in the garbage where they belong. In addition:

Bathe daily. When you wash your genitals, do not apply soap directly. It is too harsh and may dry out delicate skin. Use the foam or bubbles from your soap to gently clean yourself.

Wear cotton underwear. This allows air to circulate and discourages the bacteria that can cause unpleasant odors.

If you are experiencing vaginal itching or soreness, see your doctor and sort out the real problem. It is unlikely to be something that you can simply wash away with a douche.

If you must douche, use a simple mixture of distilled white vinegar in one pint of water, which will have less of an impact on the vaginal microflora. Even so, use this very infrequently.

Hair Care

How many different types of shampoo have you tried in your lifetime? And how often have they fallen short of what they promised to do? If you have had more than your fair share of shampoo failures, it could be because there are only a limited number of cleansing agents considered suitable for use in hair-cleaning products. If you are unsure of the truth of this statement, compare the expensive designer brands with their cheaper cousins. Often, the only genuine difference between them is the price.

The main function of a shampoo is to clean the hair. Its function is so simple that advertisers have to work doubly hard to make it sound more complicated and exciting than it actually is. Thus, using a particular brand brings with it the promise of harmony, a lust for life, nourishment, and adoration by members of the opposite sex. Some shampoos are apparently so remarkable that they not only clean your hair but give you an orgasm as well. But underneath all the fluff, a shampoo is just a bottle of highly colored, highly perfumed, detergent.

The word "shampoo" is derived from *chapo*, a Hindi word meaning to massage or knead. The first shampoos were simple solutions of soap invented by British hairdressers during the heyday of the empire. Modern shampoos, however, are usually a mixture of several different detergents and surfactants, typically sodium lauryl sulphate (SLS), *ammonium lauryl sulphate*, monoethanolamine (MEA) lauryl sulphate, diethanolamine (DEA) lauryl sulphate, and *triethanolamine (TEA) lauryl sulphate*.

Generally the strongest detergent is used in the greatest measure, then milder detergents and surfactants, which modify the harshness of the first detergent, are added. These other detergents and surfactants can also add foaming ability and conditioning properties.

For the formulator, the choice of detergent for any particular shampoo is as much a matter of aesthetics as it is about cleaning. For instance, SLS is not very soluble in cold water, and so it cannot be used to make shampoos that look clear. For these shampoos, other compounds, such as ammonium lauryl sulphate or TEA lauryl sulphate, are used. Some shampoos have extra ingredients in them to make them produce more foam, even though foam doesn't clean your hair.

Carcinogens in the Mix

As detailed on pages 99–100, a number of common ingredients in shampoos, such as 2-bromo-2-nitropropane-1,3-diol (bronopol or BNP), DMDM hydantoin, diazolidinyl urea, imidazolidinyl urea, and quaternium-15 break down into formaldehyde during storage. When formaldehyde-forming agents mix with amines, such as diethanolamine (DEA), triethanolamine (TEA), and monoethanolamine (MEA), they form carcinogenic N-nitrosodiethanolamine, or NDELA.

Nitrosamine formation is particularly problematic in shampoos, as we use them so frequently and in such great quantities. It is estimated that when you wash your hair with a shampoo contaminated with NDELA, your body absorbs more carcinogenic nitrites than if you had eaten a pound of bacon.

A further problem is that products containing the milder laureth detergents (as in sodium laureth sulphate and *ammonium laureth sulphate*) can be contaminated with the carcinogen 1,4-dioxane. Laureth compounds are part of a larger family of chemicals called ethoxylated alcohols. Many of these, including polyethylene glycol (PEG), polyethylene, polyoxyethylene, oxynol, and other eth chemicals (as in laureth) can be contaminated with 1,4-dioxane. Products containing polysorbates 60 and 80 can also be contaminated with this chemical.

The contamination of the raw materials used to create sodium laureth sulphate was noted as far back as 1978, and has been confirmed in a recent review. Yet little has been done to address the issue.

As manufacturers fall over themselves to make a more "scientific" and "improved" shampoo, the list of chemical ingredients grows. The latest published research reveals that the preservatives methylchloroisothiazolinone and methylisothiazolinone (which together are called Kathon CG) have the potential to cause nerve damage and skin cancer. Using hot water to shampoo your hair actually increases the rate of absorption of these chemicals into your body, so if you don't like cold showers, choose your shampoos carefully.

Try This Instead . . .

Hair care begins with what you eat, not what you wash with. Hair is 95 percent protein, so if your hair is limp, consider whether your protein intake is adequate.

Hair also needs to be thoroughly wet before shampooing. This helps to spread the shampoo evenly throughout the hair. For really clean hair, you need to rinse thoroughly, but in the wash-and-go culture, this is a step most of us rush through. In addition:

Read the label. Find a shampoo with the fewest possible ingredients to limit your exposure to toxic chemicals. Don't buy products that contain formaldehyde-forming agents and amines.

Use less It sounds obvious, but most of us use far too much shampoo to get the job done. Shampooing once, using half what you normally use, will clean your hair perfectly well. Always tip your head back when rinsing to avoid getting any onto your eyelids or into your eyes.

It is not easy to make a shampoo based entirely on natural ingredients. At some point, detergent must be added. But you can make mixes that are less concentrated and that expose you to fewer harmful chemicals in each wash. So:

Dilute it. Mix your shampoo with an equal amount of water, and put this mixture in an old and well-rinsed shampoo bottle. Adding a little bit of table salt (about 1 teaspoon per ½ cup of liquid) will help to thicken the mixture.

Try a variation on the diluting theme. Half fill an old shampoo bottle with your regular shampoo. Top it up with an equal amount of water or a strong herbal infusion (such as chamomile) mixed with 1 teaspoon of coconut oil (this comes as a solid but will melt in the hot infusion). Olive and jojoba oils are also good choices. Add 1–2 teaspoons of table salt to thicken the mix or, alternatively, add 1–2 teaspoons of baking soda to soften the water and aid rinsing (dissolve this in water or tea before mixing). This mixture will still foam well, and will clean and condition your hair, too. Always give it a shake before using, as the ingredients in some shampoo mixtures will separate when the mix is altered.

Use a castile soap. These come in both bar and liquid forms. Because of their high oil content, castile soaps will wash and condition your hair. Alternatively, use a pure vegetable-oil soap (these can usually only be found at specialty suppliers). These types of soaps can also be used on the body, saving you money as well as being safer.

Dandruff Shampoos

Dandruff shampoos are made with detergents to which antiflaking agents, such as coal tar, zinc pyrithizone, *salicylic acid*, and *selenium sulphide*, are added. While they can relieve itching and decrease flaking, no dandruff shampoo can control dandruff completely.

Sulphur and salicylic acid work by breaking the flakes into smaller, less noticeable pieces. It is thought that coal tar, selenium sulphide, and zinc pyrithizone can slow the production of flakes. Beyond this, little is known of how, exactly, antidandruff shampoos work.

Of all the antiflaking agents, zinc pyrithizone and coal tar are considered to be the most effective for controlling dandruff.

All antiflaking agents have some side effects. They can be irritating to both the skin and eyes. In particular, salicylic acid, an ingredient of aspirin, can be severely irritating and is poisonous if swallowed. Coal tar is a known carcinogen, and can be an irritant when inhaled or when it comes into contact with skin.

Try This Instead . . .

Dandruff is caused by a fungus and is most effectively treated from within. Effective dietary measures include cutting out sugar and yeasty foods, supplementing with B-complex vitamins and probiotics (acidophilus and bifidobacteria), and making sure that you drink plenty of water each day.

Externally, a more natural alternative is to make an effective antidandruff lotion with 1 teaspoon each of rosemary and thyme essential oils, mixed into ½ cup of apple juice and 2 tablespoons of cider vinegar. Apply this at bedtime or on days when you can let your hair dry naturally to help keep dandruff at bay.

Conditioners

Have you ever noticed how shampoo bottles always recommend that you use a conditioner afterward? This is because the detergents used in shampoos are often so harsh that you need to use a conditioner to repair some of the damage done by them. Healthy hair rarely needs conditioning. Hair damaged by detergent use (and other assaults) almost always does.

All shampoos, no matter how "mild," will strip away the protective layer of sebum (natural oils produced by the scalp) that coats your hair. Stripping the sebum away exposes the outside layer of the hair, known as the cuticle. The cuticle is made up of translucent overlapping cells that are arranged like the shingles on a roof. When these cells are disturbed, they can rub against each other and become damaged, resulting in the social horror of flyaway hair. Stripping away the sebum also leaves the cuticle (the inner part of the hair shaft) vulnerable to damage from other chemicals used on the hair.

Many shampoos contain conditioning agents that smooth down the cuticle and cover it with a synthetic version of sebum.

Conditioners, whether used separately or incorporated into your regular shampoo, do not repair hair. They cannot penetrate the hair shaft and make it stronger. Instead, they coat the hair with chemicals that temporarily glue the damaged hair shaft down—giving the illusion of healthier hair.

A typical hair conditioner will contain triethanolamine (TEA), film formers like polyvinylpyrrolidone (*PVP*), various silicones, such as *dimethicone*, humectants like propylene glycol and glycerin, quaternium compounds, preservatives like DMDM hydantoin, disodium EDTA, methylchloroisothiazolinone, and methylisothiazolinone, and fragrances.

Try This Instead . . .

The most sensible alternative is not to use a conditioner at all. You can see from the examples above that many shampoos (even the ones that are not specifically conditioning shampoos) contain some conditioning ingredients. If you follow the advice for using or making milder shampoos, you shouldn't need a conditioner.

If you do continue to use conventional conditioners, once again, the best advice is to use less. You can do this in two ways: first, use a conditioner only once or twice a week; or second, put less on your hair at each washing. This can be hard to do straight from the bottle, so try diluting it instead. To do this, half fill a well-rinsed conditioner bottle with regular conditioner, then top it up with water. Shake before use.

Alternatively, consider these more basic options:

Regular trimming. And keeping the use of hair-destroying things like rollers, curling irons, hair dryers, and lots of drying styling gels to a minimum will also help keep hair looking good.

Condition before you wash. Contrary to what we have been encouraged to do, this is the best way to keep hair soft and manageable. Rubbing good-quality oil through your hair a half hour or so before you shampoo or, better still, at night before bed will provide the same conditioning action as the hazardous ingredients in your usual conditioner.

Good choices for conditioning oils include olive oil for deep conditioning and coconut, jojoba, or almond oil for light-to-medium conditioning. Add 2 tablespoons of honey to ½ cup of oil to help "repair" split ends. Leave on for half an hour before shampooing.

After shampooing, rinse with diluted cider vinegar. This is pH neutral, and will remove detergent deposits and lightly condition the hair.

Styling Products

Most hairstyling products are used to make up for poor-quality haircuts and the damage caused by years of abusive practices, such as the use of harsh shampoos, hair dryers, heated rollers, and styling wands.

As with shampoos, many of us tend to collect half-used jars, tubes, and bottles of the stuff—a good indication that they never quite do what they are supposed to. Apart from poor performance, most styling products contain dubious chemicals, which your hair, skin, and lungs would be better off without.

Hairspray

Hairspray is essentially plastic dissolved in a solvent and put into a pressurized can or pump spray. It works by gluing strands of hair together so that they form a stronger structure that can then hold a style. Recently, it has been reported that hairspray also contains phthalates—hormone-disrupting chemicals used to keep plastics soft and pliable.

Many women find it hard to believe that hairspray is just liquid plastic. If you are one of them, try this test. Spray your usual hairspray onto your bathroom mirror and leave it to dry. If you spray a thick-enough layer, you should be able to peel it off in a single sheet. But even if you don't, you will be able to scrape off little shavings of plastic—the same stuff you deposit on your hair and into your lungs each time you use hairspray.

Hairspray also contains such ingredients as *alcohol (denatured), dimethyl ether, VA/vinyl butyl benzoate/crotonates copolymer, aminomethyl propanol, cyclopentasiloxane, dimethicone copolyol, PPG-3 methyl ether,* and fragrances.

Perhaps unsurprisingly, there is a medical condition known as hairdresser's lung—a respiratory disease that is caused by chronic exposure to hairspray. Even though the average consumer is unlikely to develop this disease, using hairspray regularly can do other nasty things to your health. Your nose is lined with tiny hairs that filter out dirt and pollution from the air you breathe. When hairspray gets into your nose and onto these little hairs, they become sticky and begin to attract and trap dust and pollution until they become saturated with dirt—at which point they can no longer filter pollutants effectively.

Other distressing side effects of hairspray use include nail abnormalities. When you spray and then style your hair using your fingers, the spray is deposited on your nails, where it can cause the new nail to grow poorly or predispose it to infection. Breathing difficulties and contact dermatitis after hairspray use are also common complaints.

Hair Gel

Like hairspray, hair gel is a type of resin or plastic. Hair gels are generally more concentrated than hairsprays, which is why you can use them to make your hair stay in so many different gravity-defying shapes. Common ingredients include polyvinylpyrrolidone (PVP), PVP/dimethyl-aminoethylmethacrylate copolymer, laureth-23, *triisopropanolamine*, *carbomer*, methicone copolymer, polyquaternium-4, propylene glycol, such preservatives as parabens, DMDM hydantoin, disodium EDTA, diazolidinyl urea, *phenoxyethanol*, *parfum*, and even synthetic colors.

Try This Instead . . .

Apart from not using it, there are very few alternatives to things like hairspray and gel. The best alternative is to stop buying hairstyling products and use the money you save on getting a really good haircut. With well-cut hair, you shouldn't need to apply lots of glue to keep your hair in place. Do this, and you may find that you and your hair live happily ever after.

Hair Today, Gone Tomorrow

Depilatories (hair removers), which come in gels, creams, lotions, aerosols, and roll-ons, are chemical razor blades. Usually, they contain a highly alkaline chemical, such as *calcium thioglycolate*, that dissolves the protein structure of the hair, causing it to separate from the skin surface. The problem is that skin and hair are similar in their composition. What damages one can also damage the other. For this reason, if you use depilatory creams, it is especially important to follow the directions, not leave them on for too long, and not reapply them too regularly.

Try reserving the use of hairsprays and gels for when you really need them, like on special occasions, when you need your hair to stay in place. In addition, when purchasing hairsprays, gels, and other styling agents:

Read the label. Try to buy products with the fewest and least toxic ingredients.

Use pump sprays in favor of aerosols. You are still at risk of inhaling the noxious chemicals in the mixture, but you will be avoiding inhaling toxic propellants as well—a small step in the right direction.

Hair Dyes

In a culture obsessed with youth and beauty, gray hairs are the enemy, and today's hair dyes are marketed as being as good for your self-esteem as they are for your hair. But underneath the advertising hype is a disturbing amount of data linking regular hair dye use with a range of different cancers.

To achieve luscious shades of chestnut brown, coppery red, mahogany, or black, permanent hair dyes must first chemically damage your hair. Under a microscope, the cuticle of human hair looks like overlapping fish scales. The pigment molecules that give hair its color are stored in the central cortex of the hair, beneath the scaly layer. Before the color can penetrate the hair shaft, the cuticle must be "opened" so that the chemicals can get into the natural pigment molecules.

Permanent hair dyes consist of two components: color and developer. The color component usually contains a range of synthetic dyes and intermediates, such as *ammonia*, *diaminobenzenes*, phenylenediamines, resorcinol, and phenols.

Mixed with the developer—usually hydrogen peroxide—the color component begins to oxidize to produce a particular color. The ammonia in the mix causes the hair shaft to swell, forcing the cuticles apart and allowing the mix to deposit the new color underneath. The process of oxidation takes time, which is why the formula usually looks one color when you first apply it and another when you rinse it off.

Toxic ingredients like *diaminotoluene* and diaminoanisole were removed from hair dye products some twenty years ago, but it is likely that a heavy past use of dyes containing these chemicals is the cause of some cases of breast cancer today. But a quick scan of the label on most hair dyes reveals that they still contain chemicals, most commonly phenylenediamines, that are just as harmful. The type of phenylenediamine used depends on the end color, thus:

* *para-phenylenediamine* (black)

* *para-toluenediamine* (brown)

- *ortho-phenylenediamine* (brown)
- *para-aminophenol* (reddish brown)
- *ortho-aminophenol* (light brown)

Other hair dye ingredients that have proven carcinogenic in at least one animal species include *4-chloro-m-phenylenediamine*, *2,4-toluenediamine*, 2-nitro-p-phenylenediamine, and 4-amino-2-nitrophenol. Coal-tar dyes have also been found to cause cancer in laboratory animals, yet no warning is required for these either.

These ingredients and their variations (usually HCl, or hydrochloride, or sulphates, such as *para-phenylenediamine* sulphate) are powerful irritants, and have been implicated in severe allergic reactions (phenylenediamines are also mutagenic, causing DNA mutations and fetal abnormalities in animals). Other irritant ingredients include hydrogen peroxide, resorcinol, and 1-naphthol. Hair dye sold in the EU containing any of these ingredients should carry a warning: *Can cause an allergic reaction. Do not use to color eyelashes or eyebrows.*

In the United States, products containing 4-methoxy-m-phenylenediamine (4-MMPD, 2,4-diaminoanisole) must also carry a warning: *Contains an ingredient that can penetrate your skin and has been determined to cause cancer in laboratory animals.* No such warning is required for this ingredient in the EU, however.

Other hair dye ingredients, such as chlorides, are highly irritating to the mucous membranes. Chloride fumes can irritate the lungs and eyes and cause burns or rashes on the skin. Hair colors also contain several penetration enhancers known to aid the absorption of other toxic chemicals into the bloodstream. These can include propylene glycol, polyethylene glycol, fatty acids, such as oleic, palmitic, and *lauric acid*, and *isopropyl alcohol*, to name but a few.

More Cancer

Both human and animal studies show that the body rapidly absorbs the carcinogens and other chemicals found in permanent and semipermanent dyes through the skin during the more than thirty minutes that dyes remain on the scalp. So, if you use permanent, semipermanent, shampoo-in, or temporary hair colors, you are increasing your risk of developing cancer.

Problems with hair dyes were first noted in the late 1970s, when several studies found links between the use of hair dyes and breast cancer. In 1976, one study reported that eighty-seven out of hundred breast-cancer patients had been long-term hair dye users.

In 1979, another study found a significant relationship between the frequency and duration of hair dye use and breast cancer. Women who started dying their hair at age twenty had twice the risk of those who began at age forty. Those at greatest risk were the fifty- to seventy-nine-year-olds who had been dying their hair for years, suggesting that the cancer takes years to develop.

A year later, another study found that women who dye their hair to change its color, rather than to mask grayness, were at a threefold risk of developing breast cancer.

Research continued and, in the early 1990s, Japanese and Finnish studies also linked hair dye use with breast cancer. More recently, a jointly funded American Cancer Society and FDA study found a fourfold increase in relatively uncommon cancers, including non-Hodgkin's lymphoma (NHL) and multiple myeloma, among hair dye users.

A more recent Harvard study suggested that compared with women who never dyed their hair, women who dyed their hair one to four times a year had a 70 percent greater risk of ovarian cancer. Women who used hair dye five times or more per year had twice the risk of developing ovarian cancer compared with women who never did so.

As if this wasn't enough, a study published in the February 2001 edition of the *International Journal of Cancer* found a link between long-term hair dye use and an increased incidence of bladder cancer.

But it is the link with otherwise uncommon cancers that causes the greatest concern, and may well be the best evidence of hair dye toxicity.

Evidence suggests, for example, that if you use hair dye, you may be increasing your risk of NHL and multiple myeloma by anywhere from two to four times over that of a nonuser. Some researchers even believe that hair dyes may account for as many as 20 percent of all cases of NHL in women.

Other data from the U.S. National Cancer Institute (NCI) shows that women who used permanent hair dyes had a 50 percent higher risk of developing NHL and an 80 percent higher risk of multiple myeloma than nonusers.

In this NCI study, other cancer risk factors, such as a family history of cancer, cigarette smoking, and herbicide or pesticide exposure, did not change the risks calculated for hair dye use. The risk increased with the number of years of use, however, and for women using black, brown, or red coloring products.

As a general rule, the darker the shade of the dye, the higher the risk of breast cancer; thus, women who use black, dark brown, or red dyes are at the greatest risk.

In all fairness, there are problems with studies into hair dye and cancer risk. Some involved small numbers of women who worked in the cosmetics industry. Historically, this group of women are exposed to the known carcinogens in hair dyes—diaminotoluene, diaminoanisole and phenylenediamines, coal-tar dyes, the dioxane found in detergents, solvents, nitrosamines, and formaldehyde-releasing preservatives—in much greater concentrations than the rest of us. Taken together, however, they do point toward an increased overall risk that may be unacceptable.

Men Are at Risk, Too

While women were once the main users of hair dyes, use among men has increased dramatically in the last few decades and, with it, the incidence of rare cancers. According to the NCI, hair dye use is responsible for a 90 percent increased risk of multiple myeloma among men.

This result echoed that of an earlier NCI study, which showed that men who had used hair dyes had a twofold risk for NHL and almost double the risk of leukemia.

No Problem?

Hair dye manufacturers continue to defend the safety of their products, suggesting that any risk is minimal. It is true that some studies dispute the cancer risk. One, which involved fifteen hundred male and female hair dye users in San Francisco, found no increased incidence of NHL. The weight of the evidence, however, suggests a need for caution.

One difficulty is that there are large variations in the chemical content of hair dyes. This means that when an association is found, it is difficult to know which ingredient or mix of ingredients is the culprit. In addition, cancer is a slow-developing disease in humans. By the time it surfaces, it is difficult to prove beyond a shadow of a doubt that one particular exposure was the cause. This is, of course, good news for manufacturers, who can continue to produce potentially toxic products with impunity and without risk of litigation—but bad news for the rest of us.

Try This Instead . . .

If you intend to keep dying your hair, consider these safer options:

Read the label. If you dye your hair, use the safer alternatives that are currently on the market. These should not contain phenylenediamines (though many so-called natural hair colors do). Never buy products that are in any way unclear about their ingredients.

Read the label again. This time look for dyes. Avoid products that use colors like Acid Orange 87, Solvent Brown 44, Acid Blue 168, and Acid Violet 73, as these are also carcinogenic.

Don't dye your hair too often. Leave the maximum amount of time between applications.

Leave hair dyes on the head for the minimum required time.

Hair colorants made entirely from plant-based ingredients are the safest choice; however, these are few and far between. Pure herbal hair dyes will need to be left in the hair significantly longer then synthetic dyes, but have the advantage of conditioning the hair while they color.

Go natural. In a world of look-alike bleached blondes and unnaturally red redheads, you'll probably be the standout.

Makeup

Many women would argue that makeup is just a bit of fun—a harmless pleasure that makes them feel good about themselves. But the makeup that women put on their faces each day—and wear for long hours at a time—is anything but a benign enhancement to beauty.

There is nothing unique about the ingredients in your favorite makeup. On the whole, these will be exactly the same as the ingredients in your face cream and bath and hair products.

By the time a woman has made up her face, she has covered her skin in *mineral oil*, a carcinogen, and preservatives, such as parabens (a sensitizer and estrogen disrupter), Kathon CG (a sensitizer, mutagen, and suspected carcinogen), and diazolidinyl urea (another sensitizer). She will also have exposed herself to synthetic colors, many of which are known carcinogens and allergens; fragrance, the ingredients of which are sensitizers, central-nervous-system disrupters, and carcinogens; plasticizers, such as polyvinylpyrrolidone (PVP), also a carcinogen; surfactants, such as triethanolamine; film formers, such as dimethicone and *polytetrafluoroethylene* (PTFE, or Teflon); talc, which is carcinogenic when inhaled and commonly contaminated with heavy metals, such as lead, and poisons, such as arsenic; synthetic waxes derived for petroleum (also potentially carcinogenic); and sunscreens, which are sensitizers as well as estrogen mimics.

Preservatives

In addition to parabens and Kathon CG (the risk of which are detailed elsewhere in this chapter), most types of makeup also contain the preservative butylated hydroxyanisole (BHA)—a chemical that is easily absorbed into the skin and has been designated a human carcinogen by the U.S. National Toxicology Program.

Eye makeup, especially mascara, can sometimes contain mercury-based preservatives, such as *phenylmercuric acetate* and *thimerosal* (the same controversial preservative used in childhood vaccines). These are toxic and damaging to the eye. Mercury-based preservatives can also be found in a wide range of toiletries, including soap-free cleansers, antiseptic sprays, makeup remover, and eye moisturizers.

Thimerosal is not always listed on the label by that name, but may instead be called by any of its many synonyms, including mercurochrome, merthiolate, sodium ethylmercurithiosalicylate, thimerosalate, thiomerosalan, merzonin, mertorgan, ethyl (2-mercaptobenzoato-S), mercury sodium salt, merfamin or [(o-carboxyphenyl)thi] ethylmercury sodium salt. After a glance at this complicated list, it's easy to see how the use of mercury in a product used on the eyes has escaped the attention of the vast majority of us.

Carcinogens

Liquid formulas like foundations are prey to the same problems as shampoos and other toiletries. That is, they often contain the same carcinogenic nitrosamines found in shampoos and foam baths. The longer the product has been on the shelf, the higher the risk of nitrosamine formation. Mascara—especially those that promise to extend lashes—can contain any number of carcinogenic plasticizers, including polyurethane.

Another common ingredient, silica, is usually touted as a natural skin-enhancing mineral—in spite of the fact that cosmetic silica is synthesized in the lab. In 2000, crystalline silica (sometimes called crystalline quartz, the same ingredient found in cat litter and scouring powders) was added to the National Toxicology Program's list of carcinogens.

While silica can be used in any cosmetic formulation, it is the easily inhaled powdered products, such as face powder and eyeshadow, that are the most risky. The concern here is that the amorphous hydrated form of silica commonly used in cosmetics can be contaminated with carcinogenic crystalline quartz. It is impossible to tell which silica-containing products are contaminated in this way, however, so using any silica-containing product is a game of chance.

Most makeup, even powder formulas, contains some form of mineral oil. Mineral oil is what binds powders together, and it also provides the basis for liquid formulations and lipsticks. Mineral oils were first recognized as carcinogens in 1987. Listed as *paraffinum liquidim* (the stuff that baby oil is made from) or *petrolatum* (petroleum jelly), these highly refined oils have a spotty history. Mineral oils are also thought to increase the photosensitivity of the skin, making it more prone to sun-induced damage and skin cancer.

Because the mineral oils used in cosmetics are highly refined, scientists cannot say conclusively how dangerous they are to humans. The thinner the oil, as in paraffinum liquidim, the more risky they are thought to be because of the high levels of volatile hydrocarbons that thin oils contain. The National Toxicology Program's "9th Annual Report on Carcinogens" notes that analyses of mineral oils used for medicinal and cosmetic purposes reveal the presence of several carcinogenic hydrocarbons known as polycyclic aromatic hydrocarbons. These include benzo[b]fluoranthene, benzo[k]fluoranthene, and benzo[a]pyrene.

Toxic Metals

Amazingly, cosmetics can also contain toxic metals, most commonly as contaminants in pigments and talc. One Finnish study that looked at eighty-eight brands of eyeshadow found that 75 percent of the products tested contained detectable levels of at least one of the following elements: lead, cobalt, nickel, chromium, and arsenic.

In this investigation, the elements found in the cosmetics were impurities in the ingredients rather than listed ingredients—a problem seen in many cosmetics. While the researchers felt that, in most cases, these levels were not enough to cause allergic reactions, another study in the U.K. found that chronic exposures to very low levels of arsenic—lower than those in the Finnish study—were capable of causing hormonal disruption.

Colors

Most of us would avoid foods that contain artificial colors. Yet, each day, women paint their faces with a range of artificial colors known to cause health problems in both the short and long term.

Artificial colors may be carcinogens (indeed, all coal-tar dyes are considered carcinogenic); others may contain hidden carcinogenic impurities in some batches, but not in others, depending on the source of the raw materials. What's more, contact dermatitis and irritation can also be caused by cosmetic pigments, such as artificial colors.

Checking for harmful dyes in cosmetics is a complex business, made more difficult by the fact that, in Europe, these colors are usually listed by their INCI (International Nomenclature for Cosmetic Ingredients) numbers—usually "CI" followed by five numbers. (This, in turn, is different again from the name given to the same ingredient when it is used as a food coloring, when in Europe it's usually an E followed by a number, as described on page 67; see table, below.)

New colors are being developed all the time, but not with an eye on safety. For example, one of the newest—FD&C Red 40 (also known as Allura Red,

CI16035, and, in foods found in Europe, as E129)—is a popular addition to eye-shadows. It was approved and has been in use since 1994 despite the fact that the safety testing was all funded and performed by the manufacturer. Nevertheless, the National Cancer Institute reports that p-credine, a chemical used in the manufacturing of FD&C Red 40, is a carcinogen.

Certain carcinogenic colors are now banned from use in both U.S. and European cosmetics; these include D&C Red 2, 3, 4, 10, and 17, FD&C Red 10, and FD&C Blue 4. Nevertheless, these still regularly appear in cosmetics that have been illegally imported from other countries.

While a single use of a single makeup product may be "safe," your total daily exposure to all colored products—soaps, shampoos, conditioners, shaving cream, toothpaste, and deodorants (and don't forget juices, cereals, pastries, coffee creamer, and even vitamins)—may add up to an unacceptable risk.

Try This Instead . . .

When it comes to makeup, it may be a case of choosing your poison carefully. If the rest of your lifestyle is relatively toxin-free, the appropriate use of

COMMON NAME	UNITED STATES	EUROPE	E NUMBER
Alizarin Cyanine Green F	D&C Green 5	CI61570	-
Pigment Orange 5	D&C Orange 17	CI12075	-
Rhodamine B	D&C Red 19	CI45170	-
Acid Red 33	D&C Red 33	CI17200	-
Pigment Red 53 sodium salt	D&C Red 8	CI15585	-
Pigment Red 53 barium salt	D&C Red 9	CI15585	-
Acetate Blue G	Disperse Blue 1	CI64500	-
Acetate Fast Yellow G	Disperse Yellow 3	CI11855	-
Brilliant Blue FCF	FD&C Blue 1	CI42090	E133
Indigo Carmine	FD&C Blue 2	CI73015	E132
Fast Green FCF	FD&C Green 3	CI42053	E143
Ponceau SX	FD&C Red 4	CI14700	E124
Allura Red	FD&C Red 40	CI16035	E129
Tartrazine	FD&C Yellow 5	CI19140	E102
Sunset Yellow	FD&C Yellow 6	CI15985	E110
Titanium dioxide	Pigment White 6	CI77891	E171

well-chosen makeup may not add significantly to your total toxic load. When you buy or use cosmetics, follow these simple guidelines to help you choose the safest ones.

Start on the inside. Beauty really does come from within. It starts with a nutritious diet, adequate rest, and periodic breaks from stress. Without these basics, no makeup in the world will make you look beautiful.

Read the label. It is essential to get into the habit of looking at the ingredients in your cosmetics. Do not rely on claims of "all natural," "organic," or "cruelty-free." These claims are meaningless. The only thing that tells the true story of the cosmetic is the ingredients list. Once you have identified an ingredient or ingredients that you wish to avoid, keep its name on a card or list that you can take with you when you shop. Remember also that price is no guarantee of safety or quality. Sometimes the cheaper brands contain fewer toxic ingredients. Only the label will tell you for sure.

But also, don't put too much faith in the label. Don't just buy a product because it was safe last time you looked. By the time you are ready to replace your eyeshadow or lipstick, it may be made from completely different ingredients. Manufacturers are continually reformulating their products, often according to what ingredients are available and least expensive at the time. In addition, many ingredients labels—for instance, those used on eyeshadows and lipsticks—list the colors for the entire range rather than the specific product you are buying. For these reasons, some products say "may include . . ." or use the symbol "+/–" before a list of ingredients, making it impossible to make sensible choices about safety.

Avoid cosmetics that are pearly, glittery, opalescent, or frosted. These are among the most dangerous since, to achieve this effect, manufacturers add such ingredients as pure aluminum, mica, and even fish scales. Used near the eye, these particles can flake off and cause corneal damage. Ingested aluminum, in particular, is linked to Alzheimer's disease. Stick to matte colors, blot well, and shine up your lips with an over- or undercoat of shea butter or natural oils.

Choose lip gloss (which has a lower volume of coloring ingredients) rather than lipstick for everyday wear, *but be aware.* Conventional lip glosses contain less color but are high in phenol, a poisonous substance that is easily absorbed into the delicate tissue of the lips (aided by the addition of petrolatum, a petroleum-derived moisturizer, as well as other wetting agents). Phenol ingestion can cause nausea, vomiting, convulsions, paralysis, respiratory collapse, and even death; minute amounts are linked to skin rashes, swelling, pimples, and hives.

Avoid all perfumed cosmetics and especially avoid lip products with a sweet taste. Often, these include saccharin (a suspected carcinogen) and phthalic anhydride (made from another suspected carcinogen, naphthalene), an irritant that can cause headaches, nausea, vomiting, diarrhea, and confusion, and has been linked to kidney and brain damage, in infants. All the more remarkable is that it is commonly used in "play" and "fun" makeup aimed at young girls.

Choose products without sunscreens. Chances are, you are wearing your makeup indoors anyway. Don't be fooled by claims of natural sunscreens. There is no such thing. The only effective sunscreens are synthetic chemicals that add to your toxic burden.

If you don't need to wear makeup, don't. Many women wear makeup for the most trivial occasions—a trip to the supermarket or bank, picking the kids up from school, weekends at home, or walks in the park. Get out of the habit. Get used to the way you look without makeup, and give your skin and your system a break. If you can't stand to go out without something on your face, stick to the basics—a swipe of carefully chosen mascara and a bit of lipstick or gloss is fine for everyday wear.

Skin Care

Moisturizers are an integral part of many women's beauty routine. While most moisturizers promise miraculous effects, they really have just one basic function—to maintain the water balance in the most superficial layers of the skin. This area of the skin, known as the stratum corneum, is made up of cells that are being constantly shed and replaced by new cells emerging from the deeper layers of the skin.

The stratum corneum is approximately 30 percent water. Two-thirds of this is bound to biological tissues and usually does not change unless there is a serious skin condition, such as eczema or psoriasis. But the remaining water content rises and falls according to what's going on in the environment—for instance, dry weather conditions, overwashing, or exposure to central heating, air conditioning, and certain chemicals.

The word is misleading since "moisturizer" would seem to indicate that it will put water into the skin. But no moisturizer, no matter how expensive or how many ingredients it contains, can do this. Even if your moisturizer could push water back into your skin, it would be quickly disseminated throughout the rest of your body rather than be held there for an indefinite period.

Moisturizing ingredients work in two ways to help slow this water loss. Humectants, such as propylene glycol, glycerin, and urea, act like water magnets, drawing moisture from the atmosphere and keeping it near the skin.

Emollients are generally fats, oils, and waxes that form a barrier on the surface of the skin. For years, moisturizing creams and lotions relied on emollients like *lanolin* and mineral oil to produce this protective barrier. Today, synthetic derivatives of vegetable oils, such as *isopropyl palmitate* and *hexyl laureate*, are more common, as are a range of synthetic film formers, such as dimethicone and *Teflon* (PTFE, or polytetrafluoroethylene).

Do They Work?

Moisturizers are mixtures of oil and water and, to keep these two opposing substances bound together and to make sure the product has a long shelf life, a cream or lotion will contain a raft of emulsifiers, stabilizers, and preservatives. To make it nice to use, it will also contain perfumes and colors. If the cream also claims other properties, such as improving wrinkles, further ingredients are added.

So, what starts out as a simple emulsion quickly becomes a cocktail of harmful ingredients, such as paraffinum liquidum, triethanolamine, propylene glycol, quaternium-15, carbomer, dimethicone, *trisodium EDTA*, BHA (butylated hydroxyanisole), parabens, and parfum. The emollients in the mix also act like penetration enhancers—ingredients that aid the absorption of other more toxic substances into the skin and eventually the bloodstream.

It's hardly surprising, then, that moisturizing creams can and do cause problems like allergic reactions, skin irritation, and contact dermatitis, characterized by redness, itching, burning, and stinging sensations. Used over the long term, they can also create the very problem they are intended to solve by actually increasing water loss from the skin.

Toxic Ingredients

Some moisturizing ingredients can actually damage the skin. Humectants, such as *alpha-hydroxy acids* (AHAs, such as lactic acid or *glycolic acid*) act like chemical peels, thinning the stratum corneum and, ultimately, accelerating water loss. If your moisturizer includes fruit acids, or AHAs, it may cause premature aging of your skin as well as increased susceptibility to damage from the sun's ultraviolet rays.

Many emollients trap dirt and sweat under the skin and some, like petrolatum, degrade the skin's natural protective barrier, making it more vulnerable to bacteria and viruses.

Film-forming ingredients like Teflon (PTFE) and dimethicone are now routinely added to body-care products without any comprehensive evaluation of their safety. Teflon contains the potential carcinogen PFOA (perfluorooctanoic acid), and some silicones are known tumor promoters and accumulate in the liver and lymph nodes. Both are nonbiodegradable.

Several of the ingredients commonly used in body lotions can make the skin more permeable, allowing more toxic ingredients to be absorbed into the body. There is also some evidence that moisturizers can make the skin more susceptible to damage caused by the synthetic detergents used in many facial and body-care products.

Particularly worrisome are the newer moisturizers that make use of nanoparticles, which slip into the spaces between skin cells before releasing their active ingredients. No research has been conducted to show how much more of these substances is absorbed into the bloodstream with these particles, so, if you want to avoid them, look for words like "liposome" or "nanosome" on the label.

While the cosmetics industry loudly trumpets the benefits of moisturizers, most of their effects are unsubstantiated and/or temporary. Healthy skin begins on the inside, and nothing you put on your skin will be as effective as sorting out your diet, your sleep, your stress levels, and your environment. Unless you have an underlying skin condition that requires medical attention, you probably don't need a regular moisturizer.

Body Lotions, Oils, and Gels

The ingredients of a typical body lotion are not much different from those of a hair conditioner. And basically, the two products perform the same function—replacing natural oils with synthetic ones, and then coating the skin with a thin waterproof layer.

While body oil may seem like a simpler alternative, many are based on mineral oil. Some, like baby oil, are 100 percent mineral oil (paraffinum liquidim), with added perfume.

Mineral oil, a by-product of the distillation of gasoline from crude oil, impedes the skin's ability to breathe, attract moisture, and detoxify. It can also slow down cell renewal and promote premature skin aging. While it is used for its lubricant qualities, which, in the short term, appear to make the skin softer, when used over the longer term mineral oil can make the skin dry out. This is because mineral oil dissolves the skin's natural oils, thereby increasing water loss (dehydration) from the skin.

Any mineral-oil derivative can be contaminated with cancer-causing polycyclic aromatic hydrocarbons (PAHs). Mineral oils may also increase the skin's sensitivity to sunlight, and have been linked to an increased risk of skin cancer. Petrolatum, paraffin or paraffin oil, and propylene glycol are all forms of mineral oil.

Among women who regularly switch toiletry brands or try new products, mineral oils have been shown to be the major cause of new skin irritation, including rashes and spots. There is no good reason for this kind of suffering to take place.

Because of the risks of mineral oils, manufacturers have switched to silicone-based oils and gels.

Silicones, such as dimethicone (or dimethiconol), *cyclomethicone*, cyclopentasiloxane, and *cyclohexasiloxane*, are synthesized from silicon metal to produce water-repellent "dry" oils and waxes. They add many of the feel-good qualities associated with modern body-care products, such as texture, silkiness, luster, and smooth application.

Silicones come in many forms. Film-forming silicones add spreadability and smoothness as well as water repellence to such products as facial cosmetics, lotions, creams, antiperspirants, and deodorants. In cosmetics like lipsticks, eyeshadows, and blushers, silicone resins and gums provide longevity to help the product stay on the skin and maintain its color; in hairstyling products, they improve control.

Used as surfactants and conditioners in hair products, silicones add foam stabilization to add shine, body, and softness to the hair. Volatile silicones (that is, those that evaporate quickly) make aesthetically pleasing and effective antiperspirants and deodorants that don't leave a residue. Highly reflective silicones enhance the shine of surfaces, such as skin and hair.

Silicones are also widely used in household cleaning products (including laundry detergents, fabric softeners, polishes, and waxes).

On the whole, silicones allow the skin to breathe better than mineral oils, but question marks still hang over their long-term safety. While they increase the feel-good factor of a product, they are poorly absorbed by the skin, which raises some doubt as to how well the ingredients suspended in them will be absorbed. Some, like dimethicone, are also cancer-causing suspects.

Try This Instead . . .

If you're going to continue to use commercial moisturizing products, choose those with the fewest ingredients and watch out especially for those that may be contaminated with carcinogens. It's the oil and wax contents of moisturizers that hold moisture next to the skin, so why not consider simple vegetable oils to maintain the skin's suppleness. They will do the same job at a fraction of the price, and you'll have the advantage of knowing exactly what you are putting on your face.

If your skin is occasionally dry, consider using natural oils after bathing or washing to temporarily seal in moisture. Natural oils contain all the nutrients natural to the plant or animal from which they come. Many, such as jojoba and emu, are amazingly similar to the oils in human skin and, as such, are nonirritating, don't clog pores, and are deeply nourishing.

Effective moisturizers can be prepared on an as-needed basis by almost anyone from a simple mixture of vegetable or biological oils (coconut, jojoba, almond, or emu) and plant butters (shea or mango), water, and glycerin. With practice, these can be made to suit different areas of the body in response to the skin's seasonal needs (heavier oils in winter, lighter ones in summer):

• almond oil	• grapeseed oil
• aloe vera	• hempseed oil
• apricot kernel oil	• honey
• avocado oil	• jojoba oil
• beeswax	• macadamia nut oil
• castor oil	• mango butter
• cocoa butter	• olive oil
• coconut oil	• rosa mosqueta oil
• emu oil	• shea butter
• evening primrose oil	• squalene
• glycerine	• wheatgerm oil

As a general rule, use lighter oils, such as apricot kernel, coconut, or jojoba oil for normal skins, and heavier oils, such as avocado and evening primrose oil, for older or drier skins. Rosehip oil is also considered a rich and nourishing oil for the face.

Face Creams

Skin has a life of its own that most of us never hear about. Getting in touch with its natural rhythms, rather than bullying it into submission with lots of creams and potions, is the most straightforward path to a better complexion.

Flip through any magazine or browse in any store and you will be confronted with a bewildering array of products that promise great skin all day, every day. But perfect unchanging skin is only the preserve of celebrities and models, who inhabit a world of perpetually good lighting, professional makeup artists, and Photoshop.

In reality, skin is a mirror, reflecting and reacting to what you eat and drink, and your exposure to environmental pollutants, allergens, cosmetic irritants, and the elements. How well you sleep and the stresses you are under are also relevant to the way your skin looks from day to day.

In real people, it is in the nature of healthy, normal skin to change on almost an hourly basis. Studies show, for instance, that:

• Production of new skin cells is highest at midnight and lowest at noon.

• Oil production in the skin is twice as high at noon as it is at 2 a.m.

• Your skin is more likely to absorb what you put onto it—for example, topical medications—at 4 p.m. than at 8 a.m.

• You're more likely to have an allergic skin reaction in the morning than later in the day.

Normal skin changes are not problems that need to be fixed, and there's no getting around the fact that if you want great skin, there are no shortcuts and no miracle products. Acknowledging this means that you can stop obsessing over the most minute and transient shifts in skin tone and color, and adopt a more sensible approach to skin care that works from the inside out.

Adjusting your lifestyle to include sleeping longer, eating better, drinking more water, and exercising more at different times of the month can help mitigate some of the natural changes that take place at skin level. But ultimately, accepting and working with these may make the difference between being at war, or making peace, with the way you look.

In spite of the fact that good skin begins on the inside, the skin-care market is overflowing with choices that promise to keep you young and wrinkle-free as well as removing dirt, oil, and makeup.

Hand and Nail Creams

Like body oils and lotions, hand and nail creams are essentially mineral oil–based. There is little difference between the ingredients of most body lotions and those that are supposed to be specifically for the hands, although hand creams tend to have even more emollients in them. Hands become dry and cracked because they are more exposed to the elements and more in use than almost any other part of the body. You also wash your hands more often, and expose them to detergents and other cleaning products more frequently every day as well.

While not as thin as facial skin, the skin on your hands is still thin enough to allow the penetration of noxious chemicals. To keep them soft and to avoid absorbing chemicals into your body, always use gloves when doing cleaning jobs, and substitute vegetable oils and vegetable oil–based creams for petroleum-based ones.

Wrinkle Creams

How skin ages is a complicated process that involves internal and external factors, some of which are within our control, but many of which are not.

Aging causes decreases in collagen and elastin, the scaffolding of the skin, causing the skin to wrinkle and sag. Gravity can also make loose skin around the eyes and jowls sag even more. Aged skin also appears more translucent because of the reduction in the number of pigment-containing cells (melanocytes). It is also thinner and more fragile, and at an increased risk of injury while being less able to repair itself. Your genetic inheritance is also influential, as are hormonal changes at menopause, although human studies have failed to conclusively link estrogen decline and wrinkly skin.

An unhealthy lifestyle will also be reflected in your skin's condition. Prematurely aging skin often mirrors the body's inefficiency in eliminating toxins and waste products. Addressing the source of the problem—for instance, through diet (see box, page 144)—rather than simply relying on topical creams and lotions is always advisable.

It has long been believed that sun exposure is the single biggest external cause of wrinkles. But is this true? Excess sun exposure can generate skin-damaging free radicals, leading to "photoaging." Ultraviolet-A (UVA) exposure is believed to be particularly harmful, as it leads to the breakdown of the skin's collagen fibers.

But it can be difficult to differentiate between genetically normal wrinkles and those caused by the sun. In addition, a recent study challenged the received wisdom by suggesting that people with very wrinkled faces were 90 percent less likely to get basal-cell carcinoma (BCC), the most common form of skin cancer, even though they had the same amount of sun exposure as cancer victims.

The key is the way that older, smooth skin repairs itself—by stimulating the production of transforming growth factor (TGF)-beta, which, in turn, suppresses the immune system and promotes blood-vessel growth, both of which are risk factors for cancer. If confirmed, this would quash the broadly accepted idea that wrinkling is an indicator of sunlight-induced damage and, therefore, of skin-cancer risk.

Smoking also increases the breakdown of collagen, as well as dries out the skin and reduces circulation, thus depleting the skin of oxygen and essential nutrients. Smoking may also lower levels of skin-protective vitamin A. Research shows that smoking twenty cigarettes a day for just a few years is equivalent to almost ten years of chronological aging—a much greater rate of damage than lifelong sun exposure.

Do Wrinkle Creams Cause Wrinkles?

Many women who scan food labels for harmful additives unthinkingly use toiletries that contain undesirable chemicals, believing that what we put on our bodies is not as influential to our health as what we put in them.

Yet, facial skin is thinner than skin elsewhere, and may absorb toxic chemicals (such as petroleum by-products; carcinogens, such as nitrosamines and formaldehyde; solvents; and estrogenic preservatives, such as parabens) at a much greater rate.

Our sun phobia means that it can be very difficult to find a commercial moisturizer that doesn't come with a sunscreen. Even some night creams now contain sunscreening agents! But increasingly, sun creams are being blamed for making us vulnerable to skin cancer. What's more, if you work outdoors, you will probably need more protection than a moisturizing cream can give, whereas if you work in an office all day, an added sunscreen is just another unnecessary chemical.

Skin Food

Diet can significantly affect the skin and its tendency to wrinkle. Researchers from Monash University in Australia studied the diets of 453 people (aged seventy years and over) from Australia, Greece, and Sweden to find out if particular foods either predicted or were associated with skin wrinkling. The findings strongly suggest that a high intake of fruit, vegetables, and fish as well as certain healthy fats can reduce skin wrinkling.

Foods and Food Properties That Protect Against Wrinkles

- higher total fat

- monounsaturated fat

- olive oil and olives

- fish (especially fatty fish)

- reduced-fat milk and milk products

- eggs

- nuts and legumes (especially lima and broad beans)

- vegetables (especially leafy greens, spinach, asparagus, eggplant, celery, onions, leeks, and garlic)

In the attempt to look younger, many women remove the superficial layers of their skin with harsh exfoliants and chemical peels, such as alpha-hydroxy acids, glycolic, *hydroxycaprylic acid*, or lactic acid, passionflower, or citrus extract. While this is widely believed to improve the appearance of sun damage, offer UV protection, and heal sunburned skin, recent evidence suggests that these chemicals and the products that contain them can actually cause premature aging as well as increased UV susceptibility.

Better Alternatives

Even among the many so-called natural alternatives, there are very few skin-care products with documented scientific evidence of benefits. Most claims made in marketing these products are based on animal studies and the "science" of guesswork.

The most important factor in a skin cream is its ability to moisturize. Min-

- whole-grain cereals
- fruit and fruit products (especially prunes, cherries, apples, and jams)
- tea
- water
- zinc-containing foods (seafood, lean meat, milk, and nuts)

Foods and Food Properties That Promote Wrinkles

- saturated fat
- meat (especially fatty processed meats)
- full-fat dairy products (especially unfermented products and ice cream)
- soft drinks and cordials
- cakes, pastries, and desserts
- potatoes
- butter

eral oils (paraffinum liquidum, petrolatum) have been largely abandoned in favor of semisynthetic lipids (fats and oils) and their constituents, including ceramide, *hyaluronic acid*, cholesterol, triglycerides, *phospholipids*, and glycerin. Synthetic humectants (ingredients that draw water to the skin) include propylene glycol and glycerin (which can be animal or vegetable in origin). Many also include silicones (dimethicone and various siloxanes).

Natural vegetable oils are more compatible with the skin, much less drying than mineral oils, and better absorbed than either mineral oil or silicones. Good examples include almond, coconut, jojoba, soy, carrot, wheatgerm, macadamia, olive, and avocado oils. Some animal-derived oils, such as squalene and emu, also make good alternatives. These oils are more than just vehicles for other ingredients; they often have skin-boosting qualities of their own—for instance, they are high in essential fatty acids, and vitamins A, D, and E. These fatty acids temporarily strengthen cell membranes, slowing down the formation of fine lines and wrinkles, and helping the skin to resist attack from free radicals. Beeswax and soy wax are good alternatives to silicones, while vegetable glycerin and honey are effective, natural humectants.

Added antioxidants may also help. A handful of studies suggest that coenzyme-Q10 (ubiquinone) smoothes wrinkles, although published research in this area is scant.

Vitamin E, either as alpha-tocopherol or as a tocotrienol, is an antioxidant that, added to a cream, can help prolong the product's shelf life. Some studies suggest it can also help to smooth superficial wrinkles if it is used continuously.

Vitamins C and E in combination probably work best against UVB damage. Vitamin E also can work synergistically with carotenoids. Other UV-protective nutrients (in the lab and in animals) include selenium, ginkgo biloba extract, and aloe vera.

Alpha-lipoic acid (ALA) scavenges both water and fat-soluble free radicals, sparing levels of vitamin C and E in the skin. ALA is rapidly available to skin cells and may also have some UV-protecting properties.

Many plant extracts, including those from cocoa and green tea, as well as rosehip oil and horsetail, are also antioxidant.

More Stuff for Your Face

The amount of stuff we put on our faces is simply staggering, and since facial skin is thinner than skin elsewhere, the potential for absorbing toxic chemicals is much greater. While most skin-care products promise to help us look younger, prolonged use can dry and age the skin considerably. It may not show when you start using it at age twenty-four, but by the time you are fifty-four, the damage will be noticeable and mostly irreversible.

Acne treatments. Teenagers often use products that boast antibacterial properties, believing that they contain some sort of magic that will wash away pimples. They won't.

Typically, such products contain:

- **Harsh detergent/surfactants**, such as sodium laureth sulphate (SLES), which can be contaminated with the carcinogen 1,4-dioxane, and/or the potential hormone disrupters cocamide DEA and triethanolamine (TEA).

- **PEG**, or polyethylene glycol, compounds are preservatives that can be contaminated with the carcinogen 1,4-dioxane. PEGs can also form carcinogens when mixed with DEA and TEA. *Pareth* is a surfactant that also belongs to the same family as PEG.

- *Phenoxyisopropanol* is an antibacterial agent, manufactured by combining carcinogenic phenol (coal tar) with the solvent *isopropanol*. It is an irritant, and allergic reactions are possible.

- **Carbomer** is a gelling agent that can be irritating to skin and eyes.

- **Parfum (or fragrance)** does not clean the face, and can be a source of skin and airways irritation.

- **Color** does not clean the skin, and is added only to appeal to the eye.

Cleansing lotions are often touted as a better way to clean makeup and grime from your face. Lotions and creams, we are told, can clean without stripping away the skin's natural oils (although products containing solvents will dissolve natural oils, usually replacing them with synthetic ones). The ingredients of most cleansing lotions are nearly indistinguishable from those of facial moisturisers. Moreover, even the simplest cleansing lotion can contain a range of suspect chemicals.

Liquid face washes are similar in their content to liquid body washes (see page 104), but contain slightly more water. Because liquids are more complex to make than solids, they generally contain more potentially harmful chemicals than detergent bars.

Exfoliating scrubs typically contain harsh detergents, emulsifiers, and abrasives. An abrasive can be anything from ground fruit pits to talc to more worrisome particles, such as aluminum oxide. Others contain skin-drying agents, such as alcohol. A simple facecloth will do the job just as well, so it's silly to invest in anything else. Exfoliants are a waste of money, may unnecessarily damage your skin through overenthusiastic use, and will certainly add to your body's toxic burden.

Toners are now accepted as the necessary intermediate step between cleaning and moisturizing. In fact, this step is an invention of the marketing world. Clean skin is as toned as it needs to be.

Many toners use alcohol to dry the skin and make it feel tighter. Others promise to close your pores, thus making your skin look younger and firmer. Unfortunately, your pore size is genetically determined, and pores neither open nor close. If they did, your face would wobble like jelly throughout the day. What toner does is put astringent chemicals on your face to lower the skin temperature. This affects the underlying tissue, which will temporarily contract, giving that characteristic tight feeling that comes after using a toner.

Try This Instead . . .

Don't use special cleansers for your face—these are not much more than a mixture of diluted dish detergent and oil. Instead:

If you have pimples, it's probably the result of hormones and a poor lifestyle. Getting plenty of sleep, drinking water rather than sodas, cutting down on the sugar and fat in your diet, investigating any food or other allergies (if the problem is really severe), and a little patience is the best way to tackle them.

Try to avoid liquid cleansers, which are more expensive and have more harsh chemicals in them.

Opt for glycerin-based soaps if you want to use a conventional bar—they are among the mildest.

Switch from detergent bars and cleansers to castile or pure vegetable oil soaps, as these will clean your face and neck without stripping them completely of the skin's natural, beneficial, and protective oils (and you won't need to invest in separate bars for your body and face, either).

Whatever you use, remember to rinse well, because film left behind by neglectful rinsing can irritate the skin.

Forget about antibacterial cleaners, since simple soap and warm water are among the best antibacterials and the most effective ways to keep your face clean. They are also less expensive and unlikely to have as many suspect chemicals in them.

To remove makeup and city grime, use almond or jojoba oil on a cottonball, then rinse with warm water. Follow with a cool rinse or mild astringent, such as witch hazel.

You can tone your face simply and easily by splashing cold water on it. If you absolutely need to buy something to "tone" your skin, buy simple products, like distilled witch hazel, or try using a weak solution of cider vinegar in distilled water.

Shaving Cream

Wet shaving with a blade is one of the oldest ways of removing unwanted hair (from any part of the body). There is now a wide variety of shaving creams or foams on the market for both men and women. They look nice, feel nice, and some even smell nice. But they can contain some not-so-nice ingredients; for example: triethanolamine (TEA) and lauramide DEA, PEG-150 distearate, BIIT and imidazolidinyl urea, parabens, quaternium-15, paraffinum liquidum, and propellants, such as isobutane and *propane.*

Try This Instead . . .

A wet shave should be a *wet* shave. Getting the hair thoroughly wet before shaving means you can use less cream or foam to get the job done. Modern shaving creams are loaded with lubricants because most men and women skip the essential wetting part of the shave. In addition:

Use a shaving soap. It won't really be a soap (unless you buy it at a specialty natural health-care store), but a detergent bar; however, you will be able to avoid the problems associated with solvents and propellants found in shaving foams. Use a brush to get lots of foam unless you have very dry skin. The shaving brush may irritate dry skin, so soap up your hands first before applying the foam to your skin.

Use shaving oil. More and more companies are making these nice oils that usually contain added essential oils to smooth and soothe the surface of the face while shaving. Opt for vegetable-oil bases rather than mineral oils.

Buy an electric shaver. The shave won't usually be so close, but it will help you avoid a lot of unnecessary exposure to harsh chemicals.

Sun Creams

Sun exposure and the use of sunscreens is one of the most complex and contradictory areas of skin health. On the one hand, exposure to the fresh air and sun is vital for a healthy body. Sunlight, for example, is an important source of vitamin D, necessary for the development and maintenance of bones and teeth. But, at the same time, too much sun exposure can raise your risk of skin cancer.

Relying on sunscreens as your sole means of protection is fraught with problems since the protection they offer is never guaranteed. In addition, most commercial sun creams contain a mixture of harsh and harmful chemicals that come with their own risks. For example, some of the chemicals in sunscreens are thought to cause disruption or permanent damage to the nervous, immune, and respiratory systems. Young children may be especially susceptible to sunscreen chemicals and their toxic side effects. Among the most harmful are *benzophenones*, which can cause allergic reactions, and *PABA*s, which have been shown to form carcinogenic nitrosamines when mixed with other chemicals.

The effectiveness of any sun cream depends on its UV absorption, its concentration, its formulation, and its ability to withstand swimming or sweating. As a general rule, the higher the sun protection factor (SPF), the greater the number of chemicals in a sun lotion or cream. It is not uncommon for sun creams to contain three or more sunscreen agents, as well as perfumes, insect repellents, and a host of other chemicals besides. Though many of the ingredients used in sunscreens have been tested individually, studies of the long-term effects of combinations of sunscreen agents, applied liberally over an extended period of time, are rare.

There are two main types of ultraviolet rays: UVA and UVB. The SPF factor in your sun cream is for UVB protection only. Most UVB rays are filtered out by the ozone layer. Those that do get through stimulate the skin's pigment to produce melanin, our natural defense against sunlight. UVA rays are not filtered out by the ozone layer and penetrate the skin at a deeper level, so they have the potential to cause more skin damage. Gauging UVA protection is a little more difficult, though most creams now put UVA information on their labels as well.

Some experts believe that when exposed to UV rays, sunscreens like oxybenzone can break down into chemicals that destroy or inhibit the skin's own natural defenses against sunlight. This leaves it vulnerable to damage by the free radicals produced by exposure to sunlight. Free radicals are the toxic by-products of metabolism. Free-radical damage to the skin is implicated in skin cancer, premature aging, and other signs of damage to the skin.

Similarly, such sunscreens as padimate-O are thought to absorb harmful UV rays. But, as scientists point out, once absorbed, this energy has to be released somewhere—usually directly onto the skin, where it is metabolized into free radicals that can actually increase the risk of skin cancer.

What's in Your Sun Cream?

There are two basic types of creams available on the market today: chemical sunscreens, which act by absorbing UV light; and chemical sunblocks, which reflect or scatter light in both the visible and UV spectrum. Both types are associated with skin irritation.

These are the most common chemical sunscreens:

- **Benzophenones** are common skin sensitizers that can provoke allergic reactions in some individuals. Common benzophenones include *oxybenzone, dioxybenzone*, and *sulisbenzone*.

- **PABA**s are formaldehyde-forming chemicals that can form carcinogenic nitrosamines when combined with amines, such as DEA, TEA, and MEA, in the

Natural Sunscreens?

Read the labels for natural and "organic" sunscreens carefully. Usually, they are simply the same old ingredients with added plant extracts and oils. Can the addition of these natural ingredients really prevent sunburn? No, of course not. For example:

- Aqua—water does not prevent sunburn.
- Glycerin—a lubricant used in moisturizers to make them feel good and go on more smoothly. It has no sun-blocking ability, but can dry the skin, making it more vulnerable to sun damage.
- Octyl palmitate—a relative of vitamin C. There is no evidence that it offers protection from the sun.
- Retinyl palmitate—also known as pro-vitamin A or pro-retinol, this has no evidence of sun protection.
- Tocopherol acetate—a relative of vitamin E; again, this has no evidence of any effect as a sunscreen.

Other ingredients, including aloe vera, carrot oil, chamomile, borage oil, and avocado oil, are used as fillers, stabilizers, or preservatives. They are seldom present in high enough quantities to protect or nourish your skin, and none has any proven sun-blocking capacity.

mixture. PABAs can cause skin irritation. Common PABAs are p-aminobenzoic acid, *ethyl dihydroxypropyl PABA*, padimate-O (ocyl dimethyl PABA), *padimate-A*, and *glyceryl PABA*.

- **Cinnamates** are common skin irritants. This group of chemicals includes *cinoxate, ethylhexyl-p-methoxycinnamate, octocrylene*, and *ocytl methoxycinnamate*.

- **Salicylates** are also skin irritants associated with a high rate of dermatitis among users. Those commonly used in sun creams include *ethylhexyl salicylate, homosalate, octyl salicylate*, and neo-homosalate.

- Other common sunscreen agents include *methyl anthranilate, digalloyl trioleate*, and *avobenzone* (butyl methoxy-dibenzoylmethane).

- The most commonly used chemical sunblocks are zinc oxide, titanium dioxide, and *red petrolatum*.

Bear in mind that in addition to sunscreens, sun creams also inevitably include all the same ingredients as body lotions, such as mineral and other synthetic oils, PEGs, TEA, and other surfactants, preservatives, and fragrances (see page 139).

Faking It

There are two ways to get a tan without exposure to the sun: using a sun bed or applying fake tan.

Sun beds produce UV radiation, just like the sun. In fact, a sun bed can be even more dangerous than the sun. It's estimated that twenty minutes in a solarium can be equivalent to approximately four hours in the sun.

Sunlight contains a mix of UVA and UVB radiation, and some of this is filtered out by the ozone layer. Sun beds produce mainly UVA radiation, which penetrates deeper into your skin. They produce less UVB radiation than the sun.

People using sun beds are less likely to use a sun cream to protect themselves against UV radiation. Goggles are essential—as with sunshine, the combination of UVA and UVB can result in eye damage by burning the cornea. Long-term exposure can result in irreversible damage and cataracts. Sunbeds can also speed up thinning of the skin, the development of wrinkles, and other changes usually associated with aging.

In the 1950s, the first self-tanning product came onto the market. There are now hundreds of cosmetic products marketed as safe and effective alternatives to direct sun exposure. But while products like these are widely promoted as a safe alternative to sun exposure, there are inevitably problems associated with them.

First of all, self-tanning lotions offer little protection from UV radiation. So, if you're taking a trip outside in the sunshine to show off your new fake tan, you'll still need to use a sun cream. Next, it's worth considering how self-tanning products work to color your skin.

The most effective products contain a chemical called dihydroxyacetone (DHA). This sugar derivative has been the staple active ingredient in self-tanners for many years. It can smell bad, and it can sometimes turn you a strange shade of orange, but, more important, it has never been fully evaluated for safety.

DHA is not a dye. It imparts temporary color to the skin through a free-radical-generating chemical reaction with the amino acids in superficial layers of the skin. The way it works is not dissimilar to the way exposure to the air can turn a cut-up apple brown.

Some products use another chemical, erythrulose, in addition to the DHA. Erythrulose works identically to DHA, but develops more slowly. The two chemicals used together may produce a longer-lasting effect.

Both dihydroxyacetone and erythrulose can cause contact dermatitis, but there is a greater irony here that won't be lost on those who have ever skimmed a women's magazine. Most antiaging creams, for instance, include ingredients that help fight the damaging skin-aging effects of free radicals, known to promote premature skin-cell death.

Using a fake tan means volunteering for this kind of damage to your skin. A 2004 laboratory study published in the journal *Mutation Research* underscored this fact with the finding that DHA interferes with the normal cell cycle in human skin, induces DNA damage, and accelerates cell death within twenty-four hours of application. This alarming study was one of only very few attempts to explore how safe fake-tan promoters are; erythrulose, for example, has never been fully evaluated for long-term safety.

Fake-tan products also suffer from the same plethora of toxic ingredients as body lotions. Often, they include numerous film formers—not just silicones, but the plasticizer tri-C14-15 alkyl citrate (which is often found in food packaging). These make application easier, but also act like plastic wrap on the skin, preventing it from eliminating toxins.

Try This Instead . . .

Recent research published in the *British Medical Journal* suggests that individuals who use sunscreens may actually be at an increased risk of developing skin cancer. This is because high-SPF creams give sun worshippers a false sense of security, encouraging them to venture out during peak periods and to stay out in the sun much longer than would normally be considered safe.

It is also because of the mix of ingredients in sun cream and the damaging effects they have on the skin. The only safe recommendation is not to rely on sunscreens as your sole method of protection. There is no doubt that sunscreens can be useful, but they should not be applied over large parts of the body for extended periods of time.

Around 80 percent of our total lifetime's exposure to the sun comes during childhood. So, it is especially important to make sure children are protected against strong sunlight. If you want to teach your children good sun-exposure habits, lead by example. Research into children's voluntary use of sun creams, for example, suggests that they copy what their parents do. Consider these simple strategies for enjoying the sun:

Get out in the sun. If you want a glow that is truly healthy, then regular, moderate sun exposure is the only way to go. This doesn't mean foolishly baking in the sun for hours, but rather enjoying the sun as a natural part of your daily routine. Studies show that we all need approximately fifteen to twenty minutes of sun exposure on our face, arms, and legs each day to produce and maintain vital supplies of vitamin D. Staying out of the sun means that many of us don't get enough vitamin D, and this has led to the reemergence of diseases like rickets and contributed to spiraling rates of depression, as well as cancers of the breast, prostate, and colon.

Keep babies under six months old out of strong sunlight. Baby sun creams with a high SPF probably have the greatest number of toxic chemicals and are definitely not suitable for the delicate and permeable skin of babies.

Limit time in the sun. It is probably best to avoid being out when the sun is at its strongest—between the hours of 11 a.m. and 2 p.m.

Cover up. When you and your children are going to be out in the sun for extended periods of time, make practical use of T-shirts, sunglasses, and beach umbrellas.

7. HOUSEHOLD PRODUCTS

In the last century or so, a greater understanding of the importance of home hygiene has been one of the most influential factors in improving health and longevity.

A clean home is a healthy home. By keeping your home clean, you are keeping levels of germs and allergens low, and this can help maintain your home as a haven where you can rest and your body can repair itself.

To maintain a clean home, most of us use an artillery of conventional detergents and antibacterial cleaners. As you cruise the aisles of your local supermarket, it may seem that there is a huge selection of different household cleaners, each with its own special formulation. But most household cleaners contain the same basic range of ingredients. You certainly don't need six specialty cleaners when one concentrated all-purpose cleaner will do most jobs around the home. Nevertheless, as a society, we are obsessed with the idea of specialty cleaning products.

As a result, we spend something in the region of $8.3 billion globally each year on household cleaners. Laundry-care products account for half of our total spendings on these products, with surface cleaners, dishwashing products, and air fresheners following close behind.

While they may remove surface dirt and sometimes germs, and, on occasion, make our homes smell nice, these products can, ironically, end up making our homes less clean than they were before. This is because the ingredients found in everyday cleaning products contaminate the air and surfaces in our homes with a horrifying mix of carcinogens, hormone disrupters, neurotoxic solvents, mood-altering chemicals, and reproductive toxins.

Any substance that comes into contact with your skin, or that you inhale, or wash down the drain and into the soil, will ultimately end up inside your body. Indeed, years of scientific research have shown that our homes are the most significant sources of exposure to toxic chemicals.

For instance, twenty-five years ago, a survey conducted by the U.S. Environmental Protection Agency (EPA) found that the highest concentrations of twenty toxic or cancer-causing chemicals—such as toluene and benzene, both human carcinogens—were up to fifty times higher indoors than outdoors.

Many of the chemicals detailed in the EPA report can be found in your favorite bottle of all-purpose cleaner, as well as in your toilet cleaner, air freshener, and dish detergent. The problem has become so great that scientists throughout the world consider household cleaning products one of the most important sources of indoor air pollution, and one of the most insidious threats to human health. They cite the fact that as our use of these cleaners in our homes, schools, and workplaces has grown over the last sixty years, the incidence of diseases like cancer and asthma has grown dramatically as well.

Your household cleaner is unlikely to be the only cause of this phenomenon, but, as you begin to become familiar with the chemicals used in everyday cleaners, you may find yourself shocked at how often your favorite bottle or spray contains two or more known cancer-causing agents.

Of course, many people who are exposed to these environmental toxins do not reach the kind of high exposures that can lead to cancer or death. Instead, they may experience an array of subtle symptoms, including headaches, rashes, or breathing difficulties, which, while less dramatic, can be extremely debilitating. But it is still worthwhile asking whether, as there is no safe dose of a carcinogen, these products should be on the shelf at all.

Although it can be hard to change your thinking about household cleaners as anything other than benign, it's worth considering some of the problems—both real and potential—that they bring with them.

- **Nobody knows how safe or unsafe they are.** If a cleaning product has made its way onto the shelves of the local supermarket, most of us assume that it must be safe. Consumer surveys show that the vast majority—some 88 percent of those asked—believe that household products have been tested for safety before they are sold, and 87 percent think manufacturers are required to list their products' ingredients on labels. Neither of these assumptions is true.

  Household cleaning products are made using a variety of industrial chemicals, often referred to as high production volume, or HPV, chemicals. According to a 1998 EPA report, "Chemical Hazard Data Availability Study: What Do We Really Know About the Safety of High Production Volume Chemicals?," 43 percent of the most widely produced chemicals have no basic toxicity data available at all, and just 50 percent have even preliminary screening data. In fact, only a measly 7 percent of HPV chemicals have a complete set of screening-level toxicity data.

In the U.K., the environmental group Friends of the Earth, in their 2000 report *Crisis in Chemicals*, noted that only 14 percent of HPV chemicals in Europe have a full set of basic safety data, 65 percent have incomplete safety data, and 12 percent have no safety data at all. What these figures mean is that no one can say for sure how safe or unsafe the chemicals in our household cleaners really are.

And of course, once again, the problem of the cocktail effect rears its ugly head. When the chemicals in your favorite cleaner are tested for safety, they are done so individually, not in combinations. Yet, in household products, combinations of multiple chemicals are the norm and, yet again, manufacturers are not required to produce independent scientific confirmation that their cleaning products are safe for people or the environment before putting them on the shelf. Like the fox that guards the henhouse, any testing that is performed is usually done by the manufacturer and, very often, the results are not made public.

• **They contain harsh and sometimes toxic chemicals.** The health and safety issues associated with cleaning chemicals are relevant to everyone. Most people these days spend as much as 90 percent of their time indoors in homes, offices, schools, and hospitals, and are in constant contact with the fumes of cleaning chemicals in the air and chemical residues on the surfaces they touch.

According to the U.S. Consumer Protection Agency, over 150 chemicals found in the home are associated with allergies, birth defects, cancer, and psychological disorders. Cleaning chemicals may be a significant contributor to indoor air pollution, causing eye, nose, and throat irritation, headaches, dizziness, and fatigue. A seventeen-year study by the EPA concluded that women who work in the home have a 54 percent higher death rate from cancer than women who work outside the home.

Knowing this, it would make sense to look on the labels of your favorite cleaners to check whether they contain any of these known toxins. Unfortunately, manufacturers of household cleaners are not required to list all the ingredients used in their products on the label—and they don't volunteer this information, as it's considered a trade secret. This means that you may never be able to identify whether your glass cleaner, dish detergent, or spot remover contains chemicals that could harm you or your family and, if so, at what concentrations.

Nevertheless, independent studies have shown that the majority of household cleaners do contain harmful ingredients (see the table below).

Many of these "bioaccumulate"—in other words, they are stored in the body—to a level where they can cause ill health. Many are also highly volatile—they easily evaporate and can be inhaled. Others that are sprayed from aerosol cans or hand pumps release a shower of microscopic, easily inhaled particles. As the other chapters in this book show, many of these chemicals can be found in other types of products as well. Using potentially toxic cleaners is simply adding to the overall burden of these toxins in your home.

• **They are ecologically unsound.** It may be only recently that we've begun to look at the impact that industrial chemicals have on human health. But there is a large and long-standing body of evidence of how these chemicals affect the environment. Over the years, volumes of data have been amassed regarding the environmental impact of the detergents, solvents, and phosphates commonly found in household products. We know what happens to animals like frogs, birds, and plants when we release these toxins into the air and waterways. We know the damaging effects of propellants and other toxic chemicals on the ozone layer.

Household Horrors

While it is not so easy to avoid chemicals present in our water supply or the pollution spewing from factories and cars, it is possible to do something about the chemicals you use in your own home. Below is a list of "red flag" chemicals commonly found in cleaning products. Their worrisome health effects provide plenty of good reasons to make the switch to the more natural alternatives given throughout this book.

SUBSTANCE	EFFECT
alcohol (including ethanol, methanol, isopropanol)	nausea and vomiting if swallowed
ammonia	fatal when swallowed
ammonium hydroxide	corrosive; irritant
bleach	potentially fatal if ingested
butyl cellosolve	damages liver, kidney, and nervous system
chlorine	number one cause of poisonings in children
formaldehyde	highly toxic; a known carcinogen
hydrochloric acid	corrosive; eye and skin irritant

hydrochloric bleach	eye, skin, and respiratory tract irritant
lye	severe damage to stomach and esophagus if ingested
naphtha	depresses the central nervous system
nitrobenzene	causes skin discoloration, shallow breathing, vomiting, and death
paradichlorobenzenes	irritates eyes, nose, central nervous system
perchlorethylene	damages liver, kidney, and nervous system
petroleum distillates	highly flammable; suspected carcinogen
phenol	extremely dangerous; suspected carcinogen; fatal if taken internally
propellants	central-nervous-system poisons; causes irregular heartbeat
propylene glycol	provokes immune response; main ingredient in antifreeze
sodium hypochlorite	potentially fatal
sodium lauryl sulphate	carcinogen; toxin; causes gene mutation
sodium tripolyphosphate	irritant
trichloroethane	damages liver and kidneys; narcotic

As our petroleum reserves diminish, another environmental concern has arisen. Many of the chemicals that are used in cleaning products are petroleum-based, contributing to the depletion of this nonrenewable resource. For instance, it is estimated that if every household in the United States replaced just one 28-ounce bottle of petroleum-based cleaner with an equivalent plant-based product, it would save 118,700 barrels of oil in one year—enough to heat 6,800 average American homes.

In and among the tons of cleaning products we pour down the drain each year are toxic substances that are not processed adequately by sewage-treatment plants or septic systems. In a May 2002 study of contaminants in stream water sampled across the United States entitled "Pharmaceuticals, Hormones, and Other Organic Wastewater Contaminants in U.S. Streams, 1999–2000: A National Reconnaissance," the U.S. Geological Survey (USGS) found persistent detergent metabolites (breakdown products) in 69 percent of the streams tested; 66 percent contained disinfectants.

The detergent metabolites detected belonged to a class of chemicals known as *alkylphenol ethoxylates* (APEs), including nonylphenol ethoxylates and octylphenol ethoxylates. These chemicals are commonly added to laundry detergents, disinfectants, laundry stain-removers, and degreasers (even some so-called natural ones) to make them more effective. Dumped or flushed into municipal wastewater, nonylphenol and octylphenol ethoxylates break down into the estrogen mimics nonylphenol and octylphenol, which are more power-fully estrogenic, and more persistent—in other words, they do not readily biodegrade in soil and water. Scientists believe that the presence of synthetic estrogens in water may be harming the reproduction and survival of salmon and other fish as well as humans.

As they circulate through the water supply, these chemicals threaten people, animals, and the environment. For instance, male fish that are exposed to APEs in rivers have been found to produce female egg-yolk proteins, and laboratory studies have shown that in humans the APE p-nonylphenol triggers the growth of estrogen-sensitive breast cancer cells.

The plastic bottles used to package cleaning products pose another environmental problem, not only because they are derived from petroleum, but also because they contribute to the mounds of solid waste that must be landfilled, and to air pollution when they are incinerated.

Wipe and Waste

The single biggest revolution in cleaning has been the invention of the wipe. The convenience of wipes is such that, in the last decade, there has been an unprecedented boom in the use of disposable cloths of all kinds. Today, in any supermarket, along with hand wipes and baby wipes, you can buy self-tan and deodorant wipes, and makeup and nail-polish-removing, blackhead-clearing, car-washing, multisurface, disinfecting, furniture, floor, fridge, and stovetop wipes.

Made from plastic, cellulose, and polyester fibers pressed together and soaked in a cleaning fluid, the global retail value of wipes in 2004 was around $4 billion and grew to approximately $5.3 billion in 2006. Personal and cosmetic wipes account for around 65 percent of this market, and even people who don't have babies are often seen buying packets of baby wipes to use as instant cleanups anywhere. For U.S. troops in Iraq, they were standard issue.

According to recent data from the Association of the Nonwoven Fabrics Industry, if someone were to load all the disposable wipes purchased in North America in 2005 onto 18-wheelers, the caravan would number nine thousand trucks, would stretch for sixty-eight miles, and would be carrying eighty-three thousand tons of used convenience cloths.

Apart from catering to the damaged psyche of a throwaway society, wipes have other disadvantages: they are expensive, can't be flushed down the toilet, and clog sewer systems when they are (even so, many manufacturers still omit relevant information on flushability on their packets). They are also very slow to biodegrade. As is the case with disposable diapers, it is likely that all the wipes we've ever used are still festering somewhere underground. The environmental impact of this has yet to be studied.

The Perils of Being Too Clean

Cleaning the house can be harmful in other, more unexpected, ways, too. For instance, by overcleaning an otherwise adequately clean home, we may be condemning our children to a future of chronic ill health.

Manufacturers of cleaning products prey heavily on parents' fears for the health of their children and loved ones. Yet, there's evidence of a link between early childhood infections and a lower risk of developing atopic diseases, such as allergies, asthma, and eczema. This idea is part of what is known as the "hygiene hypothesis"—a theory that developed out of scientists' inability to explain why rates of atopic diseases among children in developed countries were escalating out of control.

The name "hygiene hypothesis" is, of course, misleading, since hygiene per se is not a bad thing and, indeed, better hygiene is responsible for many of the gains in human health. But obsessive measures toward cleanliness, killing germs, and suppressing illnesses are clearly creating more problems than they are solving (see "Antibacterial Cleaners," page 173).

The theory goes that by "protecting" children from exposure to dirt and germs, and by preventing diseases from taking their course in childhood, we are inadvertently destroying the body's ability to respond appropriately to allergens, infection, and other stimuli that actually help the immune system to mature and function properly.

During most of our evolution, and from the moment of birth, our bodies have been exposed daily to dirt and germs. It is thought that this exposure helped to forge and maintain the immune system's sophisticated network of chemical pathways and specialized cells. According to the hygiene hypothesis, without the early input of everyday dirt and germs, the immune system cannot respond appropriately when challenged.

The idea came into being in 1989, when David Strachan, an epidemiologist at the London School of Hygiene and Tropical Medicine, noticed that children from big families—where infections were likely to circulate freely— were less likely to develop atopic disorders (such as eczema, asthma, and psoriasis).

Since then, the evidence in favor of this theory has continued to accumulate. A study by the Institute of Social and Preventive Medicine in Basel, Switzerland, published in the prestigious *New England Journal of Medicine* in 2002, looked at over eight hundred children aged six to thirteen. Researchers found that kids who lived in the dustiest environments, especially those who lived on farms, were less likely to suffer from asthma and hay fever.

As the hypothesis has evolved, scientists have found that it is not just exposure to dirt and germs that is protective. Being exposed to endotoxins—the waste products sloughed off by bacteria—also helps to "train" the immune system.

What's more, the protective effect of small exposures to these challenges has expanded to encompass not just atopic diseases, but also immune disorders, such as multiple sclerosis (MS), and type 1 (insulin-dependent) diabetes, and inflammatory bowel diseases, such as ulcerative colitis and irritable bowel syndrome (IBS).

Safer Cleaning: Getting Back to Basics

Cleaning is a necessity. It is also a science, an art, and an act of discipline. People who actually like to clean will also tell you that, on occasion, it has a spirituality all its own, that doing the dishes or scrubbing the floor can be both comforting and uplifting.

Of course, none of the information or suggestions in this book will make the regular routine of vacuuming the stairs or cleaning the bath any more appealing in itself. But making use of these simpler, greener alternatives will, in some cases, have an immediate impact on your health and environment. When you're not inhaling or absorbing risky chemicals into your body, you may find that your energy levels rise, and that nagging skin and respiratory symptoms disappear or at the very least improve. Since many of these chemicals can have a direct effect on the emotional centers of the brain, you may also find that your mood improves as well.

Sadly, it's become all too easy to rely on hazardous cleaning chemicals that end up giving us a clean, but not so healthy, home. Many of these products work very quickly and effectively, and this ease of use may leave you thinking that you are just too busy to make substantial changes in the way you take care of your home. You may be asking yourself if it will really make a difference to choose a greener way to clean your home.

Most of us sympathize with the need to keep environmental pollution to an absolute minimum, but our resolve often disappears at the supermarket, where brightly packaged products promise to transform our homes into spotlessly clean aromatherapy spas. What could green cleaning possibly have to offer that could compete with today's modern cleaning product formulations?

In fact, green cleaning brings with it a range of benefits:

- **It costs less.** By using readily available ingredients like baking soda and vinegar to clean your home, you will find you spend less on everyday cleaners.

- **Less backache.** When you make it yourself, there are no heavy bottles to carry home. Suddenly, bringing in the groceries becomes less onerous.

- **No heavy perfumes.** The fragrances used in cleaning products are significant triggers of asthma as well as headaches. Going fragrance-free may have the added effect of improving your health.

- **Self-sufficiency.** Not having to rely on commercial cleaners is emotionally freeing. Suddenly, all those commercials that try to sell you toilet cleaner as a cure for a dead-end love life seem remarkably silly.

- **A cleaner home.** Instead of washing away dirt with toxic waste or masking unpleasant smells with other smells, you will be getting your home genuinely clean.

- **Nothing dangerous under the sink.** It's a much safer way to live, especially if you have children.

- **A cleaner planet.** You'll be doing your bit—relatively effortlessly—to keep the planet in good shape for future generations.

As many of the alternatives described here are both inexpensive and freely available, you might find a little extra change in your pocket each month. This means you can give yourself a treat while congratulating yourself on keeping both your immediate and the wider environment chemical-free.

Product manufacturers are aware of the increasing interest of consumers in natural cleaning products, and there are many good alternatives if you want to buy, rather than make your own, cleaning products. Natural ingredients are usually derived from citrus, and the oils are combined with minerals, salts, sodas, and plant enzymes. Plant-based cleaners are often able to match the cleaning power of synthetically derived ingredients. Be aware, however, that many manufacturers simply add a citrus ingredient to an otherwise synthetic formulation so that a label claim can be made.

Unfortunately, there are no regulations governing this area, and many companies are free to make "natural" claims that don't stand up to any real scrutiny.

Try This Instead . . .

It's always good to know how to make basic cleaning products with safe everyday materials.

If you are unsure where to start, then begin with the basics. The best way to keep your home clean is to not let grease and grime build up in the first place. A quick regular wipedown is still the best way to prevent surfaces from getting sticky, greasy, and grimy. It will also make doing big jobs like ovens and stoves easier in the long run. Not many of us can consistently reach this level of perfection, though.

Throughout this book, you will find simple, inexpensive, and green alternatives to industrial-strength chemicals. To limit your exposure to chemicals in household cleaners, try the following options.

Dilute (and dilute again). Most liquid detergents and soaps can be made into useful all-purpose cleaners simply by diluting them. To make sure you're keeping exposure to a minimum of chemicals, try using an ecologically sound vegetable-based dish detergent or, even better, a liquid castile soap, well diluted in water.

Use hot water. Many people forget that hot water and steam are among the best, and most effective, household cleaners. In addition, it is usually the elbow grease, not the chemicals, that really gets the job done.

Use steam. A steam cleaner can be useful for really stubborn grease, and for quick cleanups on carpets. It is also a very effective disinfectant for sinks and toilets.

But effective cleaning has other rules as well. Whatever your approach, cleaning has its own set of rules. Follow these and cleaning will become, if not a source of enlightenment, at least a less burdensome chore.

Make It Yourself

Most of us are used to buying our cleaning products off the supermarket shelves. When we think of alternatives, often the first place we look is back in the supermarket—where green alternatives are often pretty thin on the ground. Why not consider making your own? The simplest (and cheapest) ingredients are often all that is needed for the majority of household-cleaning jobs.

Baking soda. Chemists call this white powder sodium bicarbonate ($NaHCO_3$). Your grandmother would probably have mixed it with water and drank it to cure heartburn. That should tell you something about how safe it is.

For cleaning, baking soda does a lot of different things:

- As a powder, it's a mild abrasive that can scratch off hardened dirt without scoring whatever it is you're trying to clean.

- It dissolves in water without leaving a gritty film like other scouring powders do.

And because it dissolves in water, baking soda gives you other benefits:

- It's a mild disinfectant with the ability to kill some bacteria and fungi.

- It helps to cut through grease.

- It softens water, thus helping your other cleaners to work and rinse off more effectively.

Vinegar. Chemists might call vinegar a dilute solution of acetic acid (CH_3COOH). When table wine turns bad, it chemically changes into vinegar. You probably wouldn't drink it as a beverage, but you might mix it with a little olive oil and put it on your salad.

Vinegar is a mild acid that cuts through grease, and disinfects by killing many types of bacteria, yeast, and molds. It is also an efficient air freshener.

Soap. Most people confuse soap with detergent. Chemists originally developed synthetic detergents as an alternative to soap where hard water (containing magnesium or calcium) or acid is present. The detergent that we buy from a store is really a synthetic that has been manufactured from a variety of mineral products like coal tar and petroleum.

On the other hand, soap—for example, traditional castile soap—is a mild detergent that is simple and is made from natural products like vegetable oils and animal fats. Used sparingly and under the right conditions, soap is gentle and a wonderful cleaning agent in that it has a minimal impact on the environment.

Borax. Borax can be bought over the counter, and, while it is an effective cleaner, it should be used with caution because it can also be toxic at high levels.

- Borax is an effective water softener and can be used in homemade products to help soap work harder and rinse away better.

- It is an effective mold and mildew remover and disinfectant.

- It can whiten clothes and help prevent odors.

Microfiber cleaning cloths. These new cloths are so useful that once you begin to use them, you will wonder why you ever bothered to waste your money on anything else.

Water is the most powerful solvent in the world. The purpose of detergents is to bring more water into contact with whatever surface you are cleaning. Microfibers effectively do the same thing. Microfibers are finer than human hair and have a superior absorbency when compared to other cloths. The combination of these properties means that microfiber cloths have a greatly increased surface area, bringing more water into contact with the cleaning surface. Used as directed, they will leave most surfaces both clean and dry.

Many manufacturers have jumped on the microfiber bandwagon recently, so you can afford to be choosy about the cloths you buy. The best ones are denser and generally more costly. They can be reused indefinitely, however, and the denser the cloth, the greater its surface area—and the more fibers there are to trap dirt.

And finally . . .

Elbow grease. There's no getting around this one. Many of the recipes in this book work just as well as the more hazardous chemicals you've been using all this time. But occasionally, using nontoxic alternatives to conventional household cleaners means that, at least some of the time, you will have to scrub harder or longer.

Clues on the Label

How do you know if the products you are using are toxic?

With any other type of product, you could check out the ingredients list on the label. But cleaning products don't generally have ingredients lists. Manufacturers have successfully pleaded their case for secrecy with the regulatory authorities. To list the ingredients would, they say, be revealing a trade secret, and this would be bad for business. This means that the concerned consumer who wants to know what's in their toilet or oven cleaner will need to learn to read between the lines.

Most countries have rules about specific safety labeling that must appear on products containing known toxins, such as methyl alcohol, turpentine, petroleum distillate products, and a variety of other common cleaning ingredients. Poisonous products, for instance, are usually marked with a picture of a skull and crossbones. In addition, the majority of commercially available cleaning products contain "signal" words on their labels, such as:

- caution
- corrosive
- danger
- flammable
- hazardous
- irritant
- warning

Household Cleaners

To fulfill the increasingly ambitious claims for their products, manufacturers rely on combinations of chemical compounds that can be harsh and highly toxic. Ask yourself, if a cleanser can instantly strip a kitchen tile of years of accumulated grease, what might it do to your skin or your body's cells or the natural environment?

Although it is impossible to avoid all the chemical culprits known to damage health, it does pay to learn which key ingredients are most problematic. As you read through the information that follows, you will notice how certain chemicals turn up again and again in a range of household cleaners. Armed with this information, you can then begin to take steps to limit what you buy or, better yet, make use of the suggestions for buying or making nontoxic alternatives. Your home will still be clean, and your health will improve immeasurably by doing so.

Air Fresheners

In spite of their name, air fresheners do not freshen the air. Instead, they are one of the most concentrated sources of poisons and pollution in the home.

These little clues on the bottle tell you that the product is dangerous. The best way to ensure that you don't use toxic, corrosive, flammable products is to make your own from safe ingredients. But if you want to buy a product at the supermarket, it's important to check for these signal words on the label of any product you buy. In addition, remember to avoid buying any product that: (a) does not clearly indicate what the active substance is; (b) does not list hazards associated with the product (like "highly irritating fumes" or "toxic when ingested"); (c) does not describe precautions you can take to avoid being harmed; and (d) does not list necessary or appropriate instructions for first-aid treatment.

Cautions are there for a reason. If the instructions tell you to use a product in a well-ventilated area, it's not because the manufacturers are concerned that you aren't getting enough fresh air. It's because the product is harmful if inhaled. Likewise, if the label recommends that you wear gloves, it's not because the manufacturers are concerned you might break a nail, but because the product is a skin irritant or is easily absorbed through the skin.

While the accepted hype is that air fresheners remove unwanted odors and re-place them with clean fresh smells, most do no such thing.

Air fresheners work in several ways. They can contain nerve-deadening agents designed to interfere with your ability to detect smells, or they can coat the nasal passages with a thin, undetectable oily film that also prevents odor de-tection. Alternatively, they can cover up one smell with another, more powerful, one. Rarely do they actually remove or break down unpleasant odors.

Air fresheners are often marketed as luxury items. And indeed, you wear a perfume and your husband has an aftershave, but, typically, they contain syn-thetic fragrances as well as solvents and fixatives that are as common in most garages as they are in luxury fragrances.

About 30–40 percent of air freshener purchases are driven by what market-ing departments call home-cleaning replacement. Time-strapped, cash-rich peo-ple may clean less often or less thoroughly, and so use air fresheners to give the impression of a just-cleaned home. The rest is driven by the promise of luxury and a quick-fix, mood-boosting experience.

Years ago, air fresheners were something that you sprayed into a room once in a while for effect. These days, you can plug them into an electric socket and have a continual release of strong perfume throughout your home. But the trend toward using continuous room perfumes means that your body never gets a break from exposure to these chemicals, and we simply don't know enough about the long-term effects of such exposure to deem this safe.

Air fresheners also provide a good example of how manufacturers leap onto current trends and use them for profit. For instance, many air fresheners now promise aromatherapy for your home. It's all nonsense, and even if your air freshener doesn't make you feel sick in the short term, it may add to longer-term problems.

Animal experiments, for example, suggest that the chemicals in air fresheners may weaken the body's defenses by making the skin more permeable. Allergic re-actions to these products can range from sneezing and watery eyes to full-scale asthma attacks. Aerosol air fresheners contain neurotoxic propellants and can be harmful to the lungs if inhaled in high concentrations or over prolonged periods of time. Solids and plug-ins produce the same symptoms, and may be poisonous to children and pets if ingested.

In 1999, a British survey of fourteen thousand pregnant women concluded that the frequent use of household aerosol sprays and air fresheners was making women and babies ill.

The study, reported in *New Scientist*, found that women who used aerosols and air fresheners most days suffered 25 percent more headaches and 19 percent more postnatal depression than those who used them less than once a week. Babies under six months had 30 percent more ear infections and more frequent diarrhea if regularly exposed to aerosols and air fresheners. Early in 2005, the same team of scientists updated their findings in the *Archives of Environmental Medicine*, with much similar results. The researchers noted that the chemicals present in many aerosols, such as xylene, ketones, and aldehydes, had already been associated with so-called sick-building syndrome, and that we now may be looking at a similar syndrome in homes.

Also in 2005, the European consumer group Bureau Européen des Unions de Consommateurs (BEUC) published a comparative study into home-fragrance safety. They looked at seventy-four different kinds of air-freshening products, including incense, natural products, scented candles, aerosols, liquid diffusers, electric diffusers, and gels, and measured the concentrations of volatile organic compounds (VOCs) and aldehydes in the air after their use.

VOCs and aldehydes are potent neurotoxins that attack both the central nervous system (the brain and spinal cord) and peripheral nervous system (responsible for relaying sensory information to the brain, but also involved in controlling organs and muscles, such as the heart, stomach, and intestines). The study found that air fresheners released toxins, such as acetaldehyde, styrene, toluene, *chlorobenzene, glycol ethers*, phthalates, and artificial musk into the air. Traces of formaldehyde and benzene were also found.

In many cases, the total VOC emissions were much higher than the "safe" dose of 200 mcg/m3 (micrograms per cubic meter). In some cases, they were as high as 4,000–5,000 mcg/m3.

Manufacturers defend their products by saying that under normal use the chemicals in air fresheners are safe. But in recent years, what constitutes normal use has changed drastically. Instead of just an occasional spray, many of us now use continuous-release devices that release fragrance chemicals into the air all day long. What's more, air fresheners are not just found in homes, but in offices and stores, and in vacuum-cleaner filters, taxis, and family cars.

As always, it is the cumulative or cocktail effect—not just from air fresheners, but because of all the perfumed products we now use—that is crucial to the development of health problems.

Your Air Freshener Is Likely to Contain . . .

Paradichlorobenzene (PDCB), naphthalene, formaldehyde, *sodium bisulphate*, glycol ethers, ethanol, and other solvents; various propellants, such as *hydrochlorofluorocarbons* (HCFCs), *butane*, propane, and isobutane; disinfectants, such as *cresol*; preservatives, such as quaternary ammonium salts; and petrochemical-based fragrances.

Try This Instead . . .

You don't need air fresheners, and the best alternative is not to buy them at all. Simply keeping your home clean and well ventilated solves most odor problems. If your house is really smelly, then you need to get to the root of the problem—often animals, blocked drains, damp conditions, gas from your oven or heater, off-gassing from new carpets, furniture or wallpaper, overfull trash cans, and cigarette smoke—rather than just masking it. To remove unwanted smells, consider some of these measures:

Buy pump sprays instead of aerosols. But don't kid yourself that these are much healthier. You will still be breathing in alcohols and perfumes as well as other chemicals. Pump sprays just mean that you avoid breathing in propellants—a baby step in the right direction.

Open a window. Fresh air is the best air freshener there is. To save money and environmental resources, we have all become accustomed to living and working in sealed premises. Unfortunately, sealing in the heat also seals in every smell, every chemical, and every gas that may be present in the environment. Unless you live in a dreadfully polluted space, opening a couple of windows to allow cross-ventilation is always the best way to get rid of a bad smell. Even in winter, this is unlikely to raise your heating bill significantly.

Buy houseplants. English ivy, spider plants, peace lilies, and philodendrons are all good choices, because they can help remove unpleasant odors and gases from your environment. (See page 43 for a full list of air-freshening plants.)

Make your own spray. A simple air freshener can be made by combining equal amounts of water and white vinegar in a spray bottle. Add 20–30 drops of your favorite essential oil (peppermint, lemon, pine, and geranium are all good choices), and shake before using. As both vinegar and essential oils can be eye irritants, don't put your face in the area you have just sprayed, and never spray directly into your face.

Make your own room freshener. Use a 7-ounce box of baking soda and 10–15 drops of your favorite essential oils. Mix these well and place in a cardboard box (you can paint or decorate this) or a small dish. Alternatively, try placing a few cotton balls sprinkled with vanilla extract in an open dish or bowl, and leave these to freshen the room. This is only a short-term solution as, after a day or so, the smell of vanilla will dissipate and stop working. Nevertheless, this is useful after parties to cut through smoky smells, and also to freshen up small spaces, such as closets and cars.

Use potpourri with caution. Most commercially prepared potpourris use petrochemical-derived fragrances. Look at the label and, if it says something like "a blend of natural aromas" or "natural" anything, it is probably not really natural at all, but nature identical. If you want to avoid these, make your own potpourri, or buy an unscented variety and scent it with your own essential oils rather than the synthetic potpourri oil blends. These won't last as long, but they will be less harmful to your health.

Be careful when buying aromatherapy candles, also marketed as natural alternatives to conventional air fresheners. Most use petrochemical fragrances instead of natural oils. Also, the candles themselves are usually made from wax derived from petrochemicals. As this burns, it can release soot containing volatile chemicals and toxic metals into the atmosphere.

All-Purpose Cleaners

All general-purpose cleaners work in essentially the same way to loosen grease and grime, and facilitate a clean rinse. For these products to live up to the promise of effortless cleaning, they usually have to be much stronger and more concentrated than necessary for everyday household use. In spite of this, few of them are significantly more efficient than simple soap and hot water for loosening everyday dirt and grime from household surfaces.

The ingredients in all-purpose cleaners are a combination of synthetic detergents, grease-cutting agents, such as solvents, and bleaches and disinfectants. Depending on the mix of ingredients, these cleaners have been shown to be irritating to varying degrees to the skin, eyes, nose, and throat, and can be corrosive if swallowed. Those that contain small amounts of phosphates are an environmental hazard.

Spray cleaners are basically the same mix of chemicals as liquid cleaners, though often in a less concentrated form. Although pump sprays don't contain aerosols, when you use them you are producing a fine mist of chemicals that is easily inhaled and quick to enter the bloodstream. So, even though the product is less concentrated, you may take in more chemicals. Amazingly, for a product that is mostly water, spray cleaners are also more expensive to buy than standard liquid formulas.

Scouring powders and abrasive creams are a traditional standby for attacking greasy deposits in the kitchen and soap scum in the bath. These products are generally made with strong bleaches or ammonia to make them work faster. When the dried bleach mixes with water, it produces *chlorine* fumes that are irritating to the eyes, nose, throat, and lungs.

Dry powders also contain crystalline silica, which is an eye, skin, and lung irritant, and is carcinogenic when inhaled. It is all too easy to inhale silica particles when you sprinkle scouring powder in the sink or bath (and some of these types of cleaners are unsuitable for certain surfaces, like plastic, because they can scratch). Once inhaled, mineral powders—whether talc, silica, feldspar, or quartz—lodge more or less permanently in the lungs.

Your All-Purpose Cleaner Is Likely to Contain . . .

Detergents/surfactants; solvents, such as ethanol, isopropanol, *butyl cellosolve*, or glycols; disinfectants, such as ammonia, *bleach* (sodium hypochlorite), *phenol*, and *pine oil*; fragrances, and colors. Abrasive or cream formulas contain fine particles of plastic, silica, calcite, feldspar, or quartz. Most also contain undisclosed preservatives, such as *quaternary ammonium compounds* and *EDTA*.

Try This Instead . . .

To limit your exposure to the chemicals in household cleaners, try the following options:

Limit your use of sprays (even pump sprays of mixtures you have made yourself) for hard-to-get-at places to reduce the number of chemicals you inhale.

For tough grease, make a strong solution containing:

½ tsp washing soda (also known as sodium carbonate,
    soda ash, or sal soda)
2 Tbsp distilled white vinegar
½ tsp liquid soap or dish detergent (or, alternatively,
    1 tsp soap flakes)
2 cups hot water

Add a few drops of essential oil if you wish. This can be used as is or put into a spray bottle to help you get at hard-to-reach places. Always wear protective gloves when working with washing soda.

Try making a simple scouring powder from 7 ounces of baking soda. That's all you need. Keep it in an airtight jar and use when you need to. It's that simple. If you like, add 10 drops of an essential oil and mix well to make a pleasant scent. Lemon, grapefruit, mandarin, tea tree, rose, peppermint, or lavender are all suitable.

To make a stain-removing scouring powder use:

8 oz. baking soda
3 oz. borax
3 Tbsp soap flakes (lightly crushed)

This will get rid of all but the most stubborn stains. To increase the bleaching power of this mixture, try adding 3 tablespoons of sodium perborate (available at health-food stores), a kind of bleach. Be sure to wear gloves when using this formula to avoid skin irritation.

An even stronger cleaner can be made with a mixture of liquid soap and trisodium phosphate (TSP). Add the following ingredients to 1½ pints of warm-to-hot water:

1 tsp liquid soap
1 tsp trisodium phosphate (TSP)
1 tsp borax
1 tsp distilled white vinegar

TSP is a strong skin irritant, so you should wear protective gloves when using it. The benefit of using TSP in this particular mixture, apart from its effectiveness against grease and mildew, is that you know what chemicals you are actually using.

Antibacterial Cleaners

Over the last decade, our enthusiasm for fighting germs at home has become unstoppable. At the supermarket, we effectively take out insurance against germs by stocking up on a bewildering array of products that boast antibacterial action. Nowadays, we can buy antibacterial hand soaps, laundry detergents, dish detergents, surface cleaners, toothpastes, mouthwashes, and hand wipes. Antibacterial agents can be impregnated into clothing, furniture, blankets, insoles, the plastic lining of refrigerators, food-storage containers, shower curtains, garbage bags, trash cans, chopping boards, and even high chairs and toys.

It is estimated that the worldwide market for antibacterial products is around $27 billion, and hospital use accounts for only 30 percent of this. U.S. consumers purchased around $540 million worth of antibacterial soaps, hand cleaners, and detergents in 2005. Indeed, some 75 percent of liquid soaps and 29 percent of bar soaps sold in the United States now contain antibacterial agents.

Hygiene per se is not a bad thing and, indeed, better hygiene in homes is responsible for keeping us out of the hospital, and better hygiene in hospitals has meant that when we are sick or in need of surgery, it is safer and the recovery time is shorter. If you have an ill or immune-compromised person in your home, taking extra care with hygiene is a necessity. But there is little that can be achieved with an antibacterial cleaner that can't be done much more simply and inexpensively with hot water and simple detergent. Also, there are now several good reasons to believe that using an antibacterial cleaner may do more harm than good.

No Protection

In 2000, the American Medical Association (AMA) issued the startling statement warning that antibacterial soaps were no more effective against germs than common soap. The AMA based its opinion on several studies that showed that while antibacterial hand soaps may initially kill more bacteria and viruses on the skin than regular soaps, within an hour or so afterward there is generally no difference in the number of germs on the skin. This is hardly surprising, given that the average adult touches around three hundred different surfaces every thirty minutes. Similarly, while antibacterial surface cleaners may initially remove more organisms than soap and water, within ninety minutes or so there is generally no difference in the numbers of bacteria and viruses that have repopulated the area.

Knowing this provides a context for the results of a widely publicized study, originating from Columbia University in 2004, entitled "Effect of Antibacterial Home Cleaning and Handwashing Products on Infectious Disease Symptoms: A Randomized, Double-Blind Trial," which showed that people who used antibacterial soaps and cleaners developed a cough, runny nose, sore throat, fever, vomiting, diarrhea, and other symptoms just as often as those who didn't use antibacterial products. The researchers also pointed out that many of these illnesses are typically caused by viruses, against which antibacterial soaps and cleaners can provide no protection.

Resistance on the Home Front

Obsessive measures aimed at killing germs are problematic because germs— that is, bacteria, viruses, and fungi—are ancient and adaptable organisms. They are programmed to survive, and, more often than not, instead of being killed by powerful chemical assaults they simply evolve and become immune to them. Constant exposure to drugs, such as antibiotics, will eventually produce an organism that no drug will kill.

WHAT CAN YOU EXPECT FROM YOUR ANTIBACTERIAL PRODUCTS?

PRODUCTS	ADVANTAGES	DISADVANTAGES
Antibacterial hand washes and sanitizers	Kills almost 100 percent of harmful germs within fifteen seconds	You are recontaminated as soon as you touch something else
Antibacterial soaps and dishwashing liquids	Prevents growth of most bacteria, fungi, and yeast	Does not kill them immediately; benefits only apply to hands, not dishes
Antibacterial sponges and scrubbers	Kills germs on sponges and scrubbers to eliminate odors	Does not destroy germs on any surfaces they come into contact with
Disinfectant sprays	Kills bacteria, fungi, and viruses; reduces surface-to-human transmission of germs	As with all antibacterial products, continued use will produce resistant organisms
Surface cleaners	Kills household germs such as Salmonella, E. coli, and Streptococcus	In some cases, they must be left on at least ten minutes to have any antibacterial effect; surfaces become "germy" again within half an hour
Triclosan/Microban-embedded products (such as chopping boards, refrigerators)	Inhibits the growth of bacteria in the products	There is no evidence to show that they protect the person using the product

This ability to adapt is what has given rise to superbugs, such as methicillin-resistant *Staphylococcus aureus* (MRSA) and other resistant strains of bacteria that have become so prevalent in hospitals that many of us now fear having to stay in these institutions in case we become infected.

Indiscriminate use of antibiotics has received heavy and deserved criticism for provoking the rise of the superbug in our hospitals. Less well publicized is the role that the exponential rise in the popularity of antibacterial household cleaners and toiletries in the last decade has had in producing antibacterial resistance at home. For years, scientists denied the impact of household antibacterials, but now the latest evidence shows that you don't need to set foot outside your home to encounter a superbug.

In 2005, researchers in Oxford, England, looked at MRSA cases in two Oxfordshire hospitals and discovered that around 25 percent of serious cases were brought into the hospitals from patients' homes. How was that possible?

The answer is that, once upon a time, we approached hygiene with simple soap and water. Today, we use a variety of synthetic antibacterial chemicals—in particular, quaternary ammonium compounds and *chlorophenols*, such as *triclosan*—to keep the bugs at bay. Unlike soap and water, which works efficiently by physically loosening dirt and germs from surfaces and bodies, and washing them down the drain, antibacterial chemicals are designed to kill. In this, they are very like antibiotics, and, perhaps not surprisingly, there is now a considerable body of scientific opinion that what is being touted on supermarket shelves as an antibacterial in household products is really an antibiotic, and that antibacterial chemicals used in the home are contributing to the growing threat posed by drug-resistant strains of bacteria.

In support of this idea, community-acquired MRSA (caMRSA)—a form of MRSA that arises in people who have had no contact with a hospital—is now being widely reported in the United States, Britain, Australia, and Canada.

Research is now showing that a whole range of antibacterial chemicals used as disinfectants in household cleaners, and as preservatives and active ingredients in personal-care products, are producing resistant strains of bacteria.

Studies from the United States and Japan have shown that household germs like *Escherichia coli* (E. coli), *Listeria monocytogenes*, *Pseudomonas aeruginosa*, *Enterococcus faecalis*, *Streptococcus pneumoniae*, and *Staphylococcus aureus* are already showing signs of resistance to common antibacterial cleaners. But worse than this, because our household cleaners work in the same way as antibiotics do, they can make bacteria resistant to true antibiotics. For instance, overuse of the common antibacterial agents *benzalkonium chloride*, chlorohexidine, and especially triclosan (a chlorophenol type of agent) not only produce resistance to these agents, but also create strong cross-resistance to penicillin-derived antibiotics as well.

The overuse of antibacterials like these in the home will eventually have the same devastating effect as overprescribing antibiotics in hospitals and clinics, producing increasingly resistant strains of bacteria that can't be killed and have the potential to make already sick people even sicker.

Bad for the Environment, Too

Most antibacterial chemicals are washed down the drain and one antibacterial in particular, triclosan, is now among the most frequently detected compounds in our waterways. It is highly toxic to aquatic life, especially algae, and through our water supply this chlorophenol works its way back into our bodies. A recent Swedish study found triclosan in the breast milk of 60 percent of the women surveyed. This is a worrisome finding, given that there are no human data to show that it is safe on ingestion.

And what happens when this antibacterial combines with chemicals in the wider environment provides further good cause for concern.

For years, manufacturers have reassured consumers that triclosan breaks down quickly in the environment. But depending on where it is and what other chemicals it comes into contact with in the environment, triclosan can break down into highly toxic compounds.

Evidence published in 2003 demonstrated that sunlight converts triclosan into 2,8-dichlorodibenzo-p-dioxin, described as a "mild" form of dioxin that nevertheless contributes to the already widespread dioxin contamination of our waterways and our bodies.

Dioxins are hormone-disrupting chemicals that mimic the action of natural estrogen. In the body, estrogen levels are generally low and finely balanced. In excess, however, estrogen is a recognized carcinogen. Estrogen mimics are particularly worrisome because they can accumulate in the environment and in the body to produce the kinds of excesses that lead to cancer, reproductive and developmental problems, and immune-system damage.

The most well-known dioxin is the highly toxic 2,3,7,8-tetrachlorodibenzodioxin (TCDD), best known as a highly toxic impurity in Agent Orange, a neurotoxic herbicide used during the Vietnam War. Most dioxins share the toxic profile of TCDD, so the concept of a mild dioxin is more of a public-relations exercise than a scientific certainty.

Moreover, triclosan in the waterways can be altered further by repeated exposure to chlorine—for instance, in water-treatment facilities. If this chlorine-exposed triclosan is then exposed to sunlight, it turns into a much more potent form of dioxin.

In 2005, research carried out at Virginia Tech University found that the chlorine in tap water and the triclosan in some soaps and other products can react together to create harmful *chloroform* gas, which can be absorbed through the skin or inhaled. If inhaled in large quantities, chloroform gas can cause depression, liver problems, and, in some cases, cancer.

Your Antibacterial Cleaner Is Likely to Contain . . .
Triclosan, phenol, benzalkonium chloride, or chlorohexidine.

Try This Instead . . .

Overuse of antibacterial products of all kinds has become a substitute for good-hygiene practices, such as washing your hands thoroughly. You can't kill all the germs on your body, nor should you want to, as some "friendly" bacteria, for instance, help to keep the numbers of more harmful bacteria in check. What you can do is ensure that you are clean enough to be healthy. Consider the following alternatives to antibacterial soaps and cleaners:

Stop using antibacterial soaps and cleaners, as regular light cleaning with eco-friendly soap or cleaner and water is better than the occasional intense cleaning with strong biocides.

Use plain soap and warm water in preference to antibacterial soap.

Rinse and wring sponges and cleaning cloths well after use, and store them where they can dry out thoroughly. Wash dish and hand towels regularly.

Don't buy antibacterial plastics, such as cutting boards and storage containers, impregnated with antibacterials like *Microban*/triclosan; these agents can leach into the stored foods.

Wipe up spills immediately, which is just common sense.

Hands are the most common vehicles for spreading germs, so wash your hands thoroughly after using the toilet, and before and after preparing food, and teach your children to do the same. Thorough hand washing is defined as 10–15 seconds of vigorous rubbing of the hands to produce a lather, followed by thorough drying. This is in stark contrast to most adults, who spend 3–5 seconds running their hands under water, and don't dry their hands thoroughly before leaving the bathroom or kitchen.

Hang hand and bath towels so that they dry thoroughly between each use. Wash all towels and facecloths regularly and dry thoroughly to remove any accumulated microbes.

Bathroom Cleaners

When cleaning your body, it's nice to know that you are doing it in a relatively clean space. What's more, in many busy households, the bathroom is sometimes the only private place and temporary refuge. For these reasons, many of us pay special attention to cleaning the bathroom even when the rest of the house is a mess.

But equally, because of the extra attention we pay to bathrooms, the smallest room in the house probably has a greater concentration of toxic chemicals in the air and on its surfaces than any other room.

While it would be easy to think of the toilet bowl as the dirtiest place in the bathroom, this is usually not the case. Your toilet bowl has a constant flush of water running through it to keep it clean. Instead, the majority of really dirty jobs in the bathroom—such as the base of the toilet, the underside of the seat and under the rim, and the soap scum that builds up in the tub or on the shower door—are usually the result of neglect. Some problems, like mildew on the tiles, are caused by poor ventilation, while others, like the mineral deposits that clog showerheads and make taps look unsightly, are due to living in a hard-water area.

There is a variety of specialty cleaners intended for use in the bathroom. But if you buy these, you may be wasting your time and money, as well as be fooling yourself regarding how much cleaner they really make your bathroom. You may also be exposing yourself to very harsh chemicals unnecessarily. Why risk it when nearly all bathroom-cleaning jobs can be done with everyday cleaners and a few special mixtures of nontoxic ingredients?

Toilet Cleaners

We have become pretty obsessed with clean toilets in recent years. Spend a night in front of the TV and you're likely to see commercials featuring animated toilet bowls singing about how happy they are now that they're using brand X, or cartoons showing flowers sprouting out of the bowl.

To keep the bowl fresh, there is a variety of liquids and powders as well as in-tank and in-bowl devices that color and fragrance the water as well as clean it and keep lime scale at bay. They are all made from roughly the same harsh ingredients. The in-tank and in-bowl types are perhaps the most risky, as every time you flush you send a microscopic spray of easily inhaled chemicals into the air in your bathroom.

Toilet bowl cleaners usually contain industrial-strength cationic detergents, such as quaternary ammonium compounds, which, in addition to thier cleaning power, also act as mild disinfectants. Cationic detergents can be toxic and poisonous to ingest, however, and may cause nausea and, in extreme cases, coma. Cationics are also more easily absorbed by the skin, which is another reason why manufacturers recommend the use of protective gloves, and advise thorough rinsing should the product come into contact with skin.

Bleach Safety

Liquid household bleaches are approximately a 5 percent sodium hypochlorite solution. Used properly, it can be a simple and effective disinfectant. Chlorine bleach fumes can also be highly irritating to the skin, eyes, nose, and throat, however. Contact with the skin can result in dermatitis. Ingestion can cause esophageal injury, stomach irritation, and prolonged nausea and vomiting.

Bleach should never be mixed with any other cleaning solution. When mixed with acids, such as ammonia, toilet bowl cleaners, drain cleaners, or even vinegar, it can release chloramine gas, which can lead to coughing, loss of voice, a feeling of burning and suffocation, and even death.

Your Toilet Cleaner Is Likely to Contain . . .

Petroleum-based detergents/surfactants; strong acids, such as *muriatic (hydrochloric) acid* or *sulphuric acid* (sodium bisulphate), oxalic acid, *sodium hypochlorite, calcium hypochlorite, sodium carbonate*, sodium metasilicate, phenols, ammonia, bleach, naphthalene, paradichlorobenzene (PDCB), *5-dimethyldantoin*, quaternary ammonium salts, colors, and fragrance.

Try This Instead . . .

Not even the darkest recesses of your toilet need attacking with this many detergents and disinfectants. Once again, it's not the cleaning products but the tools you use with them that are important. So, the first thing to do is invest in a really good-quality toilet bowl brush—one with stiff bristles—which can be stored in a unit that allows it to air-dry between uses. You can literally clean your toilet with any detergent and get the job done. A plain, diluted, vegetable-based dishwashing liquid or castile soap is ideal. Or try making a more sophisticated mixture.

Make a simple toilet cleaner with:

    4 oz. vegetable-based dishwashing liquid or castile soap
    2 cups baking soda
    4 Tbsp water
    2 Tbsp white vinegar

You can even add 1/2 teaspoon essential oil of peppermint, lemon, pine, tea tree, or eucalyptus to give it a fresh, clean scent. Mix all the ingredients together (adding the vinegar last) and put them into a thoroughly rinsed squeezable bottle. This mixture can be used both inside and outside the toilet bowl.

To remove mineral deposits add a cup of white vinegar to the toilet bowl, then toss in a handful of baking soda. Let this bubble away for ten to fifteen minutes before giving the bowl a good scrub and flush.

An overnight soak is a simple way to clean. Pour half a cup of borax straight into the bowl, use your brush to give the bowl a quick once-over, and leave it overnight.

Another overnight soak method is to place two effervescent 1,000-mg vitamin C tablets (unflavored), or a mixture of 2 tablespoons each of citric acid and baking soda, in the toilet bowl. In the morning, brush around the bowl and flush. This can help remove scum below the waterline.

If you still feel you must use conventional cleaners, make sure you put the lid down before you flush the toilet. That way, you won't be sending a spray of chemicals into the air every time you flush.

Bath and Shower Cleaners

These are usually nothing more than all-purpose cleaners (see above) plus a few extra ingredients, usually strong acids. Typically, they come as liquids, powders, and creams. Their main job is to cut through the soap scum that gets left behind on tubs, tiles, and glass shower doors, although some of the newer products act like sealants, leaving a water- and dirt-repellent film on bathroom surfaces to help keep them clean. These products contain moisture-repellent nanoparticles that are 1/10,000 the diameter of a human hair. They are sold in pump bottles and aerosol cans.

Nanoparticles have never been tested for safety, yet they are increasingly being put into household products—in an uncontrolled medical experiment using humans as guinea pigs. Recently, the results of the experiment have begun to come in, and, in 2006, the German government was the first to issue a health warning regarding the use of these novel household sprays.

Sealing sprays for glass and ceramics containing moisture-repellent nanoparticles and a propellant have provoked severe health disorders when dispensed from aerosol cans. Sprayed onto surfaces, they also dissipate into the air, where they are easily inhaled. Doctors report that once in the lungs, the combination of nanoparticles and propellants disrupts the function of alveolar and bronchial tissues and, by extension, oxygen and moisture exchange. This has led to several cases of respiratory distress and, in severe cases, to accumulation of water in the lungs (pulmonary edema), which has serious consequences.

To make using conventional bath and shower cleaners safe, never use aerosols, always wear gloves, and make sure the room is well ventilated. Never use these products around food, children, or animals. Once again, unless your bathroom is sorely neglected, you really don't need special cleaners to get the job done.

Try This Instead . . .

Use natural disinfectants. Both white vinegar and lemon juice act as mild disinfectants. Because they are acidic, they can be used to remove hard-water spots, dissolve mineral buildup, and break down filmy soap residue without leaving a film of their own. They also act as deodorizers. Use two parts water to one part vinegar or lemon juice, or use either undiluted for heavily soiled areas. Since both vinegar and lemon juice are acids, remember to wear rubber gloves if you are going to be using either for more than a few minutes. For scrubbing down the bathroom, a nylon scrubbing pad is a must.

Try a simple abrasive. Baking soda can be used on its own to provide a mild abrasive action that is safe for tiles, countertops, sinks, and tubs. Apply it with a damp cloth on surfaces or with an old toothbrush to reach hard-to-get-at places.

Consider buying shower curtains that are washable. Also wash them regularly to prevent soap and mildew buildup. If they get really scummy, spraying them with undiluted distilled vinegar before washing will help remove soap residues. If you have a glass shower door, wipe it down after each use with a superabsorbent sponge cloth or, better yet, a squeegee, which will be even more efficient. Wiping down tiles and glass doors regularly takes about thirty seconds and will prevent soap scum from building up.

Metal showerheads can be cleaned by boiling them for fifteen minutes (or until the lime scale deposits begin to soften) in ½ cup of white vinegar and 1 quart of water. This will remove all but the most stubborn mineral deposits. Scrub clean with an old toothbrush.

To clean a plastic showerhead, soak it in equal parts white vinegar and warm water for one hour, then scrub clean with an old toothbrush.

To remove mineral deposits from around taps, lay a cloth soaked in hot vinegar on the fixture that needs cleaning. Let it stand for an hour or so, then wipe or gently scrub it off.

Mold and Mildew Cleaners

Mold and mildew can make your bathroom look and smell bad, and they are also a significant cause of respiratory problems. They are mostly a problem in bathrooms that are poorly ventilated, but instead of tackling them with fresh air, we attack them with strong fungicides. Mildew removers come in many forms, including in liquids that you rub on and then rinse off, and, more recently, in sprays that you don't rinse off. They all contain the same basic ingredients. Among these are: phenol—a central-nervous-system depressor, skin irritant, circulatory-system disrupter, and suspected carcinogen; *kerosene*—which can dry the skin and cause lung inflammation; and *pentachlorophenol*—which is toxic when inhaled, absorbed, or ingested and is a known reproductive toxin associated with birth defects.

Most mildew cleaners only work in the short term. So, if you're going to use a short-term solution, why not make it a less toxic one?

Try This Instead . . .

Borax diluted in a little hot water and applied with an old toothbrush will remove mildew just as effectively. If the problem is really severe, leave the solution on for an hour or so before rinsing it off.

Think airflow, because mildew is most likely to build up in damp places. If you've got this problem, then poor ventilation may be the cause.

Carpet and Upholstery Cleaners

Most of us don't realize what effective dust and pesticide traps our carpets are. And yet, every time you tread on your carpet, you send a microscopic cloud of dust, dirt, and chemicals into the air.

Along with everyday dirt, studies show that household carpets are reservoirs for volatile organic chemicals (VOCs), such as 4-phenylcyclohexene, tetrachloroethylene, benzene, xylene, toluene, styrene, and methylbenzene, as well as tobacco smoke and heavy metals. Carpets also harbor pesticides, such as heptachlor, chlorpyrifos, *aldrin*, dieldrin, *chlordane*, *atrazine*, DDT, orthophenylphenol, *propoxur*, *diazinon*, and *carbaryl*. Infants and toddlers ingest two and a half times more of these noxious agents than adults do because they spend so much time sitting and playing on the floor. For this reason, keeping your carpet clean is probably more important than you know.

Whether carpet shampoos are the best way to keep carpets clean, however, is debatable. Carpet and rug shampoos are concentrated detergents that come in ready-to-use liquids, trigger sprays, powders, and aerosols. They are formulated to wet the surface of the carpet and take up superficial oil and grease. Applied to the carpet, they attract and trap soils, and then dry to a brittle powdery residue that can be vacuumed up.

All commercial carpet-cleaning solutions can leave behind chemical residues and odors. Whether you are using a small amount of spot-clean spray or a detergent in a carpet-shampooing machine, the basic ingredients are much the same.

Carpet shampoos typically contain water and a mixture of other ingredients like detergents and surfactants, petroleum-based solvents, such as butyl cellosolve, and preservatives. Some contain enzymes to remove protein stains, *optical brighteners*, soil retardants, such as formaldehyde, perfumes, and deodorizers.

Upholstery cleaners are similar in their formulation to carpet cleaners and can produce the same toxic effects. All commercial carpet- and upholstery-cleaning solutions leave chemical residues on your carpet and soft furnishings. This residue is perhaps the greatest risk to young children who tend to: (a) crawl around on carpets and soft furnishings; and (b) stick their hands in their mouths a lot.

Spot removers are, at best, a short-term solution for stains and, at worst, a toxic hazard. Most of these are poisonous when ingested, highly irritating when inhaled, and a cause of skin reactions in sensitive people. Typically, they contain *perchloroethylene*, *trichloroethylene*, *diethylene glycol*, ammonium hydroxide, naphthalene, and oxalic acid.

Try This Instead . . .

Regular steam cleaning is the best way to keep your carpet toxin-free. It may be expensive, but some may reason it is worth the money since the very hot water used in steam cleaners kills dust mites, fleas, bacteria, and mold, as well as providing effective cleaning power.

Throw rugs should be laundered regularly, if possible. Non-washable rugs should be shaken outside or hung on a line and beaten with an old-fashioned rug beater or old tennis racket. In between steam cleans, you can help keep your wall-to-wall carpets and area rugs clean by:

Removing shoes. Most dirt is tracked in on the bottom of shoes.

Vacuuming regularly. If possible, aim to vacuum weekly to keep the amount of dust and dirt you send into the air to a minimum.

Use a carpet sweeper. In between vacuums, these are great for picking up spills and bits of unidentifiable stuff that falls to the floor.

Spot-clean. You can spot-clean carpets and upholstery with a solution of ½ cup of borax in 1 quart of warm water. Use a stiff-bristle brush for carpets and a softer one (like a toothbrush) for upholstery stains. Vacuum well when dry.

Buy washable soft coverings (cushion and covers). Launder them regularly. If your sofas and chairs get a lot of wear, consider a washable throw for everyday protection.

Carpet Deodorizers and Fabric Fresheners

Carpet fresheners or deodorizers are mostly heavy perfumes formulated to cover up odors. Most commercial carpet-deodorizing powders are not all that sophisticated. Usually, they comprise a baking-soda base and a strong petrochemical-derived fragrance.

Fabric fresheners are similar to carpet deodorizers. These products are often marketed to smokers and pet owners as a way of removing nasty smells from their soft furnishings. They are mostly made up of surfactant, which allows the chemicals to penetrate deeply into the fabric, and perfume. They don't remove smells. Like air fresheners, they contain chemicals that alter your sense of smell.

Given that some commonly used surfactants are contaminated with carcinogens like 1,4-dioxane, it hardly seems worth the risk. Prevention is still the best way to avoid carpet and upholstery smells.

Try This Instead . . .

Make your own. You can make your own carpet deodorant by using plain baking soda fragranced with essential oils. Sprinkle this on your carpet and work it well into the pile. Leave it anywhere from fifteen minutes to overnight, depending on the strength of the odor, and then vacuum. This is less expensive than buying commercial brands and just as effective.

Disinfect carpets with borax. Sprinkle it on your carpet, work it into the pile, and wait for anywhere from two to twenty-four hours before vacuuming it up. Really moldy or foul-smelling carpets may need more than one application.
Note: Inhaling any powder can cause respiratory problems in some individuals, so make sure you use other rooms while these minerals are soaking in.

Open a window. It's still the best way to deodorize most things in your home.

Dish Detergents

While not to the same degree as laundry detergents, dishwashing liquids can still add to your total toxic load, especially if you use hot water and no protective gloves.

Because dishwashing detergents are generally made from anionic and non-ionic surfactants, they are not absorbed as well as some other types of household cleaners and are therefore considered low in toxicity. Nevertheless, anionic and nonionic detergents can still cause irritation to the skin, eyes, and mucous membranes.

Your Dish Detergent Is Likely to Contain . . .
Petroleum-based detergents, such as diethanolamine and *sodium dodecylbenzenesulphonate*, preservatives, alcohols, petroleum distillates, ammonia, salts, coloring, and perfume.

Try This Instead . . .

There are probably more urgent things to worry about than your dishwashing liquid, and, in truth, there are few good alternatives. To make using dishwashing detergents safer for the environment:

Choose vegetable-based detergents. More and more supermarkets sell at least one or two good alternatives. Just be aware that some detergents that claim to be natural can still contain other undesirable ingredients, such as colorings and perfumes. If you are unsure about an ingredient, write, e-mail, or call the manufacturer for clarification.

Use less. Adding a little borax to the water beforehand will make even the smallest amount of dishwashing liquid more effective. This is because borax is an effective water softener.

Wear rubber gloves. They will prevent irritation of the skin and prevent the absorption of contaminants in the water, including nitrosamines, dioxanes, dyes, colorings, and perfumes.

Avoid ammonia. Some dishwashing liquids contain small amounts of ammonia, so don't mix them with bleach or bleach-containing products, as this combination will form a deadly chloramine gas.

Avoid products that are colored or fragranced. This will help reduce the number of chemicals you are exposed to.

Dilute your regular brand. Most dishwashing liquids are very concentrated, and we all tend to use much too much to get the job done.

Diluting will not substantially affect the cleaning power of the product, so try mixing equal amounts of vegetable-based dishwashing liquid and water. The mixture can be thickened with approximately 1 tablespoon of salt. Store in a squirt-top bottle (any well-rinsed dishwashing detergent bottle will do). This will still foam and will still clean your dishes, but will expose you to fewer chemicals.

To make an even less toxic version of this recipe, replace conventional dish detergent with castile soap. Dr. Bronner's scent-free liquid baby soap is a good choice. That way, you can add your own fragrance with essential oils if you wish.

As an alternative to dish detergent, wash your dishes in soap flakes. And add a dash of vinegar to cut through the grease. You will not get loads of bubbles, but your dishes will be clean. You can also wash your dishes effectively in washing soda or borax (always wear gloves when using these substances).

Rinse your dishes well. Soaping them up and then leaving them to drain means that chemical residues remain on the plate and are likely to get into the next serving of food you eat from that dish.

Automatic-Dishwasher Detergents

Most automatic-dishwasher detergents are either irritants or corrosives, depending on their composition, concentration, and physical form. They are made using strong petroleum-based detergents and a strong alkali, giving them a pH value of between 10.5 and 12.0. Skin irritation or burns may result following exposure to dissolved detergents. Many also contain washing soda (sodium carbonate) and occasionally phosphates, which pollute waterways. They may also contain *sodium silicate* to prevent damage to the dishwasher, a surfactant to prevent water spots, and a fragrance.

Some of these detergents also contain dry chlorine, which becomes activated when mixed with the water in the dishwasher. This means that when you open the dishwasher, chlorine fumes are released in the steam that leaks out. These can cause eye irritation and breathing difficulty, especially for those with respiratory problems.

The average individual is unlikely to have any prolonged contact with automatic-dishwasher detergents. If you have children in the house, however, you might want to consider using a powdered variety rather than the tablet or liquid varieties. Tablets have become a significant source of poisonings among children and animals, so if you choose these, be sure to store them carefully.

Try This Instead . . .

All automatic-dishwasher detergents will leave some chemical residues on your dishes. You can cut your exposure to these by trying the following:

Choose powdered brands. Generally speaking, these contain fewer harmful ingredients than the liquid variety. Powders are also less likely to be mistakenly swallowed by young children.

Use less. The powder receptacles in dishwashers are larger than they need to be and encourage us to use more detergent than necessary in the machine. The average dishwasher only needs about 2 tablespoons of detergent in the closed cup dispenser or 1 tablespoon in the open dispenser to work well.

Use low- or no-phosphate brands. These are much kinder to the environment.

Don't use commercial products at all. Try using ½ teaspoon of pure soap powder (more will produce too many suds) mixed with 3 tsblespoons of baking soda.

Don't overdo it with normally soiled dishes. Use 2 teaspoons of borax predissolved in hot water, followed by vinegar in the rinse cycle.

Sprinkle your dishes with baking soda. Do this before loading them in the dishwasher, then add detergent to the closed dispenser only. This will cut down on the amount of detergent used, but you will still have clean dishes. (But don't put baking soda on your aluminum pans, as it will discolor them.)

Floor Cleaners

Floor cleaners are generally made from either petroleum distillates and solvents or water-based detergents. The mixture makes a cocktail that is dangerous to inhale and possibly irritating to the skin. Of the two types, water-based cleaners are much less toxic. Those containing the solvent glycol monomethyl ether are much more hazardous: if accidentally swallowed, they can cause nausea and vomiting, stomach pain, bleeding and/or chemical pneumonia.

Those that use pine oils can cause convulsions, coma, and even death if ingested. While ingesting them is unlikely because of their strong taste, parents of very young children might reason that, given good alternatives, it's just not worth the risk keeping such products in the house.

Of course, floor cleaners don't have to be swallowed to be toxic. If you have young children who tend to crawl about on the floor, they may well be picking these substances up on their hands and breathing in their fumes. Prolonged and repeated exposure of the skin and to the vapors from floor cleaners can affect the central nervous system, producing symptoms similar to drunkenness, and damage the kidneys.

You don't need anything special to clean your floors. The average household floor attracts average household grime and dust. Cleaning this off is a fairly simple task that can be made much easier if you make a habit of wiping up spills as they happen.

Your Floor Cleaner Is Likely to Contain . . .

Petroleum-based detergents, ammonia, bleach, phosphates, pine oil, or citrus oil; solvents, such as butyl cellosolve, phosphoric acid, *potassium hydroxide*, coloring, and perfume. Most contain undisclosed preservatives as well. If you use a floor polish on top of this, you will be adding plastics (possible hormone disrupters) that can damage vinyl tiles and turn them yellow over time, as well as petroleum distillates, *naphtha*, and *nitrobenzene*.

Marble Needs Special Care

Marble gives the impression of strength and grandeur, but it is really rather soft and easy to chip, break, and stain. Marble surfaces in your home should never be cleaned with spirits or acids. Even water will eventually stain and weaken marble, so it is best dealt with by using a dry soft cloth. If you absolutely have to clean marble, try doing it with a little mineral spirits and a clean cloth. Family heirlooms should only be cleaned by experts. But there is no getting around cleaning marble floors, so try using water and a weak detergent solution. If possible, wash and then thoroughly dry the floor to prevent excess moisture from seeping into the stone.

Try This Instead . . .

As with all toxic cleaners, the best alternative is to use less. Most of these products are highly concentrated, and we all tend to overestimate how much we need to use. To make using conventional cleaners safer, always wear gloves and always open a window. Or consider these alternatives:

A simple floor cleaner can be made from hot water and vinegar. Add one cup of vinegar to a full bucket of water. If your floor is really dirty, mix a small amount of liquid soap or soap flakes in with the hot water. Rinse afterward with a vinegar-and-water solution. This works well on ceramic, polyurethane-finished wood floors, and on linoleum and other vinyl tiles.

To disinfect, mop the floor with ½ cup of borax in a bucketful of hot water. To make sure the borax dissolves thoroughly, put the borax in first and then add the water, stirring until it is dissolved.

To cut grease, mix ½ cup of washing soda (sodium carbonate or sal soda) with 1 tablespoon of liquid soap, ¼ cup of distilled white vinegar, and ½ bucket of water. Washing soda is caustic, so use gloves and avoid splashing. Don't use on waxed floors, as it will damage the finish.

For wood floors, use ¼ cup of liquid soap with ½ to 1 cup of distilled vinegar or lemon juice to a bucket of water. To improve the fragrance, use a cup of strong, freshly brewed herbal tea of your choice.

For linoleum, combine 6 tablespoons of cornstarch for every cup of water, mix together in a bucket, and use it as you would any floor polish.

Glass and Mirror Cleaners

Glass and mirrors show up smudges and fingerprints more readily than other surfaces because they reflect light. No one likes a smeared, smudgy window, but the products that we use to clean our windows and mirrors are still disproportionately strong, given that they generally have a simple job to do.

Once again, this is due to manufacturers responding to what they see as consumer demand for fast-acting products. But apart from paying a premium price for something that is mostly water, you are also exposing yourself to a number of chemical hazards. As window cleaners are inevitably sprays, and because you work so close to the glass or mirror while cleaning it, you cannot help but inhale the mixture as you go, and this can be mildly irritating to the eyes, skin, nose, and throat.

Your Glass Cleaner Is Likely to Contain . . .

Solvents, such as isopropyl alcohol or butyl cellosolve, ammonia, glycol ether, *silicon*, waxes, formaldehyde, and, if it's an aerosol, propellants, such as isobutane or propane, and, sometimes, colorings and perfumes.

Try This Instead . . .

If you are stuck on using conventional products, always use them in a well-ventilated room, and choose pump sprays over aerosols.

For most glass and mirrors in the home, water is the best cleaner. Consumer reports show that water cleans mirrors and windows better than some 60 percent of the products on the market. Likewise, most homemade mixtures can equal and, in some cases, better the commercially available products. What's more, they do it at a fraction of the price of commercial brands.

Whatever you end up using to clean windows and mirrors will be made more effective and easier with the right tools. Make sure you have two lint-free cloths to do the job—one for cleaning and one for drying. Most people just use paper towels, which are equally effective, but they are also an expensive and wasteful way to clean.

Simple glass cleaner 1: Put some plain club soda in a spray bottle. Many people swear by this cleaner, which appears to work because it contains sodium citrate, which acts like a water softener and, thus, helps to clean more effectively. It won't dry as quickly as conventional cleaners but, for lightly soiled glass and mirrors, this is a perfectly adequate solution.

Simple glass cleaner 2: Mix equal amounts of water and distilled vinegar in a spray bottle. The vinegar will help cut through greasy fingerprints and also acts as a room deodorizer.

Foaming glass cleaner is for you if you like some sort of foam to show you where you've sprayed; if your windows or mirrors are particularly greasy and dirty, you can make up a stronger mixture using:

1/2 tsp liquid soap
3 Tbsp distilled white vinegar
2 cups water

Put the ingredients into a spray bottle and shake well. This works well inside the house (and is also an effective all-purpose cleaner for light cleaning), but can sometimes cause streaks on outside and car windows.

Laundry Products

Wearing clean clothes and sleeping on clean sheets is a pleasure. And in supermarkets nowadays, you can find just about everything you need to make sure that your clothes and household textiles are clean and bright. But, as with all

Toxic Softeners

Fabric softeners are made from mild detergents and cationic surfactants, such as quaternary ammonium compounds. They work by magnetic attraction. A fabric softener has a strong positive charge that forms a uniform positively charged layer on the fabric surface, making it feel softer to the touch (an excess of negative charge on fabrics is responsible for a scratchy feeling after washing and for static cling). Cationic surfactants are also used in laundry products that boast fabric-softening properties.

Fabric-softening sheets release a special resin in the dryer that deposits a waxy coating on the clothes to make them feel softer.

Along with surfactants and resins, fabric softeners deposit a range of other chemicals onto your clothes as well. According to a report by the U.S. Environmental Protection Agency, "Identification of Polar Volatile Organic Compounds in Consumer Products and Common Microenvironments," fabric softeners and dryer sheets contain an enormous number of potentially toxic chemicals. Among them are:

- **A-terpineol (alpha-terpineol)**, which is highly irritating to mucous membranes. It can also cause excitement, ataxia (loss of muscular coordination), hypothermia, CNS* and respiratory depression, and headache. Repeated or prolonged skin contact is not advised.
- **Benzyl acetate**, the vapors of which are irritating to the eyes and respiratory passages, and may cause coughing. The chemical can be absorbed through the skin, causing system-wide effects. It is a carcinogen that has been linked to pancreatic cancer.
- **Benzyl alcohol**, which is irritating to the upper respiratory tract, and can cause headache, nausea, vomiting, dizziness, a drop in blood pressure, CNS depression, and, in rare cases, death due to respiratory failure.
- **Camphor**, which is on the EPA's hazardous-waste list. It is readily absorbed through body tissues; vapors and inhalation can irritate the eyes, nose, and

cleaning products, there is a downside to having whites that are whiter than white.

Detergents were first developed when the petroleum industry tried to find a way to make money from the toxic waste materials that they generated each year. One of these was propylene. Eventually, scientists found a way of mixing propylene with benzene to produce sulphuric acid. They then added *sodium hydroxide* to the mix to neutralize this harmful acid. A sodium salt somewhat like ordinary soap was the result, and the detergent industry was born. Today's detergents are still made largely from the waste materials generated by the petroleum industry.

---

throat. It is a CNS stimulant, and is associated with dizziness, confusion, nausea, twitching muscles, and convulsions.

- **Chloroform**, which is also on the EPA's hazardous-waste list. A neurotoxin, anesthetic, and carcinogen, inhalation of its vapors can cause headache, nausea, vomiting, dizziness, drowsiness, irritation of the respiratory tract, and loss of consciousness. Chronic effects of overexposure may include kidney and/or liver damage. Its use can aggravate disorders of the kidney, liver, heart, and skin.
- **Ethyl acetate**, which is yet another item on the EPA's hazardous-waste list. It can be irritating to the eyes and respiratory tract; it's a narcotic, and exposure may cause headache and narcosis (stupor). It has also been linked with anemia, leucocytosis (an increase in white blood cells as an immune reaction), and damage to the liver and kidneys.
- **Limonene**, which is an irritant to the skin and eyes, and a possible cause of allergic reactions. It is also a carcinogen.
- **Linalool**, which is a narcotic shown to cause CNS disorders. Animal tests have proven it to adversely affect mood, muscle coordination, and spontaneous motor activity. Exposure can cause fatal respiratory disturbances. It even attracts bees (thereby posing a threat to people who are allergic to bee stings).
- **Pentane**, which is irritating to the eyes and can cause skin rashes. Its vapors may cause headache, nausea, vomiting, dizziness, drowsiness, irritation to the respiratory tract, and loss of consciousness. Prolonged and repeated inhalation of vapors may cause CNS depression.

CNS—central nervous system (the brain and spinal cord). CNS disorders include Alzheimer's disease, attention deficit disorder (ADD or ADHD), dementia, multiple chemical sensitivity (MCS), multiple sclerosis (MS), Parkinson's disease, seizures, strokes, and sudden infant death syndrome (SIDS). CNS symptoms include aphasia (loss of ability to speak or understand speech), blurred vision, disorientation, dizziness, headache, hunger, memory loss, numbness in the face, and pain in the neck and spine.

Powders and liquids contain the same basic ingredients, although liquids include extra ingredients, such as opacifiers, to make them look nice. These give the liquid a rich, creamy, opaque appearance, but do not clean your clothes. They also contain synthetic colors. Liquid detergents contain no filler at all and are more concentrated than powders. Other than that, there is no difference between types of laundry detergents. Liquid tablets and gel packs do not clean better, they don't get into the wash quicker, and they don't penetrate fabrics more efficiently. Such claims are used to justify the high price of these novelties, which are invariably much more expensive to use per wash than regular powders.

To help boost the power of your laundry powder, there are a number of wash additives on the market, including:

Pretreatments and stain removers. These are available in a variety of forms, such as pump sprays, liquids, gels, solids, or aerosols. They contain surfactants and solvents. Aerosol versions also use a variety of petroleum distillates and propellants. Most pretreatments are just liquid detergents under another name. Logic dictates that if you put detergent in a high concentration on a stain before you start to wash, you will have a better chance of getting the stain out.

Solid or stick formulas are probably best for ground-in stains because the action of rubbing them onto the fabric ensures that they are pushed deeply into the stain. They also have fewer chemicals in them. Frankly, you can substitute a liquid soap or detergent for most pretreatments, as it will do exactly the same job.

Laundry boosters. Most laundry detergents include a small amount of added bleach, but not enough to handle really tough stains. This is why there are separate bleaches that you can add to the wash to boost cleaning power. Laundry boosters used to be made with common bleach (sodium hypochlorite)—the same stuff used in swimming pools and drain cleaners.

As fabrics have become more colorful and sensitive to the effects of common bleach, however, manufacturers have come up with color-sparing bleaches based on sodium perborate or sodium chloride. Sodium perborate breaks down into hydrogen peroxide in the wash and liberates oxygen, which oxidizes, or bleaches. Sodium chloride liberates chlorine gas to oxidize or bleach stains. Chlorine is the more powerful of the two types of bleaches; it is also more irritating to the skin, eyes, and lungs. All bleaches are corrosive and harmful if swallowed.

Your Laundry Products Are Likely to Contain . . .

Petroleum-based detergents and surfactants, enzymes, bleaches, optical brighteners, builders/water softeners (pH adjusters) and processing aids, corrosion inhibitors, anti-redisposition agents, and fragrances. Powdered varieties also contain fillers—inert substances that keep the powder flowing freely. Some powders are as much as 50 percent filler. Some contain disinfectants, such as pine oil, which is highly irritating and may cause allergic reactions, as well as phenolics and coal-tar derivatives, which are carcinogenic.

Try This Instead . . .

Nearly all commercial brands of laundry detergent and fabric softener leave chemical residues on your clothes that can irritate the skin. While most are made to biodegrade within a matter of days, their manufacturing process is far from ecological. For a healthier environment, buy laundry powders and liquids that use only vegetable-based detergents. Also, for everyday stains, nonbiological detergents are perfectly adequate. Try to avoid fabric softeners altogether. Other laundry alternatives include:

Choose powders. Powders are preferable to liquids, tablets, and gel packs, and, as we all tend to use more detergent than necessary to wash clothes, use less of whichever type you buy.

Try pure soap flakes instead of detergent. Add ½ cup of borax or vinegar to the rinse cycle to remove soapy residue. Vinegar has the advantage of acting like a fabric softener and mold inhibitor as well.

Go nonbio. Biological laundry detergents are formulated with enzymes to get the most common stains out. The enzymes are obtained from selected strains of bacteria. Products that have enzymes in them can be irritating to the skin, and are a cause of allergic reactions, such as asthma and dermatitis.

Although the addition of enzymes is promoted as the best way to remove "protein" stains, such as from grass, chocolate, and blood, this is somewhat misleading. The most common clothing stains are not protein stains, but dirt and grease stains. When you use these specially formulated products, you are often paying for the expense manufacturers incurred in advertising unnecessary additives to you on TV.

Starches

Not many of us use starch in our laundry these days. Good thing, too. Laundry starches, while based on cornstarch formulas, contain a number of nasties, such as formaldehyde—a carcinogen and irritant to the eyes, throat, skin, and lungs; phenols—carcinogens that also cause CNS depression and severely affect the circulatory system, and are corrosive to skin; and pentachlorophenol—a reproductive toxin associated with fetal abnormalities and birth defects.

To remove heavy soiling add 1 teaspoon of trisodiumphosphate (TSP) to the wash. Borax and washing soda (sodium carbonate) can also remove heavy stains.

To remove perspiration and odors, pretreat with baking soda, white vinegar, or borax dissolved in water. These ingredients can also be added to the wash to freshen the load.

Make use of a clothes line if you have one. The sun's rays are the best bleaching agent in the world. Clothes that have been gently dried in the sun also tend to be naturally softer than those tumbled in the dryer.

Dry Cleaning

When you use a home dry-cleaning fluid or send your clothes out to be dry-cleaned, you are soaking your clothes in a mixture containing some of the most hazardous chemicals around. Not surprisingly, there is a large body of medical evidence showing that people who work in the dry-cleaning industry suffer from a wide range of health problems, including kidney and liver diseases, cancer of the larynx and esophagus, optic neuritis (inflammation of the optic nerve resulting in vision loss), and memory impairment.

Your Dry Cleaner Typically Uses . . .
Carbon tetrachloride, perchloroethylene, *trichloroethane*, naphthas, benzene, and toluene. The ingredients in dry-cleaning fluids, whether for home or professional use, are basically the same.

Try This Instead . . .

Take a sniff of your clothes when they come back from the cleaners. Most dry-cleaning machines are built to recapture the chemicals used in the cleaning process so that they can be used over and over again. If you can still smell any chemicals at all on your clothes, it may be time to change dry cleaners. To minimize the risk:

Buy clothes that don't need dry cleaning. Dry cleaning is a luxury that should be reserved for the most precious garments. Often, it is simply unnecessary, and manufacturers recommend dry cleaning only to cover themselves against any potential damage done through careless washing.

Air out your clothes. When you bring clothes home from the cleaners, take the plastic bag off and allow them to air out near an open window before wearing.

Wear rubber gloves. If you are using a commercial household spot remover, always wear rubber gloves and work so that the fumes are blowing away from you. Do not allow children or pets into the room while you are working. Keep the lid on the product while in use to avoid solvent being vaporized in the room. Always wash any splashes on the skin immediately with soap and plenty of water.

Never use dry-cleaning fluid in a washing machine. Also, never put articles that are damp with dry-cleaning fluid into the dryer, as most dry-cleaning fluids are flammable, and those that aren't will produce toxic gases in the dryer.

Look for dry cleaners that use the Green Earth cleaning process. This process is based on liquid silicone rather than volatile chemicals.

These days, you can buy special sheets that claim to freshen dry-cleanable clothes in the dryer. Approach these with caution. They contain powerful spot removers similar to home dry-cleaning fluids, and strong surfactants and perfumes, both of which can cause allergic reactions.

Oven and Drain Cleaners

Why do these products appear together, you might ask? Because both are made from the same strongly caustic ingredients.

There are two basic types of drain cleaners. Those used for maintenance are called buildup removers. They contain enzymes or cultured bacteria that produce enzymes, and are formulated to dissolve grease and soap scum.

The second type—drain openers—are highly corrosive and dangerous to use. This is because their main ingredients are sodium hydroxide (*lye*), a caustic that can burn the skin and cause blindness if it gets into the eyes, and sulphuric acid, a corrosive chemical that can also cause severe skin burns and blindness. Both types work by eating away at whatever is in their path. This includes your skin if you are unlucky enough to splash some on yourself. The vapors from commercial drain cleaners are also harmful.

The use of chemical drain cleaners as a preventative is not a good idea. If you have a septic tank, be aware that chemical drain openers can kill off all the beneficial bacteria necessary for the efficient working of the tank.

Even buildup removers that claim to be noncorrosive or noncaustic can contain chemicals that can be poisonous if inhaled or swallowed. Such products should clearly state their ingredients.

Try This Instead . . .

Regularly running boiling water down the drain is probably the best way to keep drains clear and running well. Since greasy deposits are a major cause of clogged drains, try not to pour grease down the drain if you can help it. In addition:

Make a foaming drain cleaner from 7 ounces of baking soda, 3½ ounces of table salt, and 7 ounces of vinegar. When the alkali (baking soda) meets the acid (vinegar), they will bubble furiously, pushing the abrasive salt through the drain. All three ingredients will work to remove deposits from the drain and clear it out. After twenty minutes or so, pour boiling water down the drain to flush it clear.

Use a drain strainer, little filters that can be used in bathrooms and kitchens to keep large particles from going down the drain and forming blockages.

Use a plunger, which can be very effective for dislodging blockages. Once you have opened the drain, use boiling water or the foaming drain cleaner described above to clear it out. Be warned, though: do not use a plunger after using chemical drain openers, as this invites hazardous splashback onto the skin and into the eyes.

Never mix commercial drain openers with anything else, not even natural alternatives. The combination could become reactive and erupt out of the sink and onto you.

Oven Cleaners

Like drain cleaners, the main ingredients of most oven cleaners are sodium hydroxide (lye), a caustic that can cause burns to the skin and blindness if it gets into the eyes, and sulphuric acid, a corrosive chemical that can also cause severe skin burns and blindness. The reason why oven cleaners are made with lye is simple. When the lye mixes with grease in your oven, it makes a crude form of soap, which then facilitates cleaning.

The majority of oven cleaners are packaged as aerosols. This means that in addition to lye and sulphuric acid, you are also being exposed to propellants. Strong alkalis can be used on cold ovens; however, there are newer types of oven cleaners that use fewer alkali chemicals. These only work in warm ovens to aid the removal of grease and grime. The vapors from both types are highly toxic.

Try This Instead . . .

Prevent messy grime from building up by lining the oven floor with a sheet of aluminum foil. This will catch most spills, and can be changed as often as necessary.

Use baking soda. This can be sprinkled into the oven while it is still warm to loosen grease, and can then be wiped away with warm water. Or you can make a spray from 3 tablespoons of baking soda dissolved in 2 cups of warm water. Spray it on, and wait twenty minutes before scrubbing it off with a fine wool pad, if necessary. Baking soda is effective for light-to-medium soiled ovens. Heavily soiled ovens may require a different approach.

Use vinegar. Using the same principles for unclogging a drain, you can spray a solution of white vinegar into your warm oven. Sprinkle with baking soda, leave it to bubble, and then scrub away.

Polishes

Nothing says clean like a nice polish on your furniture, brass, copper, and silverware, as well as shoes and car. But to achieve that nice sheen, we use a mixture of dangerous solvents and waxes derived from petroleum.

Furniture Polish

The furniture polish you use in your home comes in three basic forms: solid waxes, creams, and sprays. Each one contains different types of chemical solvents to aid the application of the polish, some of which are more harmful than others. Creams, for instance, are often water-based. But solid wax formulations can contain harsh solvents through which the oil or wax is dissolved. Spray polishes also contain harsh solvents, and require the addition of neurotoxic propellants.

Caring for wood is simple. Often, it comes down to how you treat the wood in between cleanings, rather than the polish you buy. If you don't let hot or wet things stand on the surface of the wood, and protect it from hard knocks and sharp points like pens, your furniture should stand up to everything else that everyday life throws at it.

Although wood originally came from a living thing, wooden furniture is not alive. It doesn't need nourishing or feeding. The purpose of polish is mainly to make the wood look nice, and to keep any natural moisture from being released.

If your furniture was varnished or polished in the factory, you only need to give it a good going-over once or twice a year. The rest of the time, a simple dusting is sufficient. Overuse of aerosol sprays, in particular, can leave a slight milky film on polished wood, which will be impossible to get out except by stripping and re-finishing.

Most Furniture Polishes Contain . . .

Flammable and hazardous ingredients, such as solvents, petroleum distillates, volatile organic compounds (VOCs), naphthas, nitrobenzene, phenol, ammonia formaldehyde, and benzene. The health dangers most often associated with polishes of all kinds are inhalation of fumes or vapors (especially from aerosols) and poisoning from ingestion. Polishes that look like strawberry soda or milk are especially tempting to children.

Try This Instead . . .

Unvarnished wood can be cleaned and polished easily and beautifully with very simple compounds. For instance, a dab of vinegar on a slightly damp cloth can be a very effective cleaner. A little light olive oil on a cloth will also polish and protect your wood. If you are feeling more ambitious, try making the following alternatives:

Simple furniture polish. Fill a small bottle ⅔ of the way with oil (olive or walnut are good choices, or a mixture of one of these with linseed oil in a ratio of two to one works as well). Top up the bottle with white vinegar, then add 20–30 drops of essential oil (lemon or bergamot are good choices). Shake well before each use and apply sparingly with a soft cloth. Use a second clean cloth for buffing (this is an essential step to avoid a buildup of polish). The vinegar will help to clean your furniture, while the oils will protect the wood.

Furniture wax. Use this mixture occasionally to polish and protect wood:

2 Tbsp beeswax
3 Tbsp oil
1 Tbsp white vinegar

Grate the beeswax (to help speed the melting process) into a small ceramic bowl or glass measuring cup. Add the oil and vinegar, and put the bowl into a shallow pan of boiling water. Stir it as it mixes, and, when it has fully melted, leave it to cool a bit. While the mixture is still liquid,

pour it into a small jar. Apply sparingly and leave to dry before buffing with a clean cloth.

Metal Polish

Most metal polishes contain strong acids, such as phosphoric acid and oxalic acid. They can also contain caustics, such as ammonia hydroxide, and reproductive toxins and neurotoxins, such as petroleum distillates, nitrobenzene, naphthalene, and ethanol.

The most dangerous polishes contain sulphuric acid and *hydrofluoric acid*. The hydrofluoric acid found in some rust removers and aluminum polishes can eat right through the skin down to the bone. Less toxic polishes contain detergents, trisodium phosphates, and pine oils, but these tend to be the least effective when it comes to removing tarnish.

Metal polishes are acidic because acid dissolves tarnish. Unfortunately, they can sometimes be so harsh that they damage the object you are trying to clean. They can eat through metal or metal plating. They can destroy the lacquer coatings commonly used on items, such as brassware, and leave permanent stains on the surface of every type of metal. This is especially true of the "quick dip"-type polishes.

Waxing the Car?

A typical can or bottle of car wax contains around 75–85 percent petroleum-derived naphtha. The rest of the formulation comprises wax—also usually petroleum-based. Like most petroleum derivatives, naphtha is flammable and is also an irritant and highly toxic should it be ingested or absorbed through the skin. Repeated and long-term contact may result in chapped skin and sensitivity to light. When waxing the car, wear protective gloves. When the wax is not in use, make sure the top of the can or bottle is securely closed and kept out of the reach of children.

Remember also that windshild-wiper solution is more hazardous than most of us realize. Most types are anything from 37 to 100 percent solvent, such as ethylene glycol, isopropanol, and *methanol*, with the rest being made up of detergent and water. The most toxic windshield-wiper solutions are 100 percent methanol.

Due to its hazardous nature, windshield-wiper solutions should always have a childproof safety cap. Needless to say, they should be stored away from children and pets. There are few real alternatives to their use, however, and when you're streaking along the highway on a murky, muddy, rainy day, the safety of a clean windshield is certainly a top priority. So, try to choose solutions that are detergent-based. When topping off your car, wear gloves, and avoid skin contact and inhalation. Make sure the safety cap is replaced securely.

Try This Instead . . .

Combinations of natural acids like lemon juice or vinegar and salt make good metal cleaners. Any chloride, however, such as salt or washing soda, can damage fine metals, so don't use these homemade polishes on family heirlooms. If an item is of particular value, always consider having it professionally cleaned.

For brass and copper. Rub pans with a mixture of salt and vinegar or lemon juice (or lemon rind soaked in salt) and then wash. Heating the vinegar will aid the process, since all acids are more active when hot. Give this time to work. The best way is to work the mixture all over the brass or copper item, and then let it sit for a while.

Alternatively, add ½ ounce of citric acid to 1 pint of water. (You may need to adjust the amount of acid by trial and error.) Swab this on your metal item and leave for a little while. Make sure you place the item on plenty of newspaper or other protective covering, and leave a window open. This will remove tarnish and even rust, making polishing much easier.

For bronze. Bronze should never be polished. It is easily damaged by water, and polishing will remove the patina that is part of its character. Brush very occasionally with a clean soft brush and use a cottonball to remove dirt from crevices.

For pewter. Likewise, pewter is easily damaged by metal polishes. The best way to protect it is to keep it dust-free with a clean dry cloth and, occasionally, rubbing the outside with a silver-cleaning cloth. Never rub polish on the inside of a pewter goblet or any other vessel intended to hold liquid. Pewter is absorbent, and this can make it unpleasant or even dangerous to drink from.

For silver. Some experts believe that a bit of tarnish in the crevices brings out the character and design of the piece, so don't overpolish your silver. Intricate designs are best brushed with a soft brush to get the polish into the detail.

You can make your own simple silver dip by placing a plate-sized sheet of aluminum foil into a saucepan of water and a handful of washing soda. Heat this up and place the silver in the pan for a minute or two, until the tarnish and stains are just coming off. *Do not* leave for a long time, and *do not* use this method for cleaning silver-plated items. Buff with a soft clean cloth or long-term silver cloth.

To clean the inside of a silver teapot, fill it with boiling water and add 1 teaspoon of denture cleaner and leave overnight.

Silver-plated objects should only be polished when absolutely necessary. Try using a special silver-polishing cloth for this job and remember to wear gloves.

To make your own silver-polishing cloth, mix 4 teaspoons of whiting (a fine powder that can be purchased at most hardware stores) with 2 tablespoons of household ammonia and 3 cups of water. Soak a soft absorbent cloth in this mixture, wring it out, and allow it to only dry halfway (preferably near an open window to avoid fumes filling your house), then store it in a resealable plastic bag for use as needed.

For chrome. Rather than a commercial mixture of ammonia and other chemicals, why not try straight ammonia and water. Put a dash of ammonia in water and dip a soft cloth in the mix. Rub this on the chrome, rinse, and then polish with a clean soft cloth. Make sure to wear protective gloves and try not to breathe in the fumes. If you are washing the car, be careful not to get the ammonia onto the paintwork. In the bathroom, chrome fixtures need only soap and water to clean them. Stubborn stains can be lifted by rubbing gently with a bit of baking soda on a slightly damp soft cloth.

For stainless steel. Even everyday stainless-steel pans, dishes, and cutlery can be damaged by too much polishing and scratchy sponge cleaners. To clean stainless steel, you need hot water and a little detergent—that's all. If you really feel the need for a stronger mixture, use a dash of ammonia in hot water. Drying the items immediately will prevent annoying spots from forming.

Shoe Polish

Most shoe polishes do not list their ingredients, yet many commercial shoe polishes contain a number of suspected human carcinogens that can be easily absorbed through your skin. Among them are trichloroethylene, nitrobenzene, and *dichloromethane* (methylene chloride).

Try This Instead . . .

There is no doubt that your shoes will last longer and look better when they are properly taken care of. But sadly, there are very few good alternatives to conventional shoe polish. Nevertheless, while most of us would never think that there are safety issues involved with shoe polishing, there are. To protect yourself from the nasty chemicals found in shoe polish:

Wear gloves when polishing or cleaning shoes—the chemicals in the polish are easily absorbed into your skin.

Make sure shoes are dry before wearing, as many of the vapors emitted from shoe polish interact with alcohol. The presence of alcohol in the system heightens the toxic effects of nitrobenzene. For this reason, it is wise not to wear shoes that are still wet with polish if you are going out (or staying in) drinking.

Keep shoe polish out of the reach of children.

Paints and Decorating Materials

When a building is overwhelmed with toxic chemicals, it is sometimes called a sick building. When the people inhabiting such a building become sick from chemical exposures, it is known as sick building syndrome. Studies show that in many cases of sick building syndrome, the use of chemical paints was a key factor in the damage to health.

Not so long ago, our paint contained the heavy metals lead and mercury. Although this is no longer the case, many cases of sick building syndrome have been traced to the chemicals in interior paints. Most conventional paints contain solvents and other volatile organic compounds (VOCs), and emit these toxic chemicals as gases for days, months, and even years after they've been applied. These gases can cause headaches, and irritate the eyes, nose, and throat; they are proven to increase allergies, asthma, and respiratory problems and even to weaken immunity.

The chemicals in ordinary paints can also contaminate the environment. For every ton of paint produced, the resulting waste can be anything up to thirty tons. This waste can be toxic and doesn't degrade naturally. Emulsions produce less waste than gloss or varnish, but can still cause damage. Harmful chemicals mean you shouldn't pour paint down the drain or throw it away with your trash. Your local authorities can advise you about paint disposal and recycling.

These days, many countries require paint labels to give information as to their environmental effects—for example, whether the ingredients can damage the ozone layer. Paints should also be labeled if they can cause allergies. When choosing your paint, be sure to read the label. If the information you require is not there, always contact the manufacturer.

There are, however, alternatives. Some paints contain no chemical solvents, while others just contain fewer than conventional paints. Eco-friendly paints use such ingredients as turpentine or d-limonene as alternatives to mineral spirits. Instead of plastic binders, they may use linseed oil and casein, and chalk and clay may replace fillers, such as titanium dioxide. Colors are often derived from natural earth and mineral pigments.

Your Household Paint Is Likely to Contain . . .

Acetone, ammonia, benzene, ethylene acrylate, *ethylene glycol*, formaldehyde, kerosene, *methyl alcohol*, phenol, propylene glycol, quaternary ammonium compounds, trichloroethylene, and *vinyl acetate/acrylic copolymer*.

Try This Instead . . .

Use latex (water-based) paint instead of oil-based paint. And if you can, choose low-odor paints or those based on natural ingredients and pigments—they are not only ecologically sound but also safe for the immediate home environment. Paints based on natural ingredients have the advantage of allowing surfaces and material to breathe more freely than chemical-based paint, which often creates a totally impermeable film that facilitates mold and fungus growth in homes, with adverse health effects. Most natural paint manufacturers also openly declare all ingredients used in their products, which allows allergy sufferers to check out their compatibility with the particular products.

Dispose of any leftover paint with care. You can avoid lots of excess if you calculate the amount you need carefully before you buy. Many stores will help you do this and some will take back unopened cans. Alternatively, consider donating any good leftover paint to a community organization that can make use of it.

Consider these other useful tips:

Chemical paint strippers. The worst offenders are those containing methylene chloride, trichloroethylene (TCE), and benzene (all of which can cause cancer); 1,1,1-trichloroethane (TCA) (irritating to the eyes, respiratory tract, and tissues), xylene (toxic if inhaled or consumed); or toluene (a cause of birth defects). A heat gun and a paint scraper are effective tools to remove several layers of paint. You can also use a sanding block with coarse sandpaper. Always wear safety goggles and a mask no matter what course you choose. If the paint you wish to remove is very old, it may contain lead. Inhaling the heated vapors or dust can cause lead poisoning and is very dangerous for children. In such cases it's best to get a professional in to do the job. Safe and effective water-based paint strippers are now available that are kinder to the environment and kinder to surfaces.

Paint thinners. Oil-based paints, such as glosses, require solvent thinners, such as white spirit, for cleanup. These are made of toxic chemicals, so pour the minimum amount necessary into a jar and soak the brush to remove paint. You can reuse most of the thinner if you first let the paint settle to the bottom of the jar, and then pour the clear liquid on top back into the original bottle. Wrap the remaining paint and particles in newspaper before throwing them away.

Paintbrush cleaners. Clean brushes as soon as you're done using them to avoid paint buildup. Always wash out latex paint in the sink, not in outdoor gutters. Most emulsions only require soap and water to clean. If you have difficultly with soap and water alone, you can also try to use a waterless hand cleaner, as favored by mechanics, working it into the brush before rinsing with soap and water. Paintbrushes hardened with oil-based paint can be cleaned by soaking them in hot vinegar for as long as necessary.

Spray paints. These should be avoided if at all possible. Aerosol sprays make the paint easier to inhale and the propellants in the can contribute to air pollution.

Wood preservatives. Avoid old products containing pentachlorophenol (PCP), which has been shown to cause cancer in laboratory animals, *creosote, tributyltin oxide,* or *folpet.* Wood preservatives containing arsenates are toxic to the nervous system. Burning old wood that has been treated with these preservatives releases these chemicals into the atmosphere. Seek advice from your local authorities about the best way to dispose of treated wood. When buying new wood products, especially for the garden, look for those made from woods that are naturally re-sistant to insects and wood rot, such as redwood and cedar. Alternatively, water-based preservatives are available that can seal wood and protect it from water rot and insects. Polyurethane spread under outdoor decking can prevent wood rot.

Wood stains and finishes. Use water-based stains whenever you can. Alterna-tively, look for finishes made from natural sources, such as beeswax, linseed oil, shellac, and tung oil.

8. HOME AND GARDEN PESTICIDES

No one likes the thought of sharing a living space with pests. While most of us have a clear idea of the kind of creepy crawlies we'd like to keep away—rodents, cockroaches, and flies, for instance—a pest can be broadly defined as any plant, animal, or otherwise that happens to be in the wrong place at the wrong time!

So, in addition to liberally treating our homes with commercial bug sprays, we spend billions each year trying to control the environment outdoors with a raft of garden pesticides, fungicides, and weed killers. Indeed, every year, in our obsessive bid to remove all traces of the humble dandelion from the earth's surface, we spray tons of toxic chemicals on home lawns, parks, playgrounds, golf courses, and other recreation grounds—not because dandelions are inherently bad, but purely because this little plant has taken root somewhere inconvenient. Whatever pest you are trying to control, keeping it at bay with conventional pest-control products comes at a hefty cost.

While many of us worry about the pesticides that might be lingering in or on our food these days, few give more than a moment's thought before whipping out the bug spray whenever a wasp or troop of ants invades the house. This is why the vast majority of our pesticide exposure—some 80 percent according to U.S. data—actually happens in our homes, offices, and schools, with measurable levels of up to twelve different pesticides found in the air of the average home.

In one 1995 survey, somewhere in the region of 85 percent of American homes were found to have at least three to four different pesticide products in them, including pest strips, bait boxes, bug bombs, flea collars, pesticide-containing pet shampoos, aerosols, granules, liquids, and dusts. Many household products, such as disinfectants, cleansers, and mildew removers, also contain pesticides.

The picture is much the same in the U.K. The British public spends close to $100 million on pesticide products for their homes and gardens. According to the Pesticide Action Network (PAN) U.K., British householders are dousing their homes and gardens with pesticides to the tune of 4,306 tons of pesticides each year. Worse, as much as 20 percent of these pesticides were disposed of by householders pouring them down the drain. Once in the water supply, these nasty chemicals become everyone's problem, since most water-treatment facilities cannot adequately remove these chemicals from tap water.

Of course, we don't just drink this water—we bathe and shower in it as well. It has been suggested that the amount of volatile chemicals inhaled during a fifteen-minute shower with contaminated water is equivalent to drinking about eight glasses of contaminated water. In addition, many industrial contaminants can easily pass through the skin into the body during showers, baths, and dishwashing, more than doubling the amount of chemicals that pass into your body.

Think pesticides, and the first thing that is likely to come to mind is insecticide, the stuff we use to kill ants, flies, and cockroaches. But the term "pesticide" is a blanket description for many other types of chemicals, such as bacteriocides (which kill bacteria), herbicides (which target plants), fungicides (which kill fungi), and rodenticides (the poisons laid down to kill rodents). These days, a pesticide can also be an organism, including, for example, a genetically modified crop.

Amazingly, given their widespread use, the pesticides that we use nowadays didn't even exist before World War II. In fact, many of today's most widely used types of pesticides were intended for use as chemical weapons. Organophosphates, which disable an insect's nervous system, were first developed as nerve gases. One of the most commonly used herbicides, 2,4-D, belongs to a family of pesticides known as phenoxys, which were used in World War II to destroy the Japanese rice crop. In the Vietnam War, 2,4-D was a component of the highly toxic defoliant Agent Orange.

After the war, the chemical manufacturers needed to find other uses for their products, which had been produced in massive quantities. And so they began to be applied as pesticides in agricultural production, for environmental spraying of neighborhoods for mosquito eradication, and for individual home and garden use.

Although pesticides can be helpful in the short term around your home and garden, they can be dangerous if applied or stored carelessly—for instance, within the reach of children. It's worth remembering that pesticides are chemical weapons. They are designed to kill things. For this reason, they are not really safe—even when used as directed. Regularly inhaling them, ingesting them, or getting them on your skin constitutes a cumulative assault on your health. This is because most pesticides are poisonous and persistent chemicals—they don't biodegrade in your body or the environment, so the more you use them, the more they will accumulate around and inside you.

Pesticide products are made up of a mixture of active ingredients (the chemicals that kill specific organisms) and inactive, or inert, ingredients (the chemical base in which the active ingredients are mixed; see page 215 for more on inerts). Most pesticides on the market have not undergone a complete battery of tests to find out exactly how harmful their ingredients might be to humans. What's more, while some pesticides have been subjected to safety testing, as with all the other chemicals you will find in your home, they are tested one at a time. Yet, research from Duke University in North Carolina has shown that when three pesticides (used at their "safe" levels) are combined, their toxicity is increased by a factor of several hundred.

Our enthusiasm for pesticides in the home and garden is now such that U.S. scientists have concluded that pesticide overexposure—once an occupational hazard of agricultural and factory workers—is now everybody's problem. Home use of pesticides rose 42 percent between 1998 and 2001. In the garden, herbicides are applied more intensively for lawn care than they are on most farms, with application rates of between 3.2 to 9.8 pounds per acre for lawns, compared with agricultural averages of 2.7 pounds per acre.

As our use of home and garden pesticides increases, evidence is also accumulating on the health effects of this exposure in adults and children, and, while it has long been assumed that you need to be exposed to high levels of pesticides to be damaged by them, emerging evidence says this isn't so. The weed killer atrazine, for example, is an estrogen mimic that has been shown to feminize male frogs at levels ten thousand to thirty thousand times below the presumed safe limits.

How We Are Exposed to Pesticides

Pesticides get into our bodies in a variety of ways. We can ingest them with our food and water, and they can be inhaled or absorbed through the skin when we are using sprays or foggers. While agricultural use still accounts for the major use of pesticides in the world, their applications in other areas that intersect with our lives daily has become more widespread, moving from the field to the main street to the home, without much apparent inquiry into either appropriateness or safety or, more crucially, alternatives.

Sources of common household pesticides include bathroom- and kitchen-cleaning products, wallpaper pastes, paint, wooden furniture (especially if it is made from recycled railway ties), insecticides for wood (such as woodworm treatments), and mothballs, roach, fly, and wasp sprays, pest strips, sprays for indoor plants, head-lice and intestinal-parasite treatments, swimming-pool and spa disinfectants and algaecides, and pest and weed killers used in the garden. Our irrational fear of bugs has also led to soft furnishings, carpets, and mattresses being pretreated with powerful pesticides, such as permethrin (the same pesticide implicated in the debilitating symptoms of Gulf War syndrome).

But even if you don't use pesticides in your home, you cannot avoid being exposed. If your neighbor treats his home or lawn, chances are you'll be breathing it in. If you are walking down a street where the local pest control has just sprayed, you will get it on your clothes and into your lungs. If you picnic in the park or play a few rounds of golf, you will be exposed.

Grocery stores, restaurants, hotels, hospital cafeterias, schools, and many apartment buildings and nursing homes are routinely sprayed and fumigated. Wooden playground equipment, decking, and picnic tables are treated with a variety of substances, including arsenic.

Know Your Pesticides

There are many different types of pesticides, each made from different starting materials and each with its own particular effects on the body.

A major 2004 review of the human health effects of pesticide exposure by the Ontario College of Family Physicians concluded that, while there is a widely held perception that some pesticides are safer than others, this is not backed up by the evidence. They write: "Exposure to all the commonly used pesticides—phenoxyherbicides, organophosphates, carbamates, and pyrethrins—has shown positive associations with adverse health effects. The literature does not support the concept that some pesticides are safer than others; it simply points to different health effects with different latency periods for the different classes."

Below are some of the main classes of pesticides you will come into contact with in your home and garden, as well as in the wider community.

Organochlorines

The main representatives of chlorinated pesticides are aldrin, dieldrin, chlordane, heptachlor, transnonachlor, DDT and its metabolites (DDE, DDD), endrin, hexachlorobenzene, and lindane (alpha, beta, delta, BHC). This group of chemicals also includes polychlorinated biphenyls (PCBs), originally used as electrical coolants, but which have also been used to kill bugs. These have been used extensively in agriculture, in forestry, and even in households over the last twenty years. Some organochlorines have been banned in Canada and the United States due to their persistence in the environment. They are still manufactured in Canada and the United States and exported to developing countries for use in agriculture there, however. Chlorinated pesticides are hormone-disrupting and

Railway lines, waterways, embankments, and city and suburban streets are regularly doused with bug-zapping chemicals. Even underground electric cables are treated with insecticides, such as aldrin and chlordane, to discourage any insects that may make the mistake of munching on them.

Most forms of public transportation, such as buses and underground trains, make use of pesticides by being regularly fumigated. Airlines keen to get rid of insects looking for a free ride regularly fumigate their planes. This is particularly worrisome since pesticides, while already dangerous on land, have the potential to be particularly harmful when used on planes, as up to 50 percent of the air inside the cabins is recycled. This means that passengers can sometimes find themselves sealed for hours at a stretch in a poorly ventilated chamber that has recently been gassed with no escape from the chemicals in the air. Interestingly, the symptoms of severe jet lag are very similar to pesticide poisoning.

can cause various conditions in humans, including cancer. PCB exposure can result in neurological disorders, malignant melanoma, and liver cancer.

Organophosphates

These have largely replaced organochlorines in agricultural pest control. They are often portrayed as safer than organochlorines because they break down more rapidly. Nevertheless, many organophosphates, such as parathion, malathion, diazinon, phosmet, and chlorpyrifos are highly toxic. They affect the central nervous system (CNS; the brain and spinal cord) and peripheral nervous system (nerves found outside the CNS). This particularly affects the muscles, glands, and smooth muscles that are related to organ function, and has been found to cause delayed neurotoxicity involving the cerebral cortex, brain stem, spinal cord, peripheral nerves, muscles, and eyes. Symptoms can appear thirty minutes after exposure and may last for up to twenty-four hours.

Carbamates

Including aldicarb, bendiocarb, carbaryl, propoxur, and thiophanate methyl, carbamates are used extensively in agriculture, forestry, and gardening. The immediate effects of exposure include muscle weakness, altered perception, headache, nausea, vomiting, abdominal pain, visual problems, and muscle twitches. Over the longer term, these compounds are associated with a higher risk of lung cancer, with reproductive effects including damage to testes, sperm, and DNA, and behavioral effects.

continues on following page . . .

How Do Pesticides Work?

All pesticides are lethal. Their sole purpose is to destroy plant and animal life. While we think of pesticides as being exclusively synthetic in origin, and indeed the vast majority are, there are many natural substances that can be concentrated into a pesticide mixture to the point where they become deadly to living things. Most work by interfering with the normal life-sustaining processes of the organism. Pesticides have this effect on simple organisms, such as bacteria, and they also can do the same on more complex organisms like humans. Disturbingly, the way most pesticides work is not fully understood, but most produce their toxic effects by:

• **Blocking photosynthesis.** Plants "breathe" in carbon dioxide and then use the energy from sunlight to turn the carbon dioxide into carbohydrates, or stored energy. This process is known as photosynthesis. Pesticides that disrupt this process starve plants of the energy they need to grow.

• **Interfering with metabolism.** Metabolism refers to the way a living organism transfers energy between cells. This transfer of energy is vital for the growth and survival of all living things. Pesticides that interfere with metabolism usually have to be ingested or inhaled before they become toxic to the target pest. Once inside the body, inhibitory pesticides like *rotenone* and cyanide disrupt respiratory function in animals (oxygen is necessary to fuel metabolism). In

---

Know Your Pesticides

Phenoxys

In this group of toxic chemicals, the most well known are 2,4-D and 2,4,5-T, which, when proportionately mixed, constitute Agent Orange. Extensively used in the control of terrestrial broadleaved plants, they have been proven to cause leukopenia, and non-Hodgkin's lymphoma and lung cancer. Agent Orange exposure has recently been linked to the development of type 2 diabetes.

Pyrethrins

Pyrethrins occur in nature in many plants, but today's pyrethrin pesticides are produced in the lab and known as synthetic pyrethrins (SPs). SPs interfere with the function of the insect's nervous system. They can be found in spray-on products, in flea, tick, and head-lice treatments, and also imbedded into most soft furnishings. Examples include *allethrin*, syfluthrin, *cypermethrin, deltamethrin,* and plants, herbicides that interfere with metabolism work by inhibiting seed germination or plant growth (especially at the root and shoot tips).

- **Interfering with nerve function and signaling.** Neurotoxic pesticides are most commonly used on insects, nematodes, and rodents. Organophosphate, carbamate, and pyrethroid pesticides disrupt the flow of nerve impulses, while others, such as the pesticides used in fumigants, have a narcotic effect.

- **Causing genetic damage.** Our chromosomes carry genes, and both are made up of DNA—the control center of higher organisms. Chemicals that disrupt DNA can stop the organism from reproducing or alter the way it functions in important ways. Male insects can be made sterile with such pesticides. Interfering with DNA can disrupt the rate and timing of a range of cellular functions. When the cells don't function properly, neither does the organism.

- **Causing hormone disruption.** Hormones are biochemical messengers vital to the control of reproduction and growth as well as many other biological functions of plants, animals, and insects. Some types of pesticides mimic or block the actions of hormones, such as estrogen and testosterone, thus interfering with reproduction, or mimic or block thyroid and other growth-regulating hormones, thus preventing the organism from thriving.

- **Preventing protein synthesis and causing enzyme disruption.** The cells of living organisms are made from protein. Certain pesticides can denature cell

resmethrin. Exposure to pyrethrins is associated with chronic psychiatric effects, chromosomal aberrations, rashes in licensed pet groomers, and intrauterine growth retardation, which is a major determinant of poor health in the first year of life.

Thiocarbamates

This group of fungicides includes the EBDCs (ethylene bis-dithiocarbamates) mancozeb, *maneb*, and metiram. EBDC use is becoming more widespread. When these chemicals are used on stored produce and when such contaminated fruit and/or vegetables are cooked, EBDC's active ingredients break down into ethylenethiourea (ETU). ETU can cause goiters (enlargement of the thyroid gland), birth defects, and cancer in exposed experimental animals. It has been classified by the U.S. Environmental Protection Agency (EPA) as a probable human carcinogen.

proteins or interfere with the enzymes necessary to metabolize protein and maintain healthy cell function.

Some pesticides work in more than one way and fall into more than one of these categories. Some are physically toxic—in other words, they block the cellular processes of target organisms in a purely mechanical way. Examples include spray oils that clog the respiratory mechanisms of insects, petroleum oils that dissolve protective waxes on some insects and plants, or substances that destroy the membranes of plant cells, causing them to dry out and die. Some petroleum oils can deter feeding or egg laying in some insects.

Toxic Lumber Treatments

Wood used for, among other things, playground equipment, climbing frames, patio decking, picnic tables, fencing, and shelving is treated with preservatives to help keep wood-munching bugs at bay. Wood preservatives are pesticides, and, because wood is porous, they can easily leach out of the wood and onto hands and feet, and into food. Exposure to wood treatments has been shown to raise the risk of several types of cancer:

- A 1998 study of men whose work exposed them to wood-preservation chemicals found that chlorophenol exposure may increase the risk of soft-tissue sarcoma.
- Data published in 1997 concluded there was an increased risk of non-Hodgkin's lymphoma associated with *chlorophenate* exposure among sawmill workers. Chlorophenate was widely used as a wood preservative and fungicide from the 1940s up to 1989, when its use was discontinued.
- In Germany in 1995 investigators found that women exposed to the organochlorine-, pentachlorophenol- (PCP), or lindane-based wood preservatives used in day-care centers gave birth to significantly smaller babies than nonexposed women.
- Many outdoor wood products are pressure-treated with *chromated copper arsenate* (CCA). These products constitute our biggest exposure to the toxic element arsenic. CCA is poisonous to humans, and easily rubs off treated wood. According to a 1990 U.S. Consumer Product Safety Commission study entitled "Estimate of Risk of Skin Cancer from Dislodgeable Arsenic on Pressure Treated Wood Playground Equipment," very young children, who are always putting their hands into their mouths, can ingest up to 2,016 mcg (micrograms) of arsenic per day from just playing on treated wood. To put this dosage into

Inert Ingredients

Some product labels, especially those on household cleaners and garden products, list only the active ingredients. The rest of the ingredients are considered inert, or inactive, and therefore assumed to be harmless. But the average consumer should be aware that the word "inert" on product labels is completely misleading. Far from being inactive or nonreactive, inert ingredients in pesticide products may include highly toxic chemicals.

Among the 2,300 inert ingredients used in pesticide formulations, over 1,700 of them are of unknown toxicity, 209 are hazardous air and water pollutants, 21 are known or suspected carcinogens, and 127 are listed as occupational hazards, according to a 1998 report by the Northwest Coalition for Alternatives to Pesticides. Because so-called inert ingredients are considered harmless, they are not

perspective, the maximum safe amount of arsenic for a twenty-five-pound child is 3.4 mcg/day. Arsenic is implicated in liver, lung, skin, bladder, kidney, and prostate cancers. Low but chronic exposures can produce such symptoms as stomachache, nausea, vomiting, and diarrhea.

During the lifetime of treated wood, especially if it's outdoors, the chemicals used to preserve wood can be washed away into the soil, eventually making their way into the water table. At the end of its life cycle, treated wood may be chopped up for mulch or wood chippings, and recycled back into our gardens, where it continues to pollute the soil and surrounding area for years to come.

Animals suffer from our use of wood treatments as well. In the U.K., bat populations have declined sharply as a direct result of the chemical treatment of roof timbers against pests.

Chemical treatment of wood pests in homes or workplaces is always toxic, and there are strong arguments to support the theory that such chemical treatment is less effective, more expensive, and more dangerous than alternative traditional methods.

The pests that attack wood in buildings belong to two main groups: wood-boring insects and fungal rots. Pest problems arise where the environmental conditions are comfortable for them. Dry rot, wet rot, and many wood-boring insects will only be found in damp wood.

So, solve your dampness problem and you will have gone a long way toward solving your pest problem. Consider measures to manage the physical environment in terms of dampness, ventilation, and temperature, adequate damp-proofing, replacement of severely damaged wood, and use of materials and building techniques that reduce the risk of future pest attack.

subjected to safety reviews. Interestingly, a chemical that is listed as inert in one product may be listed as an active ingredient in another.

The lack of disclosure of potentially toxic inert ingredients on product labels places consumers who wish to protect their health at a distinct disadvantage. This is especially true since inert ingredients can combine synergistically to create powerful toxins (see "The Cocktail Effect," page 28).

When most of us think of the toxicity of pesticides, we tend to think of the active ingredients—the pesticide(s) that are included to kill bugs. But, in common with many pharmaceutical drugs, cosmetics, cleaners, soaps, and perfumes, the active ingredients are usually present within a matrix of inactive or inert ingredients to improve storage, handling, application, and effectiveness.

Inert ingredients are sometimes referred to as secret ingredients because the recipe developed by chemists to meet all the requirements of storage, handling, application, effectiveness, and safety is considered a trade secret and, as such, is protected by law. What is public knowledge is the list of EPA-approved substances that can be used in pesticide products.

For years, no one paid any attention to inactive pesticide ingredients until it began to emerge that some very harmful chemicals were being added to these formulations under the misnomer of inert ingredients.

Even the notorious and harmful pesticide DDT has been used as an inert ingredient since its ban in most developed countries as an active ingredient. The EPA acknowledges that there is a complete lack of health-effect data on some 800 inert ingredients used in pesticide formulations, and at least 160 inert ingredients are known toxic chemicals, including solvents, such as chloroform, toluene, and xylene.

The Toxicity of Inerts

The term "inert" implies that a substance is nontoxic and does not interact with other chemicals or bodily systems. But determining which chemicals are inert and which ones are not is not straightforward. In theory only inert ingredients approved by the EPA are allowed in pesticide products. But in reality all inert ingredients have some level of toxicity. This toxicity can be increased by mixing with other chemicals in a pesticide product. Likewise, inerts can sometimes mix with other chemicals to form new compounds that are themselves harmful.

INACTIVE INGREDIENT	ADVERSE EFFECTS
carbon tetrachloride	Irritation of skin, eyes, nose, throat; dizziness, vomiting, abdominal pain; diarrhea; damage to kidneys, liver; CNS depression; suspected carcinogen
chlorobenzene	Eye and skin irritation, burns, and inflammation; chest pain, slow heart rate, ECG irregularities; lung, liver, and kidney damage; CNS depression; coma
chloroform	Irritation to eyes and gastrointestinal tract; damage to liver and kidneys; CNS depression; nausea, dizziness, fatigue, respiratory distress; gonadal atrophy; fetal resorption; mutagen; coma and death by cardiac arrest; suspected carcinogen
chloroethane	Irritation of eyes; abdominal cramps, nausea, vomiting; liver and kidney damage; neurological dysfunction; blood cell disorders; suspected carcinogen
cresols	Skin irritation, burns, and inflammation; irritation of eye, permanent eye damage and blindness; pneumonia; pancreatitis; CNS disorders; kidney failure
dibutylphthalate	Irritation of eyes and throat; photophobia, conjunctivitis, nausea, dizziness
diethylhexylphthalate	Eye, nose, and throat irritation; liver damage; testicular damage; CNS depression; suspected carcinogen
dimethylphthalate	Irritation of eyes, mouth, nose, and throat; dizziness, abdominal pain, nausea, vomiting, diarrhea; CNS depression; reduced respiratory rate; paralysis, coma
epichlorohydrin	Skin and eye irritation, conjunctivitis, corneal clouding; nausea, vomiting, fatigue; liver and kidney damage; inflammation of lungs, chronic bronchitis; death by respiratory paralysis; mutagenic; fetotoxic
ethylbenzene	Irritation of eyes, nose, and throat; skin irritation, inflammation, blisters, and burns; liver and kidney damage; CNS disorders; headache, sleepiness, difficulty breathing; loss of consciousness and coma
ethylene dichloride	Nausea, vomiting, diarrhea; damage to liver and kidneys; CNS depression; death due to circulatory and respiratory failure
isophorone	Irritation of skin, nose, throat, and respiratory system; lung congestion and degeneration; CNS disorders; kidney and liver damage; suspected carcinogen
methyl bromide	Eye and skin irritation; blurred vision, headache, dizziness, nausea, abdominal cramps; anorexia; bronchopneumonia, pulmonary edema; brain damage, convulsions, coma; kidney and respiratory failure

continues on following page . . .

o-dichlorobenzene	Eye irritation and cataracts; skin irritation and lesions; headache, nausea, vomiting, drowsiness; respiratory depression; anemia; kidney and liver damage; chromosomal breaks
p-dichlorobenzene	Irritation of skin, eyes, respiratory system; headache, dizziness, hyperactivity, weakness, weight loss; liver and blood disorders; kidney damage; lung congestion, difficulty breathing; mutagenic
phenol	Irritation of eyes, nose, throat; headache, dizziness, fainting, abdominal pain, nausea, vomiting, diarrhea; damage to liver, kidneys, and heart; chromosomal aberrations and damage; mutagenic
propylene dichloride	Eye and skin irritation; dizziness, disorientation, nausea, vomiting; liver and kidney damage; CNS damage; coma; hemolytic anemia; suspected carcinogen
1,1,2-trichloroethane	Gastrointestinal inflammation and congestion; liver and kidney damage; immune-function disorder; CNS depression; suspected carcinogen
toluene	Skin, eye, and respiratory irritation; abdominal pain, headache, nausea, dizziness, drowsiness, hallucinations; anemia; liver disorders and enlargement; CNS dysfunction; coma and death
trichloroethylene	Eye irritation, visual distortion; abdominal pain, nausea, diarrhea; anorexia; liver and kidney damage; peripheral nerve damage, numbness, and paralysis; blood disorders; cardiac arrhythmia; suspected carcinogen

The 'Cide Effects

Every year, millions of people worldwide (mostly in developing countries) suffer severe poisonings from pesticides. Many more are exposed to levels that are considered low but are still dangerous to health. Regular pesticide use is also associated with neurological effects, decreased immunity, and reproductive and developmental abnormalities.

Pesticides are a significant and avoidable source of toxicity today. Unlike some forms of toxic exposure in the home, it is fairly easy to identify a cause-and-effect link between pesticide use and ill health, and to track the adverse health effects from home and garden use. But there are other, equally worrisome, effects. What's more, these effects are not new.

By the late 1950s, a number of commonly used pesticides, including DDT and arsenates, had been linked with disorders ranging from leukemia to skin cancer. In 1955, rising rates of hepatitis in the United States were being linked to the increasing use of DDT and other chlorinated pesticides.

As of 1990, 117 different pesticides still in use were identified as potential causes of chronic health problems; 27 of these show strong evidence of carcinogenicity (yet only 6 of these require specific warnings on labels as to this health hazard). The other 90 pesticides cause such problems as birth defects and sterility.

There are, however, many who dispute the idea that pesticides kill people as well as bugs. They argue that daily exposure levels are low, and that such products would not be on sale if they weren't safe. But such arguments fly in the face of mounting evidence that pesticide exposure is causing deep and lasting harm to our health.

Pesticides can act as general poisons or they can target specific systems in the body, such as the immune system, the central nervous system, and the endocrine (hormonal) system. Some cause genetic damage that can be permanent and passed on to the next generation, and even subsequent generations. These important noncancer effects of pesticides have not been the focus of much study by government health authorities.

- **Acute "ill-defined" symptoms.** Typical symptoms that can occur following an acute exposure to pesticides include nausea, low energy levels, weakness, sleep problems, dizziness, headache, migraine, anxiety, depression, aching joints, mental disorientation, inability to concentrate, vomiting, convulsions, skin irritations/rashes, flu-like symptoms, allergic reactions, and asthma-like problems.

- **Chronic health effects.** These effects include cancer (in children and adults); birth defects; genetic damage; neurological, psychological, and behavioral effects; blood disorders; chemical sensitivities; reproductive effects; and abnormalities in liver, kidney, and immune function. These chronic health effects can develop following either an acute poisoning or low-level exposure over an extended period of time.

The ill-defined symptoms of pesticide exposure can, of course, be the result of a number of different conditions or diseases. Nevertheless, according to a 2003 report issued by the Health Care Without Harm organization, "Pesticide poisonings are frequently misdiagnosed or unrecognized, largely because most health care providers receive minimal training in environmental illnesses and few people know when they have been exposed to a pesticide."

Children at Risk

Concern over children's increased risk from pesticide exposure is not new. In 1989, the U.S. Natural Resources Defense Council (NRDC) alleged that as many as sixty-two hundred children might develop cancer later in life due to exposure to just eight pesticides during their preschool years. That same year, the EPA released a preliminary report suggesting that between fifteen thousand and fifty thousand infants and children in the United States each day run the risk of getting sick from potatoes on which the insecticide aldicarb has been used. But, as always, it is the link between pesticide exposure and the development of childhood cancer that has grabbed most of the headlines.

Childhood Cancer

In spite of the objections of major chemical companies, the evidence linking pesticide exposure to childhood cancer is firmly established, though not all studies show that it is the ingestion of pesticides that poses the greatest risk. Research has shown that pesticide use in the home—for instance, to get rid of termites, flies, and wasps, and in the form of no-pest strips, flea collars, and garden insecticides and herbicides—resulted in a significant increase in childhood brain cancers.

Other reports and studies have linked pesticide exposure to a wide range of malignancies in children, including leukemia, neuroblastoma, Wilms' tumor of

Increasing Our Vulnerability

Many aspects of our lifestyles make us more or less vulnerable to health problems of pesticide exposure. Certainly, women and children are more vulnerable because they tend to be smaller and so, pound for pound, receive a higher exposure than most men.

In addition, specific health conditions or individual vulnerabilities that directly increase susceptibility to pesticide effects include:

- alcoholism
- autoimmune conditions (such as lupus)
- blood disorders (such as anemia)
- chemical sensitivity
- colitis
- diabetes
- elderly (age seventy-four and over)
- heart disease
- homelessness
- immune dysfunction
- kidney disease
- leukemia
- liver disease
- lung disease (chronic)
- malnourishment
- neurological disease
- previous pesticide exposure
- pregnant and lactating women and their offspring
- prescription medications

the kidneys, and non-Hodgkin's lymphoma, as well as cancers of the brain, colorectum, and testes.

Childhood leukemia was linked to indoor and outdoor pesticide use in a 1987 study published in the *Journal of the National Cancer Institute*. The risk increased nearly four times when pesticides were used within the home at least once a week, and by more than six times when garden pesticides were used at least once a month.

In another 1995 study involving 474 children, those living in homes where no-pest strips embedded with insecticides were used had up to a threefold greater risk of developing leukemia than those living in homes without the strips. Even worse, children under age fourteen had four times the normal risk of tumors of connective tissue if their gardens at home were treated with pesticides or herbicides.

In the same study, pregnant women exposed to the pesticides used by professional exterminators in their homes were three times more likely to have a child with non-Hodgkin's lymphoma, and children directly exposed to pesticides by professional exterminators were more than twice as likely to develop the disease.

Otherwise rare cancers can also become more common with exposure to pesticides. One study at the University of Southern California found that children whose mothers used pesticides in the home once or twice a week were nearly two

- skin conditions (which increase dermal absorption)
- smoking
- youth (age thirteen or under)

Our prescription-drug culture complicates the picture further by introducing the risk of drug-pesticide reactions. About 10 percent of all prescription drugs are known to increase the toxicity of pesticides. These include:

- ambenonium
- beta-blockers (for heart conditions)
- chemotherapy
- cimetidine (Tagamet)
- cycrimine (for Parkinsonism)
- demarcarium
- digoxin
- glaucoma medications
- isoflurophate
- methimazole (Tapazole)
- myasthenia gravis medications
- neostigmine
- phenobarbital
- phenytoin
- phospholine iodide (echothiophate)
- physostigmine
- pilocarpine
- procaine (used in general anesthesia)
- propranolol (Inderol)
- pyridostigmine
- succinylcholine (used in general anesthesia)

and a half times as likely to develop non-Hodgkin's lymphoma. Those whose mothers used pesticides on a daily basis were seven times more likely to have the cancer.

Child Development and Intelligence

There is also ongoing concern regarding the toxic effects of pesticides on the developing brain and nervous system. In 1998, German researchers, for example, reported that early exposure to polychlorinated biphenyls (PCBs), which are sometimes found in pesticides, can interfere with early childhood development.

The researchers looked at both the pre- and postnatal exposure of 171 otherwise healthy infants and measured their development at seven, eighteen, thirty, and forty-two months. At all of these ages, there was evidence that PCB exposure could retard mental and motor development. The only good news in the study was the fact that where the mother breast-fed her infant for longer (even if her breast milk was a source of PCBs) and in families where parents provided a stimulating home environment, the damage done by the PCBs was significantly less.

In another 1998 study, entitled "An Anthropological Approach to the Evaluation of Preschool Children Exposed to Pesticides in Mexico," published in the journal *Environmental Health Perspectives*, children exposed to a variety of pesticides in an agricultural community in Mexico showed impaired stamina, coordination, memory, and capacity to represent familiar subjects in simple drawings. Yet another study showed that children exposed to PCBs during fetal life had IQ deficits, and hyperactivity and attention deficits, when tested years later.

Adult Exposures

Among adults exposed to pesticides, there are three major areas of concern: cancer; reproductive effects (ranging from sterility, infertility, and subfertility to birth defects, stillbirths, and miscarriage); and effects on the brain and central nervous system (neurotoxicity). It is highly likely that the link with adult diseases reflects a lifetime's exposure to pesticides beginning in childhood.

Generally speaking, ingested pesticides, like many other toxins, are stored in fatty tissue and released gradually into the bloodstream, especially during periods of stress. Also in common with many toxic exposures, the early signs and symptoms associated with chronic exposure to pesticides are often labeled "idiopathic" (of unknown origin) or "psychosomatic," a diagnosis that prevents the person from getting the help needed to get well again.

Adult Cancers

Throughout the world, studies have shown that the risk of different cancers increases with increasing pesticide exposure. In adults, the use of chlorophenoxy acid herbicides (such as 2,4-D) has been linked with an increased incidence of lung cancer, stomach cancer, and leukemia. Two studies have found a fivefold increased risk of Hodgkin's lymphoma, and other evidence suggests a five- to sixfold increased risk for non-Hodgkin's lymphoma.

In addition, many studies have shown a two- to sevenfold increased risk of soft-tissue sarcomas. One showed that farmers in Kansas using herbicides for as few as twenty days a year have six times the risk of developing lymphoma and soft-tissue sarcomas compared with nonexposed individuals. Those who mixed and applied herbicides and were exposed for twenty or more days per year were eight times as likely to develop non-Hodgkin's lymphoma.

In 1992, a Swedish investigation of 275 confirmed cases of multiple myeloma (cancer that starts in the bone marrow and spreads to various bones, especially the skull) among farmers found that exposure to chlorophenoxy acid herbicides and DDT were the most important risk factors for the disease.

Neurological Disorders

Pesticide exposure is increasingly being linked to a number of neurological disorders now common in old age. While research in this area is still in its infancy, there is a good theoretical basis for the idea that pesticide exposure can lead to degenerative disorders, such as Alzheimer's and Parkinson's diseases.

Many pesticides are designed specifically to attack and destroy the nervous systems of insects. Once disabled, the insect is not able to fly or move its legs; paralyzed and unable to feed itself, it dies. It is likely that chronic exposure to some pesticides will do much the same to the human nervous system, though research into this area is sparse.

Nevertheless, there is some evidence to suggest that people who are frequently exposed to pesticides, such as farmers and gardeners, have a higher risk of developing mild cognitive dysfunction (MCD). MCD is a somewhat more subtle disorder than dementia, though the two share some common symptoms, such as memory loss and confusion. In 2000, a study from the Netherlands found that adults exposed to pesticides on a regular basis—for instance, farmers and gardeners—had five or more times the usual risk of developing the subtle neurological impairments or learning problems considered common in MCD.

Osteoporosis

Other deleterious effects of pesticides have recently come to light. A 1999 analysis of bone density in agricultural workers published in the scientific journal *Lancet* showed that exposure to pesticides can make bones significantly more porous.

The discovery was made when British researchers assessed agricultural workers seeking litigation for ill health caused by chronic exposure to organophosphates. The men had been exposed to this type of pesticide for between three and twenty years at some point in their lives. Bone biopsies showed significant erosion of the bones in the exposed men as well as much lower bone formation at tissue and cellular levels compared with nonexposed men.

Because of a lack of data, the researchers were unable to say categorically whether the damage to the bone was a direct or indirect result of exposure to organophosphates. While the pesticide can directly enter bone and cause damage, it can also produce other symptoms (such as lethargy, fatigue, and depression) that may limit an individual's level of physical activity and, thus, have a further, indirect impact on bone health.

Diabetes

Recent research suggests that exposure to herbicides during the Vietnam War, especially Agent Orange (a mixture of the pesticides 2,4-D and 2,4,5-T), may be associated with the development of diabetes later in life.

When published, the results of this study were treated as isolated and relevant only to Vietnam vets. But the use of 2,4-D is particularly widespread even today. It is commonly used by local authorities to inhibit weed growth on roads and walking paths. It can also be purchased at garden stores for home lawn care and is often used by commercial lawn-care companies.

No one understands exactly how pesticides can cause changes in glucose metabolism or lead to diabetes, but it may be the result of some sort of hormonal effects.

Lowered Immunity

For years, nobody was sure whether pesticide exposure could damage immunity or not. Then, in 1996, scientists at the Washington, D.C.–based World Resources Institute (WRI) undertook a review of all reports of compromised immunity as a result of pesticide exposure. The conclusion was that many widely used pesticides are deeply damaging to human immune function.

Many of the studies reviewed by the WRI scientists came from the former Soviet Union, one of the few places where scientists have examined the impact of pesticides on human immunity. In one investigation of water and soil contamination in Kishinëv, in Moldova, high levels of pesticide residues on many local crops resulted in elevated rates of skin diseases, tuberculosis, tooth decay, ear infections, and acute respiratory diseases among the local children. Rates of infection in adults were also higher than expected, and laboratory testing revealed that as an individual's exposure to pesticides went up, so the levels of T cells (infection-fighting cells) went down.

The report also included data from studies of Inuit children in the northern Hudson Bay area of Canada. The children, nursed on human milk highly contaminated with organochlorine pollutants, not only suffered an increased risk of infections, but some had immune systems so depressed that they could not withstand a standard course of childhood vaccinations.

Pesticides may also interfere with thyroid function, and this, in turn, may have a debilitating effect on immunity. The mechanisms by which pesticides might affect human thyroid function are not clear, though some have hypothesized that pesticides deplete the body's mineral stores, thereby resulting in thyroid disorders.

Chronic Fatigue

In traditional Indian, or Ayurvedic, medicine, chronic fatigue syndrome (CFS) is considered the result of accumulated toxins in the body. Western medicine, too, is beginning to acknowledge the link between CFS and chemical poisoning. Pesticide poisoning, for example, can produce symptoms similar to CFS and fibromyalgia (widespread musculoskeletal pain, tenderness, and fatigue), and patients suffering from chronic fatigue have been found to have, on average, twice the levels of pesticides in their blood compared with those not suffering from CFS.

Organophosphate pesticides and insecticides, in particular, are strongly associated with CFS—a condition identical to that suffered by farm workers who regularly work with sheep dips and insecticides.

Looking for more evidence of a connection, scientists in Glasgow studied a small group of individuals who had been experiencing neurobehavioral symptoms for over a year, and who had been exposed to organophosphates—through sheep dip—for between two and five years. Their symptoms included an acute flu-like condition followed by incapacitating fatigue. In all cases, there was a long delay between exposure to the pesticides and the onset of the condition—a problem seen with many toxic exposures and one that, for a doctor who knows nothing about environmental illness, makes diagnosis difficult.

Dealing with Household Pests Naturally

Insect pests are an intimate part of every home. In the air or the cupboard, on the carpet or the counter, every home shares its resources with these tiny, often unseen invaders. But many pesticides now in use are simply not necessary. Opportunistic pests can be kept at bay with regular cleaning and attention to basic hygiene measures. Don't leave food out on countertops and, where possible, consider installing screens over windows to keep flying bugs out. The use of fungicides (for instance, in the bathroom) can be avoided by making sure rooms are well ventilated and humidity levels are kept low. Save common household bug busters like bleach for when they are really needed, as its overuse encourages stronger and more resistant species.

Pesticides are available for most common household insect pests, but these potent chemical compounds may be more harmful to you and the environment than the pests are.

Here are some natural, nontoxic ways to control household pests:

Cockroaches

Keeping a clean home is the best way to avoid cockroaches, especially in your kitchen and bathroom. Wipe up spills and crumbs immediately and vacuum regularly and thoroughly. Used vacuum cleaner bags should be thrown away in a sealed container and kept out of the house.

Common Cockroach Treatments Include . . .

Alpha cypermethrin, azamethiphos, bendiocarb, bioallethrin and *d-allethrin, bioresmethrin*, carbaryl, chlorpyrifos, chlorpyrifos methyl, *cypermethrin*, diazinon, *dichlorvos, dimethoate, d-phenothrin, fenitrothion, fenoxycarb, fipronil, flufenoxuron, hydramethylnon, hydroprene, iodofenphos, lambda cyhalothrin*, lindane, *methoprene*, permethrin, *pirimiphosmethyl*, propoxur, piriproxyfen, *resmethrin, s-bioallethrin*, and *tetramethrin*.

Try This Instead . . .

Target close, warm, moist environments. These areas are cockroach heaven. Try putting boric acid powder underneath refrigerators, near plumbing systems, and in any cracks and crevices (but avoid putting this near food or in places where children and pets can get to it since boric acid is toxic if swallowed). The roaches will track the toxic powder to their nests.

Try using catnip. Its active ingredient, nepetalactone, is nontoxic to humans and pets but repels roaches. If you have a cat-free home, try leaving small sachets in areas that cockroaches like. A strong catnip tea can be used as a spray to apply around baseboards and behind counters.

Keep a spray bottle of soap and water handy. Kill any roaches you see by spraying them directly.

Use nontoxic roach traps. Many home and garden stores sell these. Remember to inspect and replace them regularly.

Ants

According to a 2001 study by researchers at Stanford University, ants appear to invade kitchens and dining rooms to escape searing heat or excessive dampness—and there is little we can do to stop them. The study found that cold, wet conditions were those most likely to drive ants indoors, though hot dry weather also triggered small infestations.

Even if the weather is the main determinant of ant invasions, it can pay to remove the things that make life indoors cozy for ants. Keep counters and floors free of crumbs and sticky spots. Store food in sealed containers. Cut off water sources, such as drips or dishes left soaking overnight.

Common Ant Treatments Include . . .
Allethrin, bendiocarb, *boric acid*, carbaryl, chlorpyrifos, cypermethrin, *deltamethrin*, diazinon, fenitrothion, lindane, permethrin, d-phenothrin, *pyrethrin*, tetramethrin, and *trichlorphon*.

Try This Instead . . .

Be a detective. Once you find the point of entry for the ant column you can create a dry barrier, which the ants will not cross, by using simple kitchen items, such as cayenne pepper, cinnamon, or coffee grounds, or a piece of string soaked in citrus oil or lemon juice.

Try a sticky barrier. This can be made of petroleum jelly, or purchase an all-natural sticky strip. Ants will not cross any form of sticky barrier.

Create your own bait. You may not want to eat aspartame (the artificial sweetener sold as Equal and NutraSweet) because of its potential toxicity (see chapter

5), but for indoor ant control you can mix ½ teaspoon of it with ½ teaspoon of honey and ½ teaspoon of borax, and drop it in small open bottles as bait. Leave the bottles on their sides and the ants will carry the bait back to their colonies. Remember to keep this mixture away from pets and children.

Flood with boiling water or soapy water. This will effectively kill ants nesting beneath outdoor surfaces, such as patios and paved areas. This is not terribly humane, though, and should only be considered in overwhelming infestations.

Spray any ants you see with a solution of equal parts water and vinegar.

Mosquitoes

Mosquitoes can transmit serious, potentially fatal, organisms, causing such diseases as encephalitis, dengue fever, malaria, and yellow fever. They are generally most active from April through October and prefer places with still air since breezes make it difficult for them to fly. Keep windows and doors closed, especially in the early morning and early evening, when mosquitoes are most active. The best thing you can do to keep mosquitoes out is to seal any openings where they might be able to enter your home.

Common Mosquito Treatments Include . . .

d-allethrin, bioallethrin, bioresmethrin, s-bioallethrin, cypermethrin, deltamethrin, fenothrin, tetramethrin, dichlorvos, s-methoprene, permethrin, and pyrethrins.

Try This Instead . . .

Remove still water. This will take away the mosquitoes' prime breeding grounds. Change the water in birdbaths, wading pools, and pets' water bowls at lease twice a week.

Keep your gutters clean and clear of debris. Clear out anything that would stop them from draining. Remove garden items that collect water.

Plant marigolds around your house and garden. Bugs and flying insects detest the fragrance given off by marigold flowers, so they work well as natural bug repellents.

Use essential oils. Making a spray with eucalyptus oil at 30 percent concentration (that is three parts oil to ten parts water) can keep mosquitoes from biting for up to two hours. In order for it to be effective, the eucalyptus oil must have a minimum of 70 percent cineole content, the active therapeutic ingredient. Studies show this is more effective than a similar concentration of citronella oil.

Try neem oil. You can make or buy neem oil–based sprays, the active ingredient of which is a natural vegetable oil extracted from the neem tree, which is native to India. The leaves, seeds, and seed oil of the neem tree contain sallanin, a compound that has effective mosquito-repelling properties.

Houseflies

Houseflies have evolved in close association with people and their environment. While houseflies are plentiful and annoying, of greater importance is their role in the possible transmission of organisms that cause diseases and illnesses, such as typhoid, cholera, dysentery, and diarrhea.

Common Housefly Treatments Include . . .
d-allethrin, bioallethrin, bioresmethrin, s-bioallethrin, cypermethrin, deltamethrin, fenothrin, tetramethrin, dichlorvos, s-methoprene, permethrin, and pyrethrins

Try This Instead . . .

Make your own flypaper. Combine ¼ cup of syrup, 1 tablespoon of brown sugar, and 1 tablespoon of granulated sugar, and pour it into a shallow pan. Cut a brown paper bag or sheets of brown construction paper into strips and soak them in the syrup mixture. Let the paper dry overnight and then hang the strips by poking a hole at the top of each one and hanging them on a thin piece of string.

Use eucalyptus oil. Several drops on a small piece of cloth will repel flies. Refresh regularly to maintain effectiveness.

Use a fly swatter. This old-fashioned remedy is an inexpensive and effective way to kill the odd fly that invades your home.

Try small sacks of crushed mint. These can be used to repel flies by placing them around your house. You can also wrap cloves, bay leaves, and eucalyptus berries in small cloth sachets (cheesecloth is ideal) and hang them by open windows or doors.

Dust Mites

Invisible dust mites can be lurking just about anywhere in our homes—from our clothes, beds, and furniture to bookshelves, pillows, curtains, and soft toys. They aren't a problem for most people, but dust mites can sometimes trigger severe reactions in people with allergies or asthma.

Common Dust Mite Treatments Include . . .

Alpha cypermethrin, bioresmethrin, chlorpyrifos, chlorpyrifos methyl, cypermethrin, d-phenothrin, fenitrothion, methoprene, permethrin, pirimiphos-methyl, propoxur, resmethrin, s-bioallethrin, and tetramethrin.

Try This Instead . . .

Vacuum rugs, mattresses, and pillows regularly.

Keep bedrooms mite-free. Things like books, stuffed animals, throw rugs, and laundry hampers make a happy home for dust mites. Keep them out of the bedrooms of allergy sufferers.

Buy dust mite–proof bedding. You can also cover mattresses and pillows with plastic covers that prevent penetration by dust mites.

Wash dust-prone items at 130° F or higher. Bedding, soft covers, and stuffed animals need to be washed regularly in hot water to kill off dust mites.

Don't use humidifiers. Dust mites flourish in damp air and warmth, so avoid humidifiers as much as possible.

Buy filters for heating ducts. Look for those that trap dust particles smaller than 10 microns.

Wasps

Avoid swatting and squashing wasps if you find them around your home. Wasps release the chemical pheromone when crushed, which attracts other nearby wasps.

Common Wasp Treatments Include . . .
Bendiocarb, carbaryl, chlorpyrifos, dichlorvos, d-phenothrin, fenitrothion, iodofenphos, permethrin, pirimiphos-methyl, pyrethrins, resmethrin, rotenone, s-bioallethrin, and tetramethrin.

Try This Instead . . .

Don't make food accessible to them. Wasps have seasonal food preferences. In the spring and early summer, they like protein foods. Avoid leaving pet food, picnic scraps, and open trash containers outdoors. Wasps remember food sources, so they will return to search for food for a little while after you have removed their food source.

Seal possible entry points. This is the best line of defense. Check your home for cracks around windows and door frames, unsealed vents, and ripped screens. Be aware of the places where wasps always seem to hover in your home, especially in the morning, as this will provide a clue to the entry point.

Cover open food and drink containers. Open cans of soda, fruit juice, fresh fruit, and other sweet food sources will attract wasps in late summer and early fall.

Wasps like perfume. Certain fragrances can attract wasps and make them very persistent. If you are going to be outside, minimize your use of perfume and body sprays.

Try these alternatives for other common household pests:

Moths

- Cedar oil, sometimes referred to as juniper oil, is a powerful moth repellent. Put a few drops of cedar oil on pieces of absorbent cloth and leave them anywhere you store your clothes.

- You can also try making little sachets by wrapping some cedar chips in a cheesecloth square or old panty hose and placing them in closets and drawers. Lavender, rosemary, cloves, and dried lemon peels are also effective ingredients for moth-deterring sachets.

Silverfish

• Silverfish thrive on damp, warm conditions and are frequently found around kitchens and bathrooms. The best way to avoid them is to prevent damp conditions, so make sure these rooms have adequate ventilation. Vacuum thoroughly to remove sources of food and the insects' eggs.

• You can make a simple trap by wrapping the outside of a small glass with masking tape. The silverfish will climb up the rough outer surface, fall in, and become trapped because they are unable to climb back up the smooth surface on the inside of the glass. Once they are in the glass, you can drown them in soapy water.

Earwigs

• Diatomaceous earth can be used as a long-term, safe earwig repellent around the home. Place it around baseboards and window frames, where earwigs like to linger.

• A useful and reuseable trap can be made by filling a shallow pan halfway with vegetable oil. Remove dead earwigs from the oil as you find them.

• Since earwigs like dark, moist places, another simple and effective trap can be made by spraying a newspaper with water, rolling it up, and tying it loosely. Put the trap on the ground near where the earwigs are most active. After a day or so pick up the paper (and resident earwigs) and dispose in a sealed bin.

Mice

House mice are "commensal," which means that they prefer to live in structures provided by humans or close to human residences. Any home, old or new, cat or no cat, can be a "mouse house," so care must be taken to insure that they don't get too comfortable in your home—if they do they can be hard to get rid of.

Older techniques of controlling mice, such as trapping and poisoning, can also endanger companion animals and children. Live traps can be used to humanely trap and relocate mice, but unless you mouse-proof your house, you will have a continual problem.

Mice (and rats) can be very persistent in their efforts to invade your home, and when our often halfhearted attempts at rodent-proofing fail, many of us turn to poisons to control the problem. The most common chemical weapons in the battle against rodents are anticoagulant rodenticides, such as *difenacoum* and *bromadiolone*, which prevent blood clotting and cause death from internal bleeding. These rodenticides are usually incorporated in a bait of attractive food. Care needs to be taken not to place these chemical baits in areas where children, pets, or other nontarget animals can gain access, as these pesticides are designed to kill mammals.

Try This Instead . . .

If mice like your house it's because you offer food, water, and shelter. Eliminate their access to these things and your problems will be over. Mouse-proofing your house requires persistence and may take some time, though. Be patient and thorough.

Remove their food source. Grains, sugar, candies, pastas, nuts, and dry pet foods, for example, should be stored in lidded glass or metal jars, not in plastic bags and containers. Keep your bread in a breadbox, not on the kitchen counter, and remember to wash off any drips and dribbles around the mouths of syrup, honey, and jam jars before the containers are put away. Fruit with broken skin should be refrigerated, as should potatoes and onions, unless you can keep them in a mouse-proof cupboard. Drawers are virtually impossible to mouse-proof, so don't keep edibles in them. If they can't find anything good to eat, they'll move out pretty quickly.

Remove access. A mouse can squeeze through any pencil-sized opening, so regularly inspect your upper cupboards for pencil-sized cracks. Rats and mice can also run along or climb electrical wires, ropes, and cables. Check any wires or cables that enter your home, remembering that even a pencil-sized opening around a cable or wire is sufficient for mouse entry. Check for openings around pipes and seal any of these small openings with tin or lath, since mice can chew through caulking. You can also place bits of steel wool into other cracks you find. Mice can also climb vines, shrubs, and trees, so as a precaution trim the vegetation from around your home, leaving a couple of feet between your house and the vegetation. Mouse-proofing your kitchen will probably solve most of your mouse problems. The cupboard under your kitchen sink is probably the most vulnerable area in your house, so seal any openings there.

Be humane. Most good hardware shops will stock live mouse and rat traps, or will be able to order them from their suppliers.

Tending Your Garden Naturally

Whether you are growing vegetables or flowers, have a large plot of land, or just a few window boxes, chances are you have lavished a lot of care on your little patch of green. The last thing you want spoiling it are opportunistic insects, fungi, and other pests.

While the environmental problems of the world may seem beyond your control, you can make a difference right in your own backyard by adopting a more natural approach to gardening.

Pesticides can be an effective way of controlling garden pests in the short term, but they are toxic, encourage resistance among fungi and adaptable insects, and spell disaster for the environment.

Remember, the more of these products you use in your home and garden, the greater the risks. For example, in 2002, it was found that exposure to a mixture of three herbicides commonly used to kill household weeds—2,4-D, MCCP (mecoprop), and *dicamba*—increased the risk of miscarriage and reduced fertility in an animal experiment.

The levels used in this study were very low—as low as 39 parts per billion (ppb), or comparable to one drop of pesticide in five hundred bathtubsful of water. This level is seven times less than the established safe level for drinking water. Nevertheless, among the exposed animals, there was a 20 percent increase in failed pregnancy.

In many cases, there are alternatives that are often more effective in the long run, and less harmful to the environment and the applicator, than the quick-and-dirty method of commercial pest control.

Gardeners have been battling pests for centuries. Begin by learning good gardening strategies, many of which will result in fewer pest problems, then learn how to use less harmful methods for managing insect pests, weeds, and diseases in your garden before reaching for chemical controls.

Common Garden Pesticides Include . . .

The insecticides *acephate*, carbaryl, chlorpyrifos, dichlorvos (DDVP), malathion, and trichlorphon; the herbicides atrazine, *benfluralin* (Benefin), *bensulide*, 2,4-D, *DSMA* (disodium methanearsonate), *dacthal* (DCPA), dicamba, *endothall, glyphosate, isoxaben, MCPP* (mecoprop), MSMA, *pendimethalin, pronamide, siduron, triclopyr*, and *trifluralin*; and the fungicides *chlorothalonil, maneb, pentachloronitrobenzene* (PCNB; quintozene), sulphur, *triadimefon*, and *ziram*.

According to the U.S. group Beyond Pesticides, of these commonly used garden pesticides, nineteen have studies pointing toward carcinogenic effects; thirteen are linked with birth defects, twenty-one with reproductive effects, fifteen with neurotoxicity, and twenty-six with liver or kidney damage; twenty-seven are sensitizers and/or irritants; and eleven have the potential to disrupt the endocrine (hormonal) system.

Try This Instead . . .

A full discussion of how to manage a natural garden is beyond the scope of this book, but there are a number of simple things you can do in your garden to keep it beautiful, while also making it healthy and safe for your family, pets, and the environment.

First of All, Be Realistic

• Keep your garden as natural as possible by using less grass, and more trees, ground covers, flowers, and mulches.

• Choose plants that are native to the region. These plants are heartier and more resistant to pests and diseases than exotic varieties.

• Use plants that are well suited to your garden's habitat. Consider drainage, sun exposure, and soil type when making your choices.

• On sloped areas, plant ground covers instead of grass to alleviate mowing and control erosion.

Healthy Soil Makes Healthy Plants

• Test your soil for pH and nutrients. A soil test kit can be picked up in hardware or gardening stores. Add what is needed based on results.

• Add compost and organic fertilizer to your garden each year.

• For lawns, aerate soil, overseed, and top-dress with compost.

Maintain the Health of Your Plants and Lawn

• Prune plants to optimally utilize the plants' energy sources.

• Shear off dead or diseased portions, as they may attract pests.

• Mow no more than a third of a grass blade and leave clippings on the lawn.

• Water deeply, but less frequently.

• Use only slow-release fertilizers.

When Pests Become a Problem

- Use physical controls to exclude pests, such as mulch, compost, bark, grass clippings, traps, sticky wraps, pheromone bags, barriers/screens, floating row covers, seedling collars, and cheesecloth.

- Practice cultural controls, such as handpicking weeds and tilling soil in areas of weeds rather than applying herbicides.

- Practice landscape diversity. A pest that likes a certain type of plant is less likely to spread if other species are planted in between.

- A simple soap spray is one of the oldest nontoxic pesticides you can use. It can be made by mixing 1–2 tablespoons of mild liquid soap (such as dishwashing liquid) to 1 quart of water. Transfer this mix to a sprayer and use as needed.

Use natural pest control products, usually found at local garden centers or DIY stores. These include:

- **Horticultural oils**. These can be plant-based or petroleum-based. Examples of plant-based oils that can be used as pesticides include cottonseed oil and soybean oil, both of which can be effective in controlling afids and mites. Neem-seed extract can be used to discourage all types of fungi and molds as well as ants. It can also act like a growth regulator.

- **Insecticidal soap.** This can be purchased at garden centers, is a safe treatment for aphid, mite, and whitefly control, and is used by many greenhouses. It works by impairing the waxy layer of the insect's exoskeleton and eventually kills the insect.

- **Diatomaceous earth.** Derived from the fossil remains of one-celled algae, this can be used for insect and mite management.

- **Boric acid or borax.** These will kill ants and even cockroaches. Since most ants like sweets, try mixing a bit of honey or other sugar with boric acid to make a paste. Spread this on small cardboard squares and put these in the ant trail so that the ants will eat the mixture and take some back to their nest. (You can also find pesticide-free fly and wasp traps at most garden centers.)

9. PET SUPPLIES

Pets are exposed to the same chemicals in their diet and grooming supplies that people are. As consumers have become increasingly attracted to, and comfortable with, the use of natural and organic products themselves, they are becoming equally receptive to the use of natural products, including pest control and herbal supplements, for their pets. Indeed, a 1999 study led by one source, U.S. Business Research, found that 22 percent of pet owners had used some form of alternative therapy on their pet.

The pet-care industry is big business. In the United States, pet owners spend around $16 billion a year on pet products. In Europe, they spend $18 billion. Pet food accounts for about 80 percent of what we spend on our pets, but sales of a whole range of pet-care items—cat litter, flea and tick products, dietary supplements, toys, pet homes (from cages to kennels or fish tanks), baskets, feeding bowls, collars, leashes, clothing, brushes, and shampoos—are all increasing.

So, we spend a lot of money, but are we really making our pets' lives better?

Surveys show that overall pet health is declining almost as rapidly as human health. As with humans, this is a relatively recent phenomenon that began shortly after World War II.

Cats and dogs, which make up the majority of companion pets in the world, are now developing a vast list of degenerative diseases, including autoimmune diseases, allergies, heart disease, diabetes, joint and arthritic problems, and cancer. By the age of three, some three-quarters of dogs will have developed gum disease, eye problems, ear problems, untreatable infestations of fleas and other parasites, thyroid imbalances, personality disorders, and birth defects, all of which are becoming commonplace among our pets.

The problem is so acute that a relatively new phenomenon—pet insurance—has been invented to help pet owners cope with spiraling vet bills. While once, visits to the vet were rare and were usually reserved for emergencies, today they are common and our pets are being subjected to the same arsenal of modern drugs—vaccines, antibiotics, steroids, painkillers, insulin, and even antidepressants—that humans are.

The adverse effects from these drugs are as common in animals as they are in humans. Dogs given nonsteroidal anti-inflammatory drugs (NSAIDs), for example, can develop ulcers from them just as humans do.

As with humans, a pet's diet is the basis of good health. Yet recent studies have shown processed foods to be a factor in increasing numbers of pets suffering from cancer, arthritis, obesity, dental disease, and heart disease. Dull or unhealthy coats and skin problems are a common problem with cats and dogs.

Modern dogs, cats, and other animals live for years on convenience foods that come out of bags, cans, and boxes, and a growing number of vets believe that this highly processed pet food is the main cause of illness and premature death in the modern dog and cat.

Some evidence suggests that a steady diet of processed pet food can suppress an animal's immune system, and may lead to liver, kidney, heart, and other diseases. In one 1995 study at the Karolinska Institute in Sweden, young animals that were fed cooked and processed foods, while initially healthy, appeared to age more quickly and developed chronic degenerative disease symptoms. In contrast, another group of animals, raised on raw foods, aged less quickly and were free of degenerative disease.

Food is the basis of good pet health, but other factors are also influential. Everyday hygiene items, such as flea and tick collars, are also a major source of poisonings and illness among pets. Flea collars emit continuous, undetected pesticide vapors into the home, car, and around the pet. These vapors are highly toxic to the animal's skin, eyes, nose, lungs, blood, heart, liver, and kidneys. They are also harmful for the adults—and especially children—who hug, handle, pet, or otherwise enjoy the pleasure of being in close proximity to their furry friends.

Given the vast number of pet companions kept by people, it is astonishing how little relevant research there is to show how pet lifestyles, diets, and environmental exposures can contribute to illness. Such studies that have been done are usually funded by major pet-care product manufacturers and often exonerate pet products of any ill effects. The question of funding raises the specter of the same kind of unacceptable bias that regularly turns up in medical trials sponsored by drug manufacturers.

Humans are meant to be caretakers for pets but, clearly, we are failing in our duties.

Pet Food

Pet food has quite literally become a dog-eat-dog business—cat-eat-cat, too. According to a startling 2001 report from the U.S. Animal Protection Institute (API), "What's Really in Pet Food?," commercial pet foods contain mostly grain wastes and meat by-products, which can include everything from euthanized shelter animals to cancer-ridden livestock, road kill, downer animals (those unable to walk), moldy grains, and rancid restaurant grease. Feeding these low-in-nutrition packaged "scraps" to pets greatly increases their chances of developing cancer and other degenerative diseases.

According to the API report, the vast majority, around 95 percent, of our pets are fed processed pet foods. The report noted that in slaughterhouses, whatever remains of the carcass after the best cuts have been removed for human consumption goes into the can—including bones, blood, pus, intestines, bowels, ligaments, fat, hooves, horns, and beaks. Using literally every part of the carcass keeps costs down, and it is this, rather than nutrition, that motivates most pet food manufacturers. Profit is further boosted because many pet food companies are subsidiaries of big human food companies; waste from one company simply ends up as a resource for the other.

There are several problems with using rendered animal parts in processed animal foods. Using what are known as 4D animals (dead, diseased, dying, or disabled) means that whatever made the animal sick and whatever treatment was given to it before its death—for instance, medicines like antibiotics—remain in the food chain, passed on to your pet.

Commercial pet foods have other problems that are not immediately apparent from the labeling or the advertising spin. Many manufacturers cut costs by using the cheapest ingredients available at the time a food is made. As costs rise and fall, some manufacturers vary ingredients from batch to batch, resulting in changed nutrient values for each batch and possible digestive illness. Here's what's in conventional pet foods:

- **Substandard protein.** Soybean meal, wheat, corn glutens, cornmeal, whole corn, crushed corn, and ground corn are commonly used for their protein content in many pet foods. These ingredients are generally poor sources of protein compared to meat.

- **Rancid fats.** Restaurant grease has become a major component of feed-grade animal fat over the last fifteen years. Often held in fifty-gallon drums for weeks or months in extreme temperatures, this rancid grease is then picked up by fat blenders, who mix the animal and vegetable fats together, stabilize them with powerful antioxidants to prevent further spoilage, and then sell the blended products to pet food companies. Rancid, heavily preserved fats are extremely difficult to digest, and can lead to a host of animal health problems, including digestive upsets, diarrhea, gas, and bad breath.

- **Salt.** The high salt content in some pet foods can cause animals to become unnaturally high-strung and nervous. The salt content of many products can be up to thousand times more than your pet needs in one day. The excess salt can cause high blood pressure and heart disease in animals. Epilepsy is now more common in dogs than in humans.

- **Sugar.** Semimoist pet food usually contains as much as 25 percent sugar, which can come in many forms, such as sucrose, corn syrup, beet pulp, and caramel, to name but a few.

- **Humectants.** Used to keep the food moist, some can contain up to 10 percent propylene glycol. Both sugar and propylene glycol are linked to obesity, allergies, tooth decay, and other problems, like cancer. Propylene glycol is used in the making of antifreeze—and yet, it's in the food we feed our pets. Once

Cats Need Care

Cats' nutritional needs are much the same as dogs', but the way their bodies process nutrients is very different. Both cats and dogs are natural predators and both are natural meat eaters. But dogs' bodies have evolved to be omnivorous. In the wild, they will survive on a varied diet of plants and meat. Cats, however, are obligate carnivores—they die if they don't eat meat. Cats also find it difficult to process plant materials, and, with the exception of vitamin C, which cats can make themselves, felines must obtain all their nutrients—especially the amino acids arginine and taurine—from the food they eat.

In comparison to dogs, cats require three times as much protein to stay healthy, but only negligible amounts of carbohydrates. Contrary to popular belief, cats were originally desert-dwelling animals, so, while we tend to associate cats with fish, seafood is not their natural diet, and a steady diet of things like canned tuna can actually promote severe nutritional deficiencies in cats, especially of vitamins E and A. In the wild, cats will eat the whole of the animal—skin, bones, and flesh—and from this totality obtain all the nutrients necessary to remain healthy.

There is very little difference between the meat by-products that are included in catfood and those that are regularly found in dogfood. As with again, our own foods, like common salad dressings, contain propylene glycol also (just read the label). Alarmingly, a U.S. Food and Drug Administration (FDA) report in 1994 noted that propylene glycol "reduces red blood cell survival time, renders red blood cells more susceptible to oxidative damage and has other adverse effects in cats consuming the substance at levels found in semi-moist food." In January 2001, the FDA, together with the Center for Veterinary Medicine (CVM), finally banned propylene glycol in semi-moist cat-food, but it is still used in products for dogs.

- **Synthetic preservatives.** Butylated hydroxyanisole (BHA) and the related compound butylated hydroxytoluene (BHT) are used to prevent the fats and oils added to animal food from going bad. BHA and BHT have been shown to affect the nervous systems of animals—in particular, the neurological development of young animals.

- **Artificial colors.** Food colorings are still commonly used in pet foods today, despite the fact that they are not necessary and that some have been linked to medical problems.

- **Other additives.** Pet foods can contain the same mind-boggling array of potentially harmful additives that human foods have, including flavor enhancers,

dogs, vets are concerned that canned catfood may lie at the root of a range of immune diseases, such as allergies, digestive upsets, thyroid problems, adrenal and pancreatic dysfunction, tooth and gum decay, arthritis, and kidney and liver failure. A recent study of twenty-five brands of catfood found that all but one also contained cancer-causing amines—fueling speculation that a diet of processed food might well be the reason for the increasing incidence of cancer among cats.

Dry catfoods have been blamed for a range of health problems, including kidney disease, cystitis, diabetes, inflammatory bowel disease, obesity, dental problems, and autoimmune disorders. Many of these problems are related to the lack of water and the high carbohydrate levels of dry cat kibble. Cats' natural prey—for instance, a mouse or other small animal—would comprise around 70 percent water.

Our knowledge of cats' nutritional needs is relatively sketchy, but most experts in holistic pet care believe that supplementing or replacing your cat's diet of canned food with raw or lightly cooked meat will greatly improve its overall diet. To make sure your cat gets all it needs, make sure you provide a variety of meats—for example, organs, tripe, and muscle meat.

and anticaking, curing, and drying agents, as well as emulsifiers, sweeteners, solvents, stabilizers, thickeners, and texturizers.

Improving Your Pet's Diet

Dogs and cats were designed to handle raw, uncooked foods. Owners can easily mix fresh cuts of meat (not ground) with whole grains and vegetables for a balanced diet.

The meat contained in canned pet food is cooked, devoid of real nutrients, and usually full of many potentially harmful preservatives, colorings, and additives. Dry and processed canned food also lacks the natural teeth-cleaning properties of fresh raw meat. Without the natural cleansing action of the meat on the teeth, unhealthy bacteria build up in the mouth, causing infection and foul-smelling breath.

Animals require the enzymes, amino acids, and other nutrients in raw meat to stay healthy. Many skin and coat problems are a direct result of a lack of raw animal fat in the diet—fat that humans often believe is bad for their pet. Animals need a diet of at least 30 percent raw fat, and their systems are not designed to handle cooked meat or cooked fat.

Pet Grooming

Most mass-produced pet-grooming supplies contain the same contentious chemicals that you will find in human toiletries, including petroleum-based detergents, preservatives, artificial colors, and synthetic perfumes. These ingredients can cause the same kinds of skin reactions in pets as they can in humans.

Pet owners are also bamboozled by the same marketing jargon for pet supplies as found on toiletries for people, such as "all-natural," "organic," "pure," "hypoallergenic," and "aromatherapy-derived"—and should use the same common sense when faced with such claims. Indeed, many "natural" pet products are made from a raft of synthetic chemicals, with a small number of natural extracts thrown in for good measure.

If your pet is allergy-prone, check the label of your grooming products for the following potentially irritating ingredients:

- **Sodium lauryl sulphate (SLS).** Tests show that sodium lauryl sulphate can damage eyes and can be absorbed into systemic tissues, such as the brain, heart, and liver. SLS is also an irritant, and can cause eye irritation, skin rashes, hair loss, scalp scurf similar to dandruff, and allergic reactions.

Flea and Tick Control

Fleas usually gain free entry to your home through your pet or visitors' pets. Remember, for every flea on your pet, there may be as many as thirty more in its environment.

Fleas and ticks are a profitable business for the chemical-pesticide industry, as they are responsible for billions in sales every year. Pet owners are seduced into believing that these products are safe and effective, but read the warning label on conventional flea and tick products. Shampoos and dips, foggers and collars—in fact, all conventional flea and tick treatments—caution users to wear gloves, and to keep the product away from skin and mucous membranes. And yet, these chemicals are being applied in some cases all over your pet, where they can be easily absorbed, inhaled, or licked off by the pet. In addition, foggers release a great deal of toxic chemicals into the air that will then settle on carpets, furniture, and curtains.

These regular pesticide exposures are highly toxic and further weaken the overall health of your pet. Based on the very limited data available, it appears that hundreds and probably thousands of pets have been injured or killed through exposure to pet products containing pesticides.

Chronic low-dose exposures to these toxins may not kill pets or humans with the initial exposure, or even after several exposures; it takes longer for the negative effects to accumulate and disable the immune system. Because of this, the pesticide

- **DEA and MEA.** These hormone-disrupting chemicals are used as foam boosters, stabilizers, and viscosity builders or modifiers in shampoos, hand soaps, and bath products. Examples include cocamide DEA or MEA, and lauramide DEA. When mixed with formaldehyde-forming ingredients, such as 2-bromo-2-nitropropane-1,3-diol (bronopol), quaternium-15, DMDM hydantoin, and imidazolidinyl urea, they can form cancer-causing nitrosamines (see also page 99).
- **Mineral oil.** Also known as paraffinum liquidum, this coats the skin and stops it from breathing. Skin is the largest body organ and needs to release toxins freely, but mineral oil blocks this process. Mineral oil also acts like a solvent, breaking down the skin's natural oils. With every application, it will dry your pet's skin even more.
- **Talc.** Dry pet "shampoos" are often based around talc, which is carcinogenic when inhaled.

There's no magic in choosing safe pet products—just take the same care when choosing pet shampoos and other treatments as you would in choosing products for yourself.

industry continues to mislead the public and the government regulatory agencies by insisting that there is no scientific proof showing a definite cause-and-effect link between pesticide exposure and illness in either pets or humans. When industry representatives have been asked by environmental and health advocates to conduct new studies on the relationship of pesticides to cancer and respiratory and neurological disorders, their default reply is that there is no need for such studies.

But, in November 2000, a report issued by the U.S. Natural Resources Defense Council (NRDC) found that pest-control products can expose adults and children to toxic pesticides at concentrations that exceed—by as much as five hundred times—the safe levels established by the U.S. Environmental Protection Agency (EPA). The result: possible acute poisoning of pets and humans, and possible long-term problems for children, too. The risks include acute poisoning and longer-term problems like brain dysfunction or cancer.

The report found that the riskiest pet products contain a family of pesticides known as organophosphates (OPs) and carbamates. OP pesticides, which are derived from nerve gas, interfere with nerve-signal transmission. Since the neurological process they attack is common to insects, humans, dogs, and cats, these pesticides can harm more than just fleas and ticks. Carbamates disrupt the same neurological processes as OPs, and so are potentially just as harmful.

The chemical industry claims that no scientific studies have demonstrated a conclusive relationship between chemical exposure and disease, and then refuses

Is Your Home Killing Your Pets?

Our animal companions can suffer from the same range of diseases, both chronic and acute, that we do. Veterinarians, for example, report treating rising levels of cancer in animals, as well as increased numbers of poisonings and behavioral problems. Small animals, and especially cats, can be overwhelmed easily by toxins in the environment, their systems unable to metabolize or excrete poisons. This may be one reason why the incidence of feline leukemia is reaching epidemic proportions among cats.

Many pets are "indoor pets." But a small animal that spends most of its time indoors can develop health problems due to polluted indoor air. If you live in a modern home, with efficient insulation, harmful chemicals can be trapped and build up in the atmosphere. Like children, small animals can end up inhaling higher concentrations of these toxins found in household cleaners and garden pesticides in relation to their body weight. As a result, the kinds of symptoms linked with indoor pollution may appear in our pets before they appear in us. These include:

- anxiety
- burns on the mouth and esophagus
- colic

to initiate new studies on the basis that they are not needed, even though many small studies have indicated otherwise. The carbaryl class of chemicals, for instance, is associated with increased frequencies of diarrhea, coughing, breathing difficulties, and congestion. OPs can produce symptoms of headache, dizziness, nausea, fatigue, and dermatitis.

The millions of dollars spent on toxic flea control have not bought consumer satisfaction or healthy pest-free pets. This is because fleas and ticks can develop resistance to pesticides in the same way that bacteria become resistant to antibiotics. Survival of the fittest, a short lifespan, and rapid replication (multiple generations every year) have created superbugs. In fact, fleas and lice now have a longer lifecycle than they did fifty years ago. They breed more easily and even survive bouts of cold weather. As a result, it has become necessary to use stronger poisons in higher doses.

Common Flea Treatments Include . . .

Amitraz (amidine), carbaryl, chlorpyrifos, coumaphos, cythioate, diazinon, dichlorvos, fenitrothion, fenthion, fipronil (phenyl pyrazole), flumethrin, imidacloprid, iodofenphos, lufenuron (benzoylurea), malathion, naled, *permethrin*, phenothrin, phosmet, *piperonyl butoxide*, propoxur, pyrethrin/pyrethrum, S-methoprene, and tetrachlorvinphos.

- corneal damage
- cough
- excessive salivation
- foaming at the mouth
- muscle weakness
- restlessness
- seizures
- shallow breathing
- skin ulcers
- slow respiration
- vomiting

Minimizing your use of toxic household chemicals is a must if you have pets. In particular be aware of the way that aerosol sprays can cause, or make worse, animal respiratory problems. Choose cleaning products based on natural substances rather than those based on petrochemicals to reduce levels of volatile chemicals that can permeate the indoor environment and linger in a well-insulated home for long periods of time.

Try This Instead . . .

To keep your family safe, remember that you should avoid all organophosphate-based products. This is particularly important for pregnant women and families with children. Don't let children help apply flea shampoos, dusts, dips, or other products containing OPs or carbamates to their pets.

In many cases, fleas and ticks can be controlled with simple physical measures, such as brushing pets regularly with a flea comb while inspecting for fleas, and vacuuming and mowing frequently in areas where pets spend the most time outdoors.

A chronic flea infestation can serve as an early-warning sign of immune deficiency caused or exacerbated by a nutrient-poor diet. To strengthen an animal's compromised immune system, make sure your pet is getting the right vitamins and minerals to help protect against fleas and ticks. The B vitamins, particularly B_1 (thiamine) and B_6 (pyridoxine), are natural flea and tick repellents. Brewer's yeast and rice bran contain high levels of all of the B vitamins. As a first line of therapy, try adding brewer's yeast and garlic or apple-cider vinegar to your pet's food. (Note: It is not advisable to use raw garlic as a food supplement for cats.)

You can also try these natural alternatives:

Bathe and comb your pet regularly. Use natural vegetable-based soap or shampoo, not insecticides. If you find fleas on your pet's brush or comb, dip it in a glass of soapy water to remove them.

Vacuum fequently. Floors, carpets, furniture, crevices, and cracks in the areas where pets sleep and spend time should be vacuumed often, along with weekly washing of pet bedding. During heavy infestations, daily vacuuming may be necessary. Dispose of the sealed bag properly outside the home or by incinerating it.

Use cedar shampoo, cedar oil, and cedar-filled sleeping mats. These are commercially available. Cedar repels many insects, including fleas.

Make an herbal flea collar. Make up a mixture of ½ teaspoon alcohol with 1 drop each of the following essential oils: cedar wood, lavender, citronella, and thyme. Add the contents of four garlic capsules. Buy a soft flea collar (untreated), and soak the collar in this mixture until it has absorbed enough of it to be thoroughly saturated, then leave it to dry completely. This will be effective for about a month.

Tea tree oil. Add a few drops to an herbal pet shampoo to repel fleas and help heal flea-bitten skin. You can also try mixing a teaspoon of tea tree oil in 8 ounces of water and spraying this on the animal's fur. This is recommended for pets that dislike baths, which includes most cats. It is also practical for in-between baths.

Cat Litter

For litter-box-trained animals, holistic vets recommend avoiding conventional clay litters, as they are laden with silica dust, a known carcinogen. According to the kitty litter expert Marina Michaels, many "scoopable" clay litters have also been found to cause intestinal blockages in cats and kittens when inadvertently consumed while grooming.

Once upon a time cat litter boxes were homemade affairs, filled with anything at hand that the cat might dig into and use. Sand was popular if it could be easily found; garden dirt was another natural choice, since most cats were indoor-outdoor, and that was where they usually "did their business." Shredded newspaper and ashes were also common.

Then, in the late 1940s, absorbent "Kitty Litter" based on fuller's earth appeared on the market. For a long time, this was the standard for cat owners, then in the 1980s scoopable clay litters containing sodium bentonite came on the market and were an instant success. Sodium bentonite is a highly absorbent clay that is often added to kitty litter as an effective clumping agent. Mixed with liquid, it can swell to around fifteen times its original volume. Traditional clay litters had to be replaced frequently; but with scoopable litter, cat owners only had to scoop out the solids and the clumps of urine, and add a small amount of new litter. The box would last up to a month without the owner having to completely replace the used litter.

Scoopable clay litters are convenient and cost-effective for owners, but they have several downsides that can impact the health of your cat:

- The dust in clay is silica dust, a known carcinogen, which is easily inhaled into feline and human lungs.

- Cats can ingest the clay while cleaning their feet, and kittens sometimes eat litter. Sodium bentonite can form large clumps when it comes into contact with liquids. Once it reaches your cat's gut it can draw fluid out of the body, causing dehydration. It is also implicated in urinary tract problems.

- Ingested clay dust coats the digestive tract, attracting the collection of old fecal material, increasing toxicity, bacteria growth, and prohibiting proper assimilation of digested food. This can lead to stress on the immune system, leaving the animal susceptible to viral, bacterial, parasitic, and yeast infections.

- The problems can also extend to dogs, who occasionally eat "litter box snacks."

Try This Instead . . .

An effective alternative to conventional kitty litter is a wheat-based litter, which has the same scoopable, flushable, and biodegradable qualities of regular kitty litter. Failing that, you can look for recycled and pelletized paper, or litter made from recycled pine wood waste.

10. CHEMICALS: A TO Z

The number of chemicals we encounter each day is staggering, and it would take several full volumes just to list them all. Some chemicals turn up in our homes more frequently than others, however, and this A-to-Z list provides a snapshot of their potential effects. Listed below each chemical name is either its common name or a common synonym you can find on the labels of the products you buy.

Not everyone will experience the reactions listed here. Indeed, that is the frustrating thing about chemical research. We know so little about who is likely to react, and why and to what extent. For this reason, this glossary tries to be as comprehensive as possible in terms of recognizing adverse reactions.

Some background information may help you to understand what you read here. For instance, hazardous chemicals can be absorbed into the body through:

- the respiratory tract via inhalation

- the skin via dermal contact

- the digestive tract via ingestion (Ingestion can occur if a chemical is deliberately put into food, or because of eating or smoking with contaminated hands or in contaminated areas.)

A chemical may have serious effects by one route of exposure and minimal effects by another.

In addition, chemicals can produce both local and systemic (widespread) effects. With a local effect, the chemical does not need to be absorbed to produce an effect. Instead, it takes place at the point of contact, which may be the skin, the mucous membranes, the respiratory tract, the gastrointestinal system, or the eyes. Such chemicals are known as irritants because they can cause inflammation of the skin and the mucous membranes in the eyes, nose, or respiratory tract.

A systemic effect is an adverse health effect that takes place at a site distant from the body's initial point of chemical contact due to the chemical being absorbed into the body. Substances with systemic effects often have "target organs" in which they accumulate and exert their toxic effect, such as the kidneys, liver, or heart. Some substances that cause systemic effects are cumulative poisons. These substances tend to build up in the body as a result of numerous chronic exposures. Chemicals that cause systemic effects can further be classified as:

- **Reproductive toxins**, which cause impotence or sterility in men and women.

- **Carcinogens**, substances that can cause cancer.

- **Mutagens**, anything that causes a change in the genetic material of a living cell. Many mutagens are also carcinogens.

- **Teratogens**, any agent that interferes with the developing embryo and can cause birth defects on exposure during pregnancy.

- **Neurotoxins**, which affect the nervous system, including diseases associated with nervous system damage, such as multiple sclerosis, Parkinson's disease, Alzheimer's disease, and sudden infant death syndrome (SIDS).

When exposure involves several substances simultaneously, the resultant systemic toxic effect may be significantly greater with the combination than with the cumulative toxic effect of each substance alone. This is called synergy. Good examples of this include exposure to alcohol and chlorinated solvents, or smoking together with asbestos.

Glossary

acephate

An insecticide found in a variety of commercial garden products, in common with other organophosphates, this can cause a host of symptoms, including changes in heart rate, central-nervous-system impairment, blurred vision, gas-

trointestinal problems (cramps, heartburn, hyperperistalsis), and breathing difficulties. With long-term use, it is a fetal toxin and hormone disrupter.

acesulfame K
E950, acesulfame potassium, Sunette, Sweet One

An artificial sweetener used in foods and medicines, acesulfame K is about
two hundred times sweeter than sugar. It has a bitter aftertaste, so it is usually
combined with sugar or the other popular sweetener *aspartame* to mask its bitter-
ness. Each of these chemicals carries its own health risks, and it is possible that
the combination may be more damaging than if either is taken individually. Acesulfame K has been shown to cause cancer in animals, which means that it may
also pose a cancer risk in humans.

acetamide MEA
N-2-hydroxyethylacetamide

A wetting agent/humectant used in cosmetics, such as lipsticks and cream
blushers, to retain moisture. In the short term, acetamide can cause mild skin irritation. No studies are available on the effects of long-term exposure in humans,
but chronic ingestion has produced benign and malignant liver tumors in rats and
an increased incidence of malignant lymphomas in mice. It may be contaminated
with harmful impurities linked to cancer and other health disorders (see *monoethanolamine*).

acetone
dimethyl ketone, methyl ketone

An industrial denaturant and solvent used in the manufacture of waxes,
plastics, varnishes, aerosol paints, explosives, and chloroform. It is also found in
a staggering number of domestic products, including furniture polish and cleaners, surface cleaners, laundry presoaks and starches, shoe polish, garden insecticides, pet flea and tick products, premoistened wipes, nail-polish remover, and
perfumes. Used to extract flavors, aromas, and perfumes from herbs, spices, and
flowers, it can also be found in the marking inks used on meats, and is used in
some skin-cleaning formulas for its ability to dissolve fats and grease.

Used on the skin, it can produce skin rashes, dryness, and irritation. Inhaling
acetone even for short periods can provoke nose, throat, lung and eye irritation,
headaches, light-headedness, and fatigue. Chronic exposure can damage the kidneys and liver.

acrylates

These are film formers, emulsifiers, and surfactants that help cosmetics and
body-care products stick to the skin and can make it feel softer. Their safety has

not been thoroughly investigated. Although they are presumed to be nontoxic, they can be irritating to the skin and eyes.

alcohol, denatured
ethanol, ethyl alcohol

A solvent used extensively in the manufacture of varnishes, artificial flavorings, perfumes, and inks. It is a fuel and gasoline additive and, medicinally, it is used as an antiseptic. But it can also be found in pizza crusts in the United States, where it is used to extend handling and storage time. The starting material for denatured alcohol is ethyl alcohol (ethanol), the alcohol commonly found in beer, wine, and spirits; denatured, or industrial, alcohol is ethanol to which poisonous or nauseating substances have been added to prevent its use as a beverage. It's clear and colorless, and highly flammable. Used on the skin, it can cause dryness and irritation over time. Ingestion of small amounts of denatured alcohol can cause behavioral changes and impaired vision; large amounts can cause nausea, vomiting, coma, and death.

aldrin

An organochlorine insecticide, aldrin breaks down to a related compound, *dieldrin*, in the body and in the environment. Those who are chronically or occupationally exposed to moderate levels of this compound can experience headaches, dizziness, irritability, vomiting, and uncontrolled muscle movements. Aldrin builds up in the body after years of exposure, and is toxic to the nervous system as well as a suspected carcinogen and hormone disrupter. Aldrin is banned or restricted in around fifty countries, including the U.K. and United States, though it is still used in some countries for termite control.

alkyl compounds

Alkyl compounds are used as surfactants and detergents found in cosmetics, toiletries, household goods, and pesticides. They are problematic in many ways. One common type, the alkyl benzyl sulphonates (ABS), include linear alkyl benzene sulphonates (LAS) and linear alkyl sodium sulphonates, both of which are slow to biodegrade. LAS are the most common surfactants used in household products.

Another type, *alkylphenols*, are hormone disrupters. One member of this family of chemicals is the spermicide nonoxynyl (used on condoms, and in spermicidal foams and gels), which may give some idea of their powerful biological toxicity.

alkylphenols

nonylphenol, nonylphenoxy ethoxylates, alkylphenol polyglycol, poylethylene glycol, alkyl aryl ethers

These surfactants and detergents are found in household cleaners, laundry detergents, cosmetics, pesticides, paints, and varnishes. Although still used in commercial products in the United States, they are confined to industrial detergents in the U.K. They can easily get into the water supply and food chain, and are hormone disrupters believed to be contributing to reproductive problems in men, such as low sperm counts, damaged sperm, and testicular cancer. Many alkylphenols are toxic to aquatic organisms and are implicated in the feminization of male fish.

allethrin

d-allethrin

Used almost exclusively in homes and gardens for control of flies and mosquitoes, and in combination with other pesticides to control flying or crawling insects, it is also used to control lice in humans and animals. Allethrin is a synthetic *Pyrethrin*, a botanical insecticide extracted from chrysanthemum flowers. It is harmful if swallowed, its vapors can worsen chronic respiratory diseases, such as asthma, and skin contact can cause dermatitis. It is a suspected mutagen and immunotoxin, and harmful to birds, fish, crustaceans, and aquatic insects.

alpha cypermethrin

A pyrethroid insecticide used against a wide range of insects, including ants, roaches, spiders, and crickets, it is also used in agriculture on cereals, vegetables, and fruit, and on foods during storage. It can be irritating to the skin and eyes. Longer-term exposure can cause headache, dizziness, nausea, vomiting, diarrhea, excessive salivation, and fatigue. It is a suspected hormone disrupter.

alpha-hydroxy acids

Alpha-hydroxy acids, or AHAs, come from a variety of sources, including citrus fruits, such as grapefruit and papaya. *Lactic acid* is also an AHA.

In their more concentrated form, AHAs are used by dermatologists to remove the top layers of the skin, usually as a treatment for skin disorders and wrinkles. Patients like to call such procedures facial peels, but dermatologists call them chemical burns. While not used in skin products at anywhere near such concentrations, AHAs still burn the skin slightly. The glow you get from products containing AHAs is actually a mild irritation caused by the chemical burning. Some people react more than others to this burning, and AHAs are reported to be a major cause of adverse reactions to soaps, shampoos, and moisturizers.

alum
potassium alum

Alum usually refers to synthetic *aluminum*-containing crystals produced in the lab for commercial use as natural deodorants. A powdered form is used as an astringent to prevent bleeding from small shaving cuts. The styptic pencils sold for this purpose contain aluminum sulphate or potassium aluminum sulphate. Similar products are also used on animals to prevent bleeding after nail clipping.

alumina
aluminum oxide
See *aluminum*

aluminum
E173

One of the most abundant minerals on the planet, aluminum has many uses in household products. It is a color additive in cosmetics (especially eyeshadows) and in foods. It is also a common ingredient in antacids, and in deodorants and antiperspirants (most commonly as aluminum chlorohydrate, aluminum zirconium, aluminum chloride, alumina, aluminum sulphate, and aluminum phenosulphate).

The human body has no dietary requirement for aluminum, and, if ingested in large doses, it is considered toxic, carcinogenic, and mutagenic. Applied to the skin (for instance, in deodorants), it is an irritant, and, with a lifetime's use, has been associated with an increased risk of Alzheimer's disease (a common form of dementia). Products containing aluminum zirconium compounds have been shown to cause granulomas (small nodules of chronically inflamed tissue) under the arms with prolonged use.

aluminum chloride

An industrial fungicide that is a suspected neurotoxin and reproductive toxin.

aluminum chlorohydrate
See *aluminum*

aluminum phenosulphate
See *aluminum*

aluminum sulphate
See *aluminum*

aluminum zirconium tetrachlorohydrex gly
See *aluminum*

4-amino-2-nitrophenol
p-aminonitrophenol

Used as an oxidizing agent in permanent and semipermanent hair dyes, it has also been linked to bladder cancer in animal and human studies.

aminomethyl propanol
2-amino-2-methylpropanol

A thickener and gelling agent used in cosmetics, this is a skin irritant, and can also be contaminated with harmful impurities. As an amine, it can mix with other chemicals in the product, on the skin, or in the body after absorption to form carcinogenic nitrosamine compounds. (See also chapter 6.)

ammonia
ammonia, anhydrous

A cleaning and bleaching agent commonly found in glass cleaners, all-purpose cleaners, disinfectants, floor cleaners, furniture and metal polishes, drain cleaners, oven cleaners, and toilet-bowl cleaners, ammonia is toxic by all routes of exposure. Its fumes, even at the low levels contained in most household products, are irritating, and, in some cases, damaging to the eyes, nose, and lungs. On contact with the skin, it can cause redness and even burns. Ammonia must never be mixed with *bleach*, as the combination results in toxic chloramine gas.

ammonium laureth sulphate
This surfactant is found in shampoos and foaming bath products. Although considered mild, it can be irritating to sensitive skin. Laureth compounds can be contaminated with 1,4-*dioxane*, a known carcinogen. Since consumers have no way of knowing which laureth compounds are contaminated, avoidance is the safest option.

ammonium lauryl sulphate
ammonium dodecyl sulphate

A surfactant found in shampoos and foaming bath products, it can be mildly irritating to the skin.

aroma
Added to foods and tobacco products, an aroma is just flavoring by another name (and flavorings are simply perfumes by another name). Health effects of aroma include allergic reactions; some of these may mimic common dental prob-

lems, such as bleeding gums, mouth ulcers, and gingivitis. Like fragrances, aromas can affect the central nervous system to produce headaches, mood swings, fatigue, dizziness, and nausea, among other symptoms. Aromas are generally petroleum derivatives and can be contaminated with cancer-causing substances.

aromatic hydrocarbons

A family of petroleum-derived chemicals often used as solvents, common aromatics include *toluene*, *xylene*, *coal tar*, *naphthas*, styrene, and *benzene*. Widely used in cosmetics, perfumes, and household cleaners, they are also used in printing, fiberglass-reinforced products, glues, and veneers. Aromatic hydrocarbons derive their name from the pleasant, slightly sweet odor attributed to many of them.

They are powerful neurotoxins, however, and symptoms of overexposure include fatigue, confusion, dermatitis, and chemical pneumonia. Aromatic hydrocarbons are readily absorbed through the skin and subsequently affect the lungs, skin, blood, eyes, kidneys, and nervous system. Some are associated with reproductive hazards. Benzene, for instance, suppresses production of blood cells and can cause leukemia. See also *polycyclic aromatic hydrocarbons*.

arsenic

A pesticide primarily found in treated wood in the form of chromated copper arsenate, it is used for picnic tables, decks, and playground equipment. Because wood is porous, the arsenic can easily be transferred onto hands and from there into mouths, especially with children. Ingesting small amounts of arsenic can cause nausea and vomiting, decreased production of red and white blood cells, abnormal heart rhythm, damage to blood vessels, and a sensation of pins and needles in the hands and feet. Ingesting high levels can result in death. Exposure to arsenic can increase the risk of lung, skin, bladder, liver, kidney, and prostate cancers.

aspartame
E951, NutraSweet, Equal, Benevia

An artificial sweetener made from the amino acids aspartic acid and phenylalanine, and methyl alcohol, since its discovery in 1969 it has become a staple ingredient in breakfast cereals, chewing gum, colas and other sodas, yogurt, breath mints, juice, and manufactured desserts.

All regulatory authorities believe aspartame is safe. Nevertheless, it has been dogged by health concerns from the outset. During storage and when heated, it quickly breaks down into its component parts, each of which is considered toxic. Aspartame's two major constituents, phenylalanine and aspartic acid, can cause brain damage in very high doses. Even at the low levels permitted in foods, aspartame can be toxic to people who suffer from phenylketonuria (PKU). Relatives of those who have PKU may also be genetically sensitive to aspartame.

Neurotoxicity is the major concern, however, and, indeed, is cited as the number one problem in a recent lawsuit against the manufacturer. According to the U.S. Food and Drug Administration (FDA), aspartame is associated with headache, dizziness, loss of balance, mood swings, nausea, memory loss, muscle weakness, blurred vision, fatigue, weakness, skin rashes, and joint and musculoskeletal pain, even when consumed in only moderate amounts. Aspartame is believed to cause or worsen epileptic seizures, fibromyalgia, multiple sclerosis (MS), lupus, attention deficit disorder (ADD), diabetes, thyroid problems, Alzheimer's disease, chronic fatigue, depression, and eye conditions such as macular degeneration, diabetic blindness, and glaucoma.

The most recent evidence suggests that regular consumption of aspartame at levels considered safe considerably raises the risk of rare tumors known as lymphomas.

a-terpineol
alpha-terpineol

A synthetic fragrance found in perfumes, colognes, laundry detergents, fabric softeners, air fresheners, aftershaves, hairsprays, and deodorants, it is highly irritating to mucous membranes. Inhalation can cause excitement, loss of muscle coordination, hypothermia, central-nervous-system and respiratory depression, and headache.

atrazine

Among the most widely used industrial herbicides in the world, this is the one most commonly found as a residue on foods and in the water supply. It is also used for weed control on noncrop land, such as railways, roadsides, and industrial areas. Atrazine can cause irritation to the skin and eyes. Over the long term, it is a hormone disrupter, carcinogen, and reproductive toxin. In the environment, atrazine has been shown to feminize male frogs at doses well below the accepted "safe" levels.

avobenzone
butyl methoxy-dibenzoylmethane

A broad-spectrum synthetic sunscreen ingredient that can protect against the entire range of the sun's UVA rays, studies suggest that it is a potential hormone disrupter.

azamethiphos

An organophosphate insecticide used to control cockroaches, beetles, spiders, and flies, symptoms of exposure include headache, dizziness, nausea, vomiting, abdominal cramps, diarrhea, blurred vision, and muscle twitches.

azo dyes

A large category of dyes used in foods and cosmetics as well as for dying textiles, such as cotton, silk, wool, viscose, and synthetic fibers, these are considered easy to use, relatively cheap, and able to provide clear, strong colors. There are approximately two thousand azo dyes on the market.

The majority of these dyes are water-soluble and are, therefore, easy for the body to absorb. Absorption takes place through inhalation and swallowing of dust, as well as through skin contact. In humans, azo dyes can cause allergic reactions, such as hives. Many are considered neurotoxic and carcinogenic. Azo dyes can cause cross-reactivity with the *phenylenediamine* colorants used in hair dyes. This means that if you are sensitive to one type of dye, you can, over time, develop sensitivity to the other. Azo dyes, which frequently are washed down the drain, may also be toxic to aquatic organisms and cause long-term damage to aquatic environments.

bendiocarb
carbamic acid, methyl-, 2,3-(dimethylmethylenedioxy) phenyl ester

A carbamate insecticide used to control mosquitoes, flies, wasps, ants, fleas, cockroaches, silverfish, ticks, and other pests in homes, industrial plants, and food storage sites, this is highly toxic, especially to the central nervous system, if it is ingested or absorbed through the skin. Symptoms of bendiocarb poisoning include weakness, blurred vision, headache, nausea, abdominal cramps, chest discomfort, pupil constriction, sweating, muscle tremors, and decreased pulse. Persons with asthma, diabetes, or cardiovascular disease are at special risk with any kind of exposure.

benfluralin
benefin

An herbicide used primarily on turf, including lawns and golf courses, to control grasses and other weeds, it is a skin sensitizer, and can be irritating to the skin and eyes. In animal studies, it affects the circulation and the liver.

bensulide
phosphorodithioic acid

An organophosphate herbicide used on vegetable crops, such as carrots, cucumbers, peppers, and melons, in cotton, and on turf to control annual grasses, such as bluegrass, crabgrass, and broadleaf weeds, it is a central-nervous-system disrupter that can provoke chest tightness, nausea, abdominal cramps, diarrhea, headache, dizziness, weakness, blurring and teary eyes, loss of muscle coordination, and face muscle twitches.

benzaldehyde

Various benzaldehyde compounds are used as synthetic fragrances; 4-methoxy benzaldehyde, for instance, has a sharp, bitter almond-cherry fragrance, while 4-hydroxy-3-methoxy benzaldehyde (or vanillan) has a vanilla fragrance. Benzaldehydes can be irritating to the mouth, throat, eyes, skin, lungs, and gastrointestinal tract, causing nausea and abdominal pain. In laboratory studies, they have been linked to kidney damage, cellular mutations, and central-nervous-system disruption.

benzalkonium chloride
alkyl benzyl dimethylammonium chloride

A *quaternary ammonium compound* used typically as a disinfectant and preservative, this is found in disinfecting hand soaps, mouthwashes, and aftershaves, as well as in dishwashing detergents, disinfectants, and cleaners. It can be an irritant to the eyes and skin if used in high concentrations. Its wide use is causing new strains of resistant bacteria. Laboratory studies suggest it may cause reproductive defects and act as a mutagen.

benzene

A carcinogenic solvent derived from petroleum, this is found in lacquers, varnishes, oven cleaners, detergents, furniture polish, air fresheners, spot removers, nail-polish remover, and perfumes. Irritating to mucous membranes and poisonous when ingested, harmful amounts may also be absorbed through the skin through the use of everyday products. It may cause sensitivity to light as well as skin rashes and swelling. Benzene is a carcinogen as well as a powerful bone-marrow poison, destroying the marrow's ability to produce blood cells.

benzoates

A large family of naturally occurring and synthetic chemicals used as preservatives in foodstuffs and cosmetics, they are commonly encountered as *sodium benzoate, benzoic acid, benzoyl peroxide,* and *parabens* (see individual listings). Benzoates are universally associated with allergic reactions, especially in those suffering from asthma. They often cause gastric irritation, numbing of the mouth, and urticaria (nettle rash or hives).

benzoic acid
E210, carboxybenzene

A food and cosmetic preservative and member of the larger family of *benzoates,* this is used to inhibit the growth of mold, yeast, and some bacteria. It is also used as a pesticide. Although it occurs naturally in many plants, most commercial benzoic acid is synthetic. People who suffer from asthma, rhinitis, or urticaria may find their symptoms get worse after consuming benzoates.

benzophenones

Used as fixatives in perfumes, some benzophenones, such as dioxybenzone, oxybenzone, sulisobenzone, and benzophenone-3, absorb ultraviolet light and are therefore used as a sunscreening agent, especially for UVA protection. In sensitive individuals, they can provoke allergic reactions and photosensitivity.

benzoyl peroxide

Found in products to treat acne, benzoyl peroxide loosens and removes the top layer of skin and kills bacteria on the skin. It can cause contact dermatitis and sensitization, and is not to be used in cases of acne rosacea. Animal studies suggest that, when applied topically, it can promote the formation of skin tumors in animals. In foods, it is used as a bleaching agent for flours, and in blue cheeses, such as gorgonzola, and milk.

benzyl acetate

A synthetic fragrance with a floral, fruity aroma, this is found in perfumes and air fresheners and in a range of fragranced household products, including dryer sheets. Also used as a flavoring and aroma in foods and beverages, its vapors are irritating to the eyes and respiratory passages, and may cause coughing. It can be absorbed through the skin, thus causing systemic effects. Long-term use has been linked to pancreatic cancer.

benzyl alcohol
benzenemethanol

A solvent and synthetic fragrance found in a wide variety of fragranced household products, including perfumes and air fresheners as well as foods, when applied topically it is irritating to the skin and mucous membranes. When inhaled, it is irritating to the upper respiratory tract and can cause headache, nausea, vomiting, dizziness, a drop in blood pressure, central-nervous-system depression, and, in rare cases, death due to respiratory failure. Consumption of large doses may cause vomiting, diarrhea, and central-nervous-system depression. This is also a potential carcinogen.

benzyl cinnamate
See *cinnamates*

benzyl salicylate
See *salicylates*

beta-hydroxy acids
βHAs

Derived from many natural sources, BHAs, like *salicylic acid*, are often found in antiaging creams and other types of cosmetics, where they are used to burn off the top layers of skin. BHAs are similar to *alpha-hydroxy acids*, but are thought to be marginally less irritating to the skin.

bioallethrin

See *allethrin*

bioresmethrin

A member of the synthetic pyrethroid family, this is a broad-spectrum insecticide that is effective against flies, mosquitoes, and other flying pests in households, and is also widely used in commercial, industrial, food-storage, and public-sector settings. In household aerosols and sprays, it is usually formulated in combination with *pyrethrum*, *bioallethrin*, *tetramethrin*, and *piperonyl butoxide*. It is a hormone disrupter and is highly toxic to fish, bees, and aquatic invertebrates.

bisphenol A

A ubiquitous plasticizer that is the building block for polycarbonate plastic (used to make food and beverage containers and babies' bottles), but also in the manufacture of epoxy resins and other plastics; it is also used as an inert ingredient in pesticides (although not in the United States), and as a fungicide, antioxidant, and flame retardant. Bisphenol A is a hormone disrupter that mimics the effects of estrogen in the body. Studies link regular exposure to this chemical to insulin resistance, miscarriage, and diseases of the prostate, including cancer.

bleach

See *sodium hypochlorite*

borax
sodium borate

This mild alkali agent is used in cosmetics and toiletries as a water softener, preservative, and texturizer. Mildly irritating when used externally, it should not be applied to broken skin. If ingested, it can produce such symptoms as nausea, persistent vomiting, abdominal pain, and diarrhea.

boric acid
E284

An antimicrobial, preservative, and pesticide commonly used to control fungus on citrus fruits, this is highly poisonous. Regular exposure has been linked to fetal malformations. Severe poisonings have occurred from topical use and ingestion. For instance, when used externally, it can be absorbed through wounds or grazes and, at the low doses sometimes used in mouthwashes, it can result in chronic intoxication, leading to confusion, lethargy, anorexia, and hair loss.

bromadiolone

The active ingredient in certain rodenticides, this is an anticoagulant that causes the animal to bleed to death internally once it is ingested. This is toxic to all animals, including humans.

brominated vegetable oils
443

These are vegetable oils to which bromine—a heavy volatile, corrosive, non-metallic liquid element—has been added. These are used in soft drinks, citrus-flavored beverages, ice creams, and baked goods. Blending these high-density oils and other low-density oils (used as flavorings) makes the finished product easier to cook with and improves the texture of prepackaged foods. Adding them to fruit juices gives a slightly cloudy look that makes them appear natural. Animal studies suggest these oils accumulate in the body, producing fatty deposits in the liver, heart, and kidneys. The spleen, pancreas, lung, aorta, and skeletal muscle may also be affected. Growth retardation and impaired metabolism have also been reported, and, worse, all attempts to remove brominated vegetable oils from the bodies of animals once they have been stored have proved impossible. They are in your body for life. Banned in Belgium, Sweden, and Britain, they are still allowed and used in the United States and Canada.

bromonitrodioxane

Used as a disinfectant in household cleaners, and as a biocide in shampoos and other hair products, this *formaldehyde* releaser can cause allergic contact dermatitis, and mix with other chemicals in the product to produce carcinogenic nitrosamines. (See also chapter 6.)

2-bromo-2-nitropropane-1,3-diol
bronopol

A preservative found in toiletries, cosmetics, and household cleaners, it is a *formaldehyde*-forming chemical that can react with nitrosating ingredients in the mix to form carcinogenic nitrosamines. (See also chapter 6.)

bronopol
See *2-bromo-2-nitropropane-1,3-diol*

1,3-butadiene

A plasticizer found in containers for foods and cosmetics, this is also a common toxin in car exhausts, and an occasional contaminant in cosmetic ingredients, such as *acrylates* and *isobutane*. Breathing in low levels of 1,3-butadiene can irritate the eyes, nose, and throat. Inhaling high levels for a short time can cause central-nervous-system damage, blurred vision, nausea, fatigue, headache, decreased blood pressure and pulse rate, and unconsciousness. Long-term exposure is carcinogenic. Animal studies suggest that inhalation can cause birth defects, and liver and kidney damage.

butane
E943a

A propellant used in foods, cosmetics, and household and garden sprays, chronic exposure can produce a range of central-nervous-system symptoms, such as headache, breathing difficulties, mood swings, nausea, vomiting and dizziness, and symptoms mimicking drunkenness. Butane is a highly flammable volatile organic chemical (VOC) popular with solvent abusers because it produces a quick high; however, it can also produce convulsions, coma, and a quick death. VOCs also accumulate in human breast milk. While butane doesn't damage the earth's ozone layer, it does contribute to the formation of ground-level ozone, or smog, which can cause serious breathing problems. See also *isobutane* and *propane*.

butyl benzyl phthalate
BBP

A widely used plasticizer that humans are most likely to come in contact with through food-packaging materials, BBP has been associated with adverse effects on the central nervous system in humans and is classified by the U.S. Environmental Protection Agency (EPA) as a possible human carcinogen, based on limited evidence that it produces leukemia in female rats. It is also a suspected estrogen mimic.

butyl cellosolve
butoxyethanol, 2-butoxy-1-ethanol

A solvent and grease cutter commonly found in heavy-duty all-purpose cleaners, degreasers, and window cleaners, inhalation of this chemical can cause headaches and nausea. It is also easily absorbed through the skin into the bloodstream and can damage internal tissues as well as the liver, kidneys, and central nervous system.

butylated hydroxyanisole
E320, BHA

An antioxidant added to foods to keep fats from becoming rancid, this is also used as a yeast defoaming agent. BHA is found in butter, meats, cereals, chewing gum, baked goods, snack foods, dehydrated potatoes, and beer. It is also found in animal feeds, food-packaging, cosmetics, rubber, and petroleum products. Studies show it can provoke an allergic reaction in some people and may trigger hyperactivity. There are serious concerns over its potential carcinogenicity and estrogenic effects.

butylated hydroxytoluene
E321, BHT

Although commonly used in toiletries and prepackaged foods, BHT is most widely used as an antioxidant in rubber and plastic, and in liquid-petroleum products, such as gasoline and motor oil. Exposure through the skin or through ingestion can trigger contact allergies and dermatitis. Some evidence suggests BHT is a potential carcinogen and reproductive toxin. Once in the bloodstream, BHT can accelerate the breakdown of vitamin D (necessary to maintain immunity, and healthy bones and teeth).

butylene glycol

Used in cosmetics as a humectant, solvent, and fragrance fixative (keeping the scent strong), this can also be used as a preservative. It has a similar toxicity to *ethylene glycol*, which, when ingested, may cause depression, vomiting, drowsiness, coma, respiratory failure, convulsions, renal damage, kidney failure, and death. It is a *formaldehyde* former and penetration enhancer. It is widely used even though it has not been granted GRAS (generally recognized as safe) status because of concerns (based on animal data) of reproductive and mutagenic effects.

butylparaben
See *parabens*

C13-14 isoparaffin

A solvent and lubricating agent derived from petrochemicals, this is a relative of mineral oil used to make the product go on smoothly. It may cause skin irritation and increase photosensitivity of the skin.

calcium benzoate
See *benzoic acid*

calcium hypochlorite
See *sodium hypochlorite*

calcium sulphite
See *sulphites*

calcium thioglycolate
calcium mercaptoacetate

This depilatory (hair-removing) chemical has never been fully assessed for safety by any relevant group or association.

camphor oil
Japanese white oil, camphor tree

Used as a flavoring for beverages, baked goods, and condiments, it is also used in embalming fluid, in the manufacture of explosives and lacquers, and as a moth repellent and fragrance in household products. Readily absorbed into the bloodstream through all routes of administration, this was banned for topical use as a liniment for sore muscles and colds in the United States in 1980 because of reports of poisonings through skin absorption and accidental ingestion. Vapors and inhalation can irritate the eyes, nose, and throat. On the EPA hazardous waste list, it is a central-nervous-system stimulant that is associated with dizziness, confusion, nausea, twitching muscles, and convulsions.

caprylic/capric triglyceride
fractionated coconut oil

An emollient and solvent derived from plants, vegetable oils, and dairy fats, this is commonly used in soaps and skin-care formulas. It is also sometimes used as a synthetic flavoring in foods. There are no known safety concerns.

carbaryl

A carbamate insecticide used mostly against caterpillar pests on apples, but also on citrus fruit, mangoes, bananas, strawberries, nuts, vines, olives, soybeans, cotton, rice, tobacco, and grains, it is also used to treat lice in humans and livestock. Inhalation or ingestion at high doses can be toxic to the nervous and respiratory systems, resulting in nausea, stomach cramps, diarrhea, excessive salivation, sweating, blurring of vision, and lack of coordination and convulsions. Over the long term, carbaryl is considered a reproductive toxin and potential human carcinogen.

carbolic acid
See *phenol*

carbomer

A gelling agent, this is a synthetic polymer (a plasticlike material) used to thicken, stabilize, and promote the shelf life of cosmetic products. No adverse effects are known; however, this agent is poorly studied.

carbon tetrachloride

A toxic solvent that produces cellular destruction throughout the body, especially in the liver, kidney, and central nervous system, this is toxic by all routes of exposure: inhalation, absorption, skin contact, and oral ingestion. In 1970, the Food and Drug Administration (FDA) classified carbon tetrachloride as a substance so hazardous that no warning label could be devised that would adequately protect the consumer. It was subsequently banned from use in household products, although it remains in use in industry, and as a fumigant and dry-cleaning solution.

carboxymethyl cellulose

A synthetic gum used in creams and lotions as an emulsifier and stabilizer, this has been shown to cause cancer in animals when ingested. Its toxicity with topical applications is unknown.

carrageenan
E407, chondrus extract, Irish moss

Used as a thickener and emulsifier in a wide variety of foods and also in toothpastes, carrageenan is part of a naturally occurring family of carbohydrates extracted from red seaweed. Because it can contain traces of monosodium glutamate, it has the potential to trigger allergic reactions. Ingestion has been associated with stomachaches.

Most recently, there have been concerns that it is a carcinogen. This could be because inferior products can be contaminated with *ethylene oxide*; however, it can also be because of the way some high-molecular-weight carrageenans break down in the body into more dangerous low-molecular-weight carrageenans and poligeenans. In animals, carrageenan has been associated with cancer of the gastrointestinal tract, and laboratory studies using human breast cancer cells suggest that it can act as a trigger for breast cancer.

cetearyl alcohol
cetyl stearyl alcohol, emulsifying wax

An emollient, moisturizer, and emulsifier that can be animal, vegetable, or petrochemical in origin, it closely resembles human sebum (the waxy substance that protects the skin). Although it is largely nontoxic, in sensitive individuals it can cause contact dermatitis, hives, and skin sensitization.

chlordane

Although now widely banned, chlordane is a persistent organochlorine insecticide that continues to contaminate soil and water. Used primarily to control termites and as a broad insecticide on a range of crops, chlordane affects the nervous, digestive, and immune systems, and damages the liver. Headaches, irritability, confusion, weakness, vision problems, vomiting, stomach cramps, diarrhea, and jaundice have occurred in people who breathed air containing high concentrations of chlordane or accidentally swallowed small amounts of this chemical. Tests show it can kill birds and fish.

chlorhexidine

This is an antimicrobial used in mouthwashes, sprays, and dental gels to prevent and treat the redness, swelling, and bleeding gums associated with gingivitis. It is considered effective but, with regular use, it can discolor teeth and is implicated in rising rates of resistant bacteria.

chlorine
E925, sodium hypochlorite, chlorine dioxide, hydrochloric acid

Used in the processing of fish, vegetables, and fruits, and as a flour-bleaching agent, this is also used as a bleach and disinfectant in a wide range of household cleaners, including laundry bleach, dishwasher detergent, and tile cleaners.

Chlorine in food destroys nutrients and yet, in some areas, it is routinely added to tap water to make it "safer" to drink—even though there is growing evidence that chlorinated drinking water causes bladder and rectal cancers. In addition to its direct toxic effects on living organisms, chlorine also reacts with organic materials in the environment to create other hazardous and carcinogenic toxins, including trihalomethanes (THMs) and *chloroform*, and organochlorines, an extremely dangerous class of compounds that cause reproductive, endocrine, and immune system disorders.

THMs can be removed from tap water with an adequate home-filtration system that uses activated carbon to filter the water. As a household cleaner, chlorine vapors are powerfully irritating to the eyes and respiratory tract. Chlorine and its related compounds are also environmentally damaging, break down slowly in the ecosystem, and are stored in the fatty tissues of wild animals. (See also *sodium hypochlorite*.)

chlorobenzene
benzene chloride, chlorobenzol

A solvent used in dyes, pesticides, and perfumes, this is also used for degreasing vehicle parts. It is harmful if swallowed, inhaled, or absorbed through skin. In the short term, it is a skin irritant; over the longer term, it is considered a possible carcinogen.

chloroethane
ethyl chloride

A chlorinated solvent used for cleaning and degreasing, it is also used in the production of cellulose, dyes, and medicinal drugs, as well as to numb skin prior to medical procedures, such as ear piercing and skin biopsies, and in the treatment of sports injuries. Toxic to the nervous, cardiovascular, gastrointestinal, and musculoskeletal systems, this is a recognized carcinogen and suspected reproductive toxin.

chlorofluorocarbons
CFCs
These are aerosol propellants, such as trichloromethane and dichlorodifluoromethane, used to disperse cleaning solvents and degreasers, paints, pesticides, and cosmetics. Once in the atmosphere, CFCs stay there for a long time (several decades) and are the main cause of stratospheric ozone depletion, and, therefore, are important contributors to the phenomenon of global warming.

chloroform
Used as a solvent for fats, oils, waxes, and resins, and as a cleaning ingredient, exposure may cause respiratory irritation and skin allergies. Chloroform is a neurotoxin, anesthetic, and carcinogen. Inhalation of vapors may cause headache, nausea, vomiting, dizziness, drowsiness, irritation of the respiratory tract, and loss of consciousness. Chronic exposure to chloroform can aggravate some medical conditions, such as kidney disorders, liver disorders, heart disorders, and skin disorders. Studies have shown it causes liver and kidney cancer in animals.

chlorophenate
A fungicide and wood preservative not widely used today, but still present in older woods, evidence suggests that exposure increases the risk of non-Hodgkin's lymphoma.

chlorophenols
Because of their broad-spectrum antimicrobial properties, chlorophenols have been used as preservative agents for wood, paints, vegetable fibers, and leather, and as disinfectants. In addition, they are used as herbicides, fungicides, and insecticides, and as intermediates in the production of pharmaceuticals and dyes. Chlorophenol exposure is irritating to the skin and eyes. Prolonged exposure is toxic to the liver and immune system, and is a suspected trigger for cancer.

4-chloro-m-phenylenediamine
See *phenylenediamines*

chlorothalonil
Chlorothalonil is a broad-spectrum organochlorine fungicide used to control fungi that threaten vegetables, trees, small fruits, and grass. Exposure can

cause severe eye and skin irritation. Very high doses may cause a range of symptoms, including loss of muscle coordination, rapid breathing, nosebleeds, vomiting, hyperactivity, and death. In animal studies, female mice developed tumors in the fore-stomach area (attributed to irritation by the compound), and males developed both cancerous and benign kidney tumors. No studies on humans have been performed to date.

chlorpyrifos
Dursban
A broad-spectrum organophosphate insecticide, this was originally used primarily to kill mosquitoes, although it is no longer registered for that use. Chlorpyrifos is effective in controlling cockroaches, grubs, flies, termites, fire ants, and lice. It is also a skin and eye irritant. Short- and long-term exposure may affect the cardiovascular, respiratory, and central nervous systems.

chromated copper arsentate
CCA
See *arsenic*

cinnamates
A family of sunscreening agents that includes octocrylene, octyl methoxycinnamate, and cinoxate, cinnamates are derivatives of cinnamon and are chemically related to balsam of Peru, tolu balsam, coca leaves, cinnamic aldehyde, and cinnamic oil. People with sensitivities to these chemicals may have an allergic reaction to sunscreens containing them. The cinnamates are much less potent than many other chemical sunscreens and require the addition of other UVB absorbers to achieve higher SPFs. Laboratory studies suggest that some cinnamates may act like estrogens in the body.

cinnamyl alcohol
A synthetic fragrance with a sweet balsam, hyacinth odor, this is a common skin and eye irritant.

cinoxate
See *cinnamates*

citral
A synthetic lemon fragrance used in perfumes, household cleaners, and air fresheners, and in foods, citral is an allergen and irritant; it has estrogenic effects and has been found to cause enlargement of the prostate gland in animals.

citric acid
E330

A food acid naturally derived from citrus fruit, and used in foods and cosmetics; as a flavoring, it is found in sodas and soft drinks, ice creams and ices, sweets, baked goods, and chewing gum. It is also used as a pH (acid to alkaline) adjuster in beverages, as a preservative in cured meats, and as a color preserver in canned vegetables. Prolonged exposure damages tooth enamel. Citric acid may interact with any protein in the food to which it is added, freeing up glutamic acid, which can trigger allergies in some people (see *monosodium glutamate*). In cosmetics, it is a preservative and also an *alpha-hydroxy acid*, used to strip off the top layers of the skin (supposedly revealing "younger" skin underneath). Like all AHAs, citric acid can cause irritation. As AHAs become more popular in cosmetics like soaps, shampoos, and moisturizers, they have also become a major cause of adverse skin reactions.

citronellol

A synthetic fragrance and flavoring, in perfumes it provides a sweet, roselike odor. As an artificial flavoring in foods, it is used in berry, citrus, cola, fruit, rose, and floral flavors for beverages, ice creams, sweets, baked goods, chewing gum, and gelatine deserts. It is also used as a pesticide to combat mosquitoes and other flying insects. Applied topically, it can be a severe skin irritant.

coal tar

The black residue obtained by the distillation of coal, this is often found in antidandruff treatments and in products used to treat seborrhoeic dermatitis and psoriasis. It is found in some bath soaps, and may cause photosensitivity in some, and, with prolonged use, also make itching worse. The EPA classifies coal tar as a human carcinogen.

cocamide dea
cocamide diethanolamine

Found in dishwashing liquids, shampoos, and cosmetics, cocamide DEA is a strong detergent, foam stabilizer, and thickener. It can irritate the skin. It also belongs to a family of fatty acids called alkanolamines, which are considered hormone-disrupting chemicals. While not carcinogenic on its own, it has the potential to form carcinogenic nitrosamines when mixed with *formaldehyde*-forming ingredients. (See also chapter 6.)

cocamide mea
See *cocamide DEA*

cocamidopropyl betaine

A detergent that is a strong allergen and skin and eye irritant, this is also a penetration enhancer—allowing other chemicals in the mix to be more easily absorbed through the skin. It can be contaminated with *diethanolamine* (DEA), which, when combined with *formaldehyde* (released by other ingredients during storage), produces carcinogenic nitrosamines. (See also chapter 6.)

coumarin

A naturally derived fragrance, coumarin is a common skin sensitizer. Several types of coumarin have already been banned in the European Union because of their potential to cause serious skin reactions and photosensitization. In animals, it causes lung and liver cancers, and is damaging to the kidneys. According to the International Agency for Research on Cancer (IARC), coumarin is "rapidly and extensively absorbed after topical or oral administration to human subjects." Human data show it to be liver toxic. It may also cause central-nervous-system disruption.

creosote

Used in medicines to treat skin diseases, such as psoriasis, and also used as animal and bird repellents, insecticides, restricted pesticides, animal dips, and fungicides, creosote is a widely used wood preservative. As an antimicrobial agent, it can be found in heavy-duty household cleaners and disinfectants.

Once made by distilling tar extracted from beechwood, it is now largely derived from *coal tar*. The Environmental Protection Agency (EPA) has determined that coal tar–derived creosote is a probable carcinogen.

cresol
2-methoxy-4-methylphenol

A disinfectant (and relative of *phenol*) that attacks the central nervous system, respiratory system, liver, kidneys, pancreas, spleen, skin, and eyes, it can enter the body via the lungs or the skin. Repeated or prolonged exposure to low concentrations of cresol can produce chronic systemic poisoning. The symptoms of poisoning include vomiting, difficulty in swallowing, diarrhea, loss of appetite, headache, fainting, dizziness, mental disturbance, and skin rash.

crystalline silica

Also known as silicon dioxide (SiO_2), it is the basic component of sand, quartz, and granite rock. An abrasive mineral-based powder found in highly popular brands of all-purpose cleaners, when inhaled, it is an eye, skin, and lung irritant. Crystalline silica has been classified as a human lung carcinogen. Additionally, breathing crystalline silica dust can cause silicosis, a fibrotic lung disease (producing scar tissue in the lungs), which can be progressive and disabling and, in severe cases, fatal. (See also *silica*.)

cyclamate
E952, Natreen, Cologran

An artificial sweetener thirty-five times sweeter than sugar with a sweet-sour taste, in tabletop sweeteners, cyclamate is often found blended with *saccharin*. It is allowed in the EU, where it's widely used in "budget" fruit drinks, and so is mainly consumed by children. In the United States, the FDA banned it in 1969 after evidence emerged linking it to bladder cancer in animals. The ban is still in force. It is still widely used in Europe, Australia, and New Zealand, however, though the noose has been gradually tightening around cyclamate as a food additive. The U.K.'s Food Standards Agency (FSA), for instance, now advises parents to drastically limit children's exposure to this chemical.

cyclohexasiloxane
See *silicones*

cyclomethicone
See *silicones*

cyclopentasiloxane
See *silicones*

cypermethrin

A pyrethroid insecticide that has wide uses in cotton, cereals, vegetables, and fruit, and for food storage, cypermethrin is a skin and eye irritant, and central-nervous-system toxin. Symptoms of poisoning include abnormal facial sensations, dizziness, headache, nausea, anorexia, fatigue, vomiting, and increased stomach secretion. The Environmental Protection Agency (EPA) classifies it as a possible carcinogen. It may also suppress immune function.

2,4-D
2,4-dichlorophenoxy acetic acid

An herbicide used in agriculture, industry, and household garden products, exposure to this phenoxy compound can cause eye and skin irritation. One single application to grass that is tracked indoors can be expected to linger in carpet for up to a year. Studies have linked 2,4-D to non-Hodgkin's lymphoma, childhood leukemia, and childhood brain cancer. Recently, exposure to lawns treated with 2,4-D has been associated with cancer in dogs.

d-allethrin
See *allethrin*

d-limonene
See *limonene*

d-phenothrin
This synthetic pyrethroid insecticide, used to control bedbugs, flies, gnats, mosquitoes, cockroaches, and lice, is also a skin, eye, and respiratory tract irritant. With prolonged exposure, headache, dizziness, anorexia, and hypersalivation can occur. It is toxic to fish and bees.

dacthal
DCPA, dimethyl tetrachlorolerephthalate

A chlorinated herbicide used in agriculture (on fruits and vegetables), and in public and domestic settings, this is often found in home weed-and-feed preparations. It is also poorly studied for its effects on humans or the environment in spite of the fact that in the United States, DCPA and its breakdown products became the most commonly detected pesticide residues in an Environmental Protection Agency survey of drinking-water wells conducted during 1988–1990.

DDE
1,1-dichloro-2,2-bis(p dichlorodiphenyl)ethylene

DDE is a breakdown product of DDT present in the environment and in the body. Exposure can cause headache, dizziness, nausea, vomiting, incoordination, tremor, mental confusion, anxiety, and a sensation of tingling or crawling on the skin. It is a carcinogen and hormone disrupter.

DDT
dichlorodiphenyltrichloroethane

DDT is an organochlorine insecticide. Its once widespread use on crops has been halted due to its extreme toxicity to humans and wildlife; however, it is still used widely to control mosquito-borne malaria. DDT is a persistent neurotoxin, and traces of it regularly turn up in foods grown in DDT-contaminated soils. Chronic exposure damages the nervous system, liver, kidneys, and immune system in experimental animals. It is a reproductive toxin, hormone disrupter, and carcinogen.

dea-cetyl phosphate
See *diethanolamine*

dea-oleth-3 phosphate

This surfactant, found in cosmetics and toiletries, is a relative of *polyethylene glycol* (PEG). It can be carcinogenic in itself as well as contaminated with the carcinogen 1,4-*dioxane*. (See also *diethanolamine*.)

DEET
N-diethyl-m-toluamide

An insecticide found in a variety of commercial products used on clothing, household pets, and furnishings, it is the active ingredient in most mosquito repellents, and is unusual in that it is licensed to be applied directly to human skin. It is, however, an irritant that can produce a variety of skin reactions, including rashes, blisters, and mucous membrane irritation, and numb or burning sensations of the lips. DEET is also a neurotoxin that can produce insomnia, mood disturbances, and impaired cognitive function and seizures. In addition, several cases of toxic encephalopathy in children have been linked to the use of this agent. Symptoms of toxic encephalopathy include agitation, weakness, disorientation, ataxia, seizures, coma, and death.

deltamethrin

A pyrethroid insecticide found in a variety of commercial garden products as well as indoor-use products to control mosquitoes, flies, fleas, and cockroaches, this is considered the most powerful of the synthetic pyrethroids. Like all pyrethroids, it can produce a variety of symptoms linked to disruption of the central nervous system, including headache, dizziness, sweating, rapid heartbeat, tingling skin, and hypersalivation; it is irritating to the skin, eyes, and respiratory tract. It is also highly toxic to fish, bees, and other beneficial insects.

diaminobenzenes

Color developers found in permanent and semipermanent hair dyes, they work by a process of oxidation and, if absorbed, can be powerful mutagens. See also *phenylenediamines*, which belong to this family of chemicals.

diaminophenol

Oxidizing coloring agent for general-use hair dyes, this can cause allergic reactions and should never be used to dye eyelashes or eyebrows.

diaminotoluenes

Intermediates in the synthesis of dyes used for textiles, furs, leathers, spirit varnishes, and wood stains and pigments, these were once widely used in hair dyes, but were removed from use by many countries after they were found to cause liver cancer in rats.

diammonium EDTA
Diammonium ethylenediaminetetra acetate

A stabilizer used in cosmetics and household cleaners, laundry products, and pesticides to prevent the ingredients from binding with trace elements (particularly minerals and metal impurities), which change the texture, odor, and consistency of the product. The technical term for such ingredients is a "chelating agent." If ingested or absorbed into the body, chelating agents can concentrate these impurities in the body. (In the environment, they concentrate heavy metals and other contaminants in soil and the water supply.) Diammonium EDTA can be irritating to the mucous membranes and skin, leading to allergies, asthma, and skin rashes.

diazinon

An organophosphate insecticide used to control cockroaches, silverfish, ants, and fleas in the home and on pets, it is often found in formulations mixed with other pesticides, such as pyrethrins, *Lindane*, and disulphoton.

Symptoms associated with high-level exposure to this chemical include weakness, headaches, tightness in the chest, blurred vision, excess salivation, sweating, nausea, vomiting, diarrhea, abdominal cramps, and slurred speech. Diazinon is also known to be toxic to birds and fish.

diazolidinyl urea

A broad-spectrum antibacterial preservative used in cosmetics and personal-care products, this has particularly good activity against *Pseudomonas species*. It is a *formaldehyde*-releasing preservative that can form carcinogenic nitrosamines when mixed with nitrosating agents in the product. (See also chapter 6.) It is also a sensitizing agent that can provoke contact dermatitis.

dibutylphthalate
See *phthalates*

dicamba

A *benzoic acid* herbicide found in weed-control products, this chemical can cause irritation to the lungs, eyes, and skin in humans. Acute exposures can produce such symptoms as vomiting, muscle weakness, slowed heart rate, shortness of breath, mood swings, incontinence, cyanosis (bluing of the skin and gums), muscle spasms, and exhaustion. Long-term exposure can cause damage to the liver.

1,2-dichloroethane
ethylene dichloride

An industrial-strength solvent found in paint, varnish, and finish removers, and degreasers, this is also a skin irritant, a narcotic, and is toxic to the liver and kidneys, as well as to the nervous and immune systems. A probable human carcinogen and mutagen, it may cause systemic effects, and is regarded as a priority pollutant (one that regulatory authorities urgently need to study to fully understand its toxicity) in many countries.

dichloroethane
See *1,2-dichloroethane*

dichloromethane
methylene chloride, methylene dichloride
A powerful industrial solvent mainly used as a paint stripper and a degreaser. In the food industry, it is used to decaffeinate coffee, and to prepare extracts of hops and other flavorings. It is also used as a fumigant pesticide for stored strawberries and grains. Chronic exposure may be carcinogenic, as it has been linked to cancer of the lungs, liver, and pancreas in laboratory animals. It is a mutagen and teratogen, causing birth defects if exposure occurs during pregnancy.

dichlorvos
DDVP
Organophosphate insecticide used in household and garden pesticide products and in dog flea collars, this is also given to dogs to kill intestinal worms. Exposure can quickly produce symptoms of tightness of the chest, wheezing, blurred vision, tearing, runny nose, headache, sweating, twitching, nausea, vomiting, abdominal cramps, and diarrhea.

dieldrin
This organochlorine insecticide is no longer used in most countries because of its toxicity, although some countries do still use it for termite control. Surveys of dairy products, meat products, fish, oils, fats, and certain vegetables, such as root vegetables, regularly reveal traces of dieldrin in our food.

Dieldrin can form as a breakdown product of another pesticide, *aldrin*, and because of its extreme persistence, it can be found everywhere in the environment. Symptoms of exposure to the two substances are basically the same and include headaches, dizziness, irritability, vomiting, and uncontrolled muscle movements. Dieldrin is toxic to the nervous system and is a suspected carcinogen and hormone disrupter.

diethanolamine
DEA
A solvent, emulsifying agent, detergent, dispersing agent, and humectant found in cosmetics and body-care products, this is irritating to the skin and mu-

cous membranes. DEA is used in relatively few products, but DEA-containing compounds, including *cocamide DEA*, cocamide MEA, DEA cetyl phosphate, *DEA-oleth-3 phosphate*, DEA lauryl sulphate, lauramide DEA, myristamide DEA, and oleamide DEA, are very widely used.

While DEA by itself is not harmful, it can react with other ingredients known as *formaldehyde* formers in the product to form a potent carcinogen called nitrosodiethanolamine (NDEA). NDEA is readily absorbed through the skin, and has been linked with health problems, such as stomach, esophageal, liver, and bladder cancers. Related compounds, such as TEA lauryl sulphate and *tri-ethanolamine*, can also mix with other ingredients to form NDEA in cosmetics. (See also chapter 6.)

diethylene glycol

A solvent belonging to a family of chemicals called *dioxanes* (not to be confused with the pesticide *dioxin*), this is commonly found in glass cleaners. Diethylene glycol has not been fully assessed by any relevant body or group; however, *dioxanes* are thought to be carcinogenic, and research suggests that they are immune-system suppressants.

diethyl phthalate

See *phthalates*

diethylhexyl phthalate

See *phthalates*

difenacoum

A rodenticide that works by preventing the animal's blood from clotting, it kills the animal by causing internal hemorrhaging. It is acutely toxic to humans and other animals, causing the same kind of effects as it does in rodents.

digalloyl trioleate

This sunscreening agent is poorly studied in humans or animals, so its potential toxicity is not clear.

dimethicone

A film-forming, antifoaming agent and skin conditioner based on silicone and found in toiletries and cosmetics, this chemical makes the product more spreadable and can make the skin feel smoother, but it also traps other substances (including other ingredients in the product) beneath it. Because film formers do not allow the skin to breathe properly, they may exacerbate skin irritation caused by sweat or other substances in the product. See also *silicones*.

dimethicone copolyol

A more waterproof form of *dimethicone* that sticks to skin and hair better, this is a silicone-based polymer that is used as a conditioner in hair-care products and as a skin protectant. It is not considered toxic, but, with prolonged use, it can make the skin look dull. See also *silicones*.

dimethoate

An organophosphate insecticide used to control mites and other insects, repeated exposure can cause impaired memory and concentration, disorientation, severe depression, irritability, confusion, headache, speech difficulties, delayed reaction times, nightmares, sleepwalking, drowsiness or insomnia, and flu-like symptoms. This is also a potential carcinogen and reproductive toxin.

dimethyl ether
dimethyl oxide, wood ether, methyl ether

Found in hairsprays and other toiletries in pressurized containers, this is a relative of *propylene glycol*, and is a solvent that is easily absorbed through the skin. Once in the body, it can bioaccumulate and is known to be a reproductive toxin. It is also a solvent and a fuel used in welding, and finds use as a refrigerant. It has an anesthetic effect in high concentrations.

5-dimethyldantoin

A caustic found in toilet-bowl cleaners, it forms hypochlorite in water, which is corrosive to skin and mucous membranes.

dimethylphthalate
See *phthalates*

dimethylpolysiloxane
See *silicones*

dioctyl adipate
adipic acid

A plasticizer and solvent found in bath oils, eyeshadows, foundations, colognes, blushers, nail-polish removers, perfumes, moisturizers, and fake-tan preparations, this is also an element in the plastic wraps used for prepackaged foods, especially meats. Studies show it can migrate from the wrapping material into food. Applied topically, it can be irritating to the skin and eyes. With regular ingestion, it is considered a possible human carcinogen, based on animal studies that show an increased incidence of liver tumors.

dioxane

diethylene dioxide, diethylene ether, diethylene oxide

Found primarily as a contaminant in toiletries and household products, dioxane is a hazardous air pollutant and carcinogen. It is often a contaminant in ethoxylated surfactants, detergents, foaming agents, emulsifiers, and solvents., These ingredients are identifiable by the prefix "PEG" or words like "polyethylene," "polyethylene glycol," and "polyoxyethylene," or syllables such as "-eth-" or "-oxynol-."

dioxins

polychlorinated dibenzo-p-dioxins (PCDDs)

Dioxins are the toxic by-products of several types of industry: during incineration of organic waste containing chlorine (that is, plastics), and during manufacture of paper, wood preservatives, and chlorinated aromatics, such as 2,4,5-trichlorophenol (an intermediate in the manufacture of the herbicide 2,4,5-T). Found in bleached paper products, including disposable diapers, tampons, panty liners, toilet paper, milk and juice cartons, and paper containers for microwaveable food, they are also used in some pesticides and herbicides. More than 90 percent of all human exposure to dioxins comes from food, mainly from animal fat.

Tetrachlorodibenzo-p-dioxin (TCDD) is the most-well-researched dioxin and arguably the most toxic. When scientists refer to the toxic effects of dioxins, they usually mean TCDD. Many PCDDs are known to be toxic, hormone disrupting, and carcinogenic.

dioxybenzone

A chemical used in sunscreen to block UVB, it is a derivative of *benzophenone*.

disodium EDTA

E386, disodium ethylenediaminetetra acetate

A preservative and antioxidant used in foods, cosmetics, and household cleaners. In foods, it promotes color retention in tinned vegetables, and is found in cereals, fruit pie fillings, and salad dressings. In cosmetics and other formulations, its purpose is to prevent the ingredients in a given formula from binding with trace elements (particularly minerals and metal impurities) and thereby changing the texture, odor, and consistency of the product.

The technical term for such ingredients is "chelating agent." If ingested or absorbed into the body, chelating agents can concentrate these impurities in the body. In the environment, they concentrate heavy metals and other contaminants in soil and the water supply. Applied topically, disodium EDTA is irritating to the

eyes and skin, and acts as a penetration enhancer, allowing other active ingredients, and more harmful chemicals, to penetrate deeper into the skin and eventually reach the bloodstream.

dmdm hydantoin
diemethylol dimethyl hydantoin

A water-soluble preservative used in cosmetics, this can act as a *formaldehyde*-
releasing agent. This should not be combined with DEA or DEA-containing
compounds, as this can cause the carcinogenic substance NDELA to form. See
also *Diethanolamine*.

DSMA
disodium methanearsonate

An *arsenic*-based weed killer. Fatal if swallowed.

EDTA
ethylenediamine tetraacetic acid, ethylene-diaminotetra acetate

A preservative that stabilizes the bleach and foaming agents in detergent
products, preventing them from becoming active before they are immersed in
water. It is also used as a water softener. Unfortunately, it binds with toxic metals
in the environment and carries them back into our drinking-water supply and
into foods, especially fish and shellfish. EDTA can be irritating to the skin and
mucous membranes, and may cause allergic reactions. Liquid detergents are
more prone to contamination and therefore use more of this preservative than
the powdered variety.

endosulphan

The use of this chlorinated hydrocarbon insecticide is widely restricted. It
is poisonous to a wide variety of insects and mites, and can be used as a wood
preservative as well as on a wide variety of food crops, including tea, coffee,
fruits, vegetables, rice, and grains. It is a nervous system stimulant that can produce such symptoms as lack of coordination, imbalance, breathing difficulty,
gagging, vomiting, diarrhea, agitation, temporary blindness, convulsions, and
loss of consciousness. Toxic to the liver and kidneys with long-term use, it is a
suspected mutagen and reproductive toxin. It is poisonous to birds, fish, and
bees.

endothall

A dicarboxylic acid herbicide used to control weeds on land and in water, this
agent is very irritating to the eyes, skin, and mucous membranes. In humans, ingestion can damage the lungs and gastrointestinal tract.

enzymes

Enzymes are living organisms that are added to a diverse spectrum of consumer products, such as laundry detergents. Most laundry detergents are formulated with enzymes that act as stain removers. These products are called biological detergents. Enzymes are obtained from selected strains of bacteria. Products that have enzymes in them can be irritating to the skin, and cause allergic reactions, such as asthma and dermatitis.

Enzymes are also added to prepackaged foods to improve flavor, texture, and digestibility. Although enzymes occur naturally in foods, the ones used in commercial food production are synthesized in the lab and often genetically engineered. To date, there have been no reports of consumer allergies to enzyme residues in food, but then, there has been little formal research into adverse effects. Like all proteins, enzymes can cause allergic reactions when people have been sensitized through exposure to large quantities. Those that have been genetically engineered may be more likely to provoke allergic reactions. Use the table below to identify added enzymes in foods.

MARKET	ENZYME	PURPOSE/FUNCTION
Dairy	rennet* (protease)	Coagulant in cheese production
	lactase	Hydrolysis of lactose to create lactose-free milk products
	protease	Hydrolysis of whey proteins
	catalases*	Removal of hydrogen peroxide
Brewing	cellulases, beta-glucanases, alpha amylases*, proteases*, maltogenic amylases*	For liquefaction, clarification, and to supplement malt enzymes
Alcohol production	amyloglucosidase	Conversion of starch to sugar
Baking	alpha-amylases*	Breakdown of starch, maltose production
	amyloglycosidases	Saccharification
	maltogen amylase (Novamyl)	Delays process by which bread becomes stale
	protease*	Breakdown of proteins
	pentosanase	Breakdown of pentosan, leading to reduced gluten production
	glucose oxidase	Stability of dough
Wine and fruit juice	pectinase	Increase of yield and juice clarification
	glucose oxidase* beta-glucanases*	Oxygen removal

MARKET	ENZYME	PURPOSE/FUNCTION
Meat	protease* papain	Meat tenderizing
Protein	proteases, trypsin, aminopeptidases	Breakdown of various components
Starch	alpha amylase*, glucoamylases, hemicellulases*, maltogenic amylases*, glucose isomerases*, dextranases, beta-glucanases*	Modification and conversion (for example, to dextrose or high-fructose syrups)
Inulin	inulinases	Production of fructose syrups

Enzymes marked with an asterisk (*) are produced using GM technology. Other genetically engineered enzymes in food production include alpha-acetolactate decarboxylase (brewing), chymosin (cheese), alpha-glucanotransferase (starch), lipase (fats, oils), phytase (starch), pullulanase (brewing, starch), and xylanase (baking, starch).

epichlorohydrin
A major raw material used in the manufacture of epoxy and phenoxy resins, it is also used as an insecticide and fungicide. Skin contact can cause burns, and contact with eyes may cause permanent damage. It is a carcinogen, and a reproductive and central-nervous-system toxin; long-term exposure may, in addition, lead to liver or kidney damage.

ethyl acetate
This solvent, flavoring, and fragrance is found in foods, toiletries, and household products. In foods, it is used to flavor beverages, ice creams, baked goods, chewing gums, and desserts. It is also used in the decaffeination of green coffee beans and tea leaves. In the home, it can be found in air fresheners and dryer sheets. It is a mild skin and respiratory tract irritant, and central-nervous-system depressant. Its vapors damage the lungs, liver, heart, and central nervous system. It can have narcotic effects and has also been linked with anemia and leucocytosis (an increase in the number of white blood cells, an immune system reaction), and with damage to liver and kidneys.

ethyl acrylate
This solvent and synthetic flavoring is used in foods and as a fragrance ingredient (though this latter use is restricted in many countries). It is also used in the

manufacture of water-based latex paints and adhesives, textile and paper coatings, leather finish resins, and in the production of acrylic fibers. Highly irritating to the eyes, skin, and the mucous membranes, ethyl acrylate is a potential human carcinogen, and is toxic to the liver and kidneys as well as the immune and gastrointestinal systems.

ethyl alcohol
ethanol
See *alcohol*

ethyl dihydroxypropyl PABA
See *PABA*

ethyl linalool
See *linalool*

ethylbenzene
A solvent found in natural products such as *coal tar* and petroleum, this is also found in manufactured products, such as inks, insecticides, and paints. People exposed to high levels of ethylbenzene in the air can experience dizziness, throat irritation, tightening of the chest, and a burning sensation in the eyes. Animal studies have shown effects on the nervous system, liver, kidneys, and eyes on exposure to fumes.

ethylene dichloride
EDC, 1,2-dichloroethane, glycol dichloride
A solvent and an intermediate in the manufacture of *trichloroethane* and fluorocarbons, it is also found in paint varnish and finish removers, and pesticides. In foods, it is used in the production of spices.

It is highly toxic whether taken into the body by ingestion, inhalation, or skin absorption. In laboratory tests, exposure has led to stomach, breast, and skin cancers in animals. Chronic (long-term) exposure to ethylene-dichloride vapors produced effects on the liver and kidneys in animals. Men occupationally exposed to EDC have been rendered sterile.

ethylene glycol
A solvent and humectant often found in windshield-wiper solutions, this chemical can cause damage to the internal organs, especially the kidneys, heart, and nervous system, through skin absorption; inhalation can cause dizziness, drowsiness, and respiratory failure.

ethylene oxide

This industrial chemical is an intermediate in the production of *ethylene glycol* and other chemicals. Ethylene oxide is a common indoor pollutant that is toxic by inhalation and ingestion. Symptoms of overexposure include headache and dizziness, progressing with increasing exposure to convulsions, seizure, and coma. It is also an irritant to the skin and the respiratory tract, and inhaling the vapors may cause the lungs to fill with fluid several hours after exposure.

Laboratory animals exposed to ethylene oxide throughout their lives have had a higher incidence of liver cancer.

ethylhexyl-p-methoxycinnamate
See *cinnamates*

ethylhexyl salicylate
octyl salicylate
See *salicylates*

ethylparaben
See *parabens*

eugenol

A synthetic flavoring in foods and a fragrance in cosmetics, it is also used as a fungicide and insecticide. A skin irritant and allergen in cosmetics, if ingested it may cause vomiting and gastric irritation. It is poorly studied with regard to human safety, but is known to cause tumors in rats.

farnesol

Used both as a pesticide and perfume, this agent may cause skin and eye irritation. Little data are available on its toxicity in humans.

fenitrothion

An organophosphate insecticide used to control a variety of boring insects, such as beetles, as well as flies, mosquitoes, and cockroaches, it is irritating to the eyes. Symptoms of longer-term exposure in humans include general malaise, fatigue, headache, loss of memory and ability to concentrate, anorexia, nausea, thirst, loss of weight, cramps, muscular weakness, and tremors. It is a carcinogen, and an immune system and reproductive toxin.

fenoxycarb

A carbamate insecticide used to control fire ants, fleas, mosquitoes, and cockroaches, long-term animal studies suggest it is toxic to the liver. But, overall, this pesticide is poorly studied with regard to its effects on human health.

fipronil

A phenyl pyrazole insecticide used for ant and cockroach control as well as in flea and tick products, pets treated with fipronil have experienced skin irritation and hair loss; dogs appear to be more prone to these effects than cats. In other animal studies, this chemical has proven carcinogenic and, on this basis, it is classified as a possible human carcinogen.

flufenoxuron

A benzoylurea insecticide that is irritating to the eyes, skin, and mucous membranes, long-term exposure can cause nausea, vomiting, diarrhea, headache, confusion, and electrolyte depletion.

fluoride
sodium fluoride, sodium monofluorophosphate

Added to toothpastes and to water to prevent dental caries, in chemical tables, fluoride falls somewhere between arsenic and lead in terms of its toxicity. When containers of fluoride arrive at the doors of toothpaste manufacturers, they come with a skull and crossbones on the front. Fluoride is a systemic poison and there is enough of this substance in half a tube of family toothpaste to kill a small child.

Fluoride works best applied topically, but toothpaste rarely stays on the teeth long enough to be totally effective. Its benefits are highly contested and continually overstated. Ten years ago, fluoride was touted as reducing the incidence of dental caries by 40–60 percent; today, the revised figure is 18–25 percent. Levels of caries tend to be lowest in nonfluoridated areas, and better diets and conscientious brushing are likely to be the major factors in improved dental health.

While there is very little concrete evidence that fluoride genuinely protects teeth, there is plenty of evidence to show that regular exposure can cause harm.

Studies have shown a clear relationship between oral cancers and fluoride intake in both animals and humans. Benign squamous papilloma, for instance, which appears as a white patch on the inside of the mouth and is the precursor of squamous cell carcinoma, can be triggered by fluoride exposure.

Fluoride can cause sensitivity or allergic-type reactions and is now suspected in a host of illnesses, including gastroesophageal reflux disease (GERD), bone problems, diabetes, thyroid malfunction, and mental impairment. Fluoride exposure from toothpaste, supplements, and water before the age of six is also an important risk factor for dental fluorosis, which mottles and discolors teeth.

folpet

A carboximide fungicide found in many commercial garden products, this is irritating to the skin, eyes, and mucous membranes. Animal studies suggest that long-term exposure can trigger cancer in the duodenum.

formaldehyde
E240, paraformaldehyde

This disinfectant, germicide, fungicide, defoamer, and preservative is not used in foods, but can be used to disinfect containers, pipes, and vessels in the food industry. It is widely used in household products, such as deodorizers, disinfectants, furniture polishes, detergents, personal-care products (including shampoo), and cosmetics (including nail polish and hardeners). Formaldehyde vapors are common indoor pollutants, and are suspected human carcinogens that also alter your sense of smell and can cause respiratory irritation. Anyone with asthma, lung infections, or similar ailments can be severely affected by exposure to formaldehyde. It can also cause stuffy nose and itchy or watery eyes, nausea, headache, and fatigue. Some preservatives used in cosmetics and household products break down into formaldehyde during storage. Examples include *2-bromo-2-nitropropane-1,3-diol, diazolidinyl urea, DMDM hydantoin, imidazolidinyl urea*, and quaternium-15.

g-methylionone

This synthetic fragrance is a known contact allergen that is commonly found in household cleaners, laundry detergents, and dishwashing liquids, as well as cosmetics.

g-terpinene

A synthetic fragrance commonly found in cologne, perfume, soap, shaving cream, deodorant, and air freshener, it can trigger asthma. As a central-nervous-system disrupter, it can cause such symptoms as headache, mood swings, depression, incoordination, and lethargy.

geraniol

This synthetic fragrance is found in cosmetics, soaps, detergents, creams, lotions, and air fresheners. It is also used as a synthetic flavoring agent in beverages, ice creams, and sweets, and is sometimes found in "natural" pesticides to repel mosquitoes, flies, cockroaches, ants, gnats, and ticks. It is irritating to the skin and eyes, and a sensitizer and neurotoxin.

glutaral
glutaric dialdehyde, glutaraldehyde

An antimicrobial, bactericide, fungicide, and virucide sometimes found in household and garden products, this agent is also used as a preservative in cosmetics. Inhalation can damage mucous membranes, act as a sensitizer, and trigger allergic reactions. It is harmful if absorbed through the skin.

glycerides

Formed from a mixture of fatty acids and glycerol, glycerides have a variety of uses. In cosmetics, they are often used as emulsifiers and emollients in soaps and detergents, as well as moisturizers. In foods, they also act as emulsifiers and defoaming agents. They can be added to bakery products to improve softness, and are found in beverages, spreads, shortening, and desserts. Generally presumed to be safe, but full safety data are lacking.

glycerin
E422, glycerol

A form of alcohol used as a solvent, humectant (water magnet), and lubricant in cosmetics, glycerin can be processed from plants or animals. Prolonged contact can dry the skin (in common with other humectants, such as *PEGs*) as glycerin draws moisture from the closest, most abundant source. If you live and/or work in a dry environment, the nearest source of moisture will be your skin. In foods, glycerin is used to keep soft foods, such as bakery goods, confections, chewing gums, and sauces, moist. It is generally considered safe.

glyceryl PABA
See *PABA*

glyceryl stearate

An emulsifying wax made from hardened vegetable oil and *glycerin*, with the addition of vegetable stearic acid, this is generally considered safe, although it can provoke allergic reactions or contact dermatitis in some individuals.

glycol ethers

Widely used industrial solvents, these can be used alone or in combination; they can be found in such products as paints, varnishes, dyes, stains, inks, cleaners (for degreasing, dry cleaning), perfumes, and cosmetics, as well as jet fuel, deicing additives, and brake fluids. Glycol ethers enter your body when they evaporate into the air you breathe, and are rapidly absorbed into your body if the liquid contacts your skin. Overexposure can cause anemia, intoxication similar to the effects of alcohol, and irritation to the eyes, nose, or skin, and they can damage the kidneys, liver, and central nervous system. In laboratory animals, low-level exposure to certain glycol ethers has caused birth defects and infertility in males. There is evidence that workplace exposure can reduce human sperm counts. Common glycol ethers include:

- diethylene glycol
- diethylene glycol dimethyl ether

- diethylene glycol monobutyl ether
- diethylene glycol monomethyl ether
- dipropylene glycol
- dipropylene glycol monomethyl ether
- ethylene glycol diethyl ether
- ethylene glycol dimethyl ether
- ethylene glycol monobutyl ether
- ethylene glycol monoethyl ether
- ethylene glycol monoethyl ether acetate
- ethylene glycol monomethyl ether
- ethylene glycol monomethyl ether acetate
- ethylene glycol monopropyl ether
- glycol monoethyl ether
- propylene glycol monomethyl ether
- propylene glycol monomethyl ether acetate
- triethylene glycol dimethyl ether

glycolic acid
See *alpha-hydroxy acids*

glyphosate
An organophosphate herbicide found in a variety of commercial garden products, it has a generally low toxicity, but chronic exposure in animals to high doses of glyphosate has led to birth defects, and damage to blood and the pancreas.

hexyl laurate
dodecanoic acid, lauric acid
This synthetic flavoring and fragrance remains largely unevaluated for its effects on humans.

hexylcinnamaldehyde
See *cinnamates*

hexylene glycol

Used as a humectant, plasticizer, solvent, and emulsifier in cosmetics, this can cause skin irritation in some individuals. Vapors can be irritating to the eyes and lungs. In animals, repeated ingestion or skin applications have been shown to affect the kidneys and liver.

homosalate

See *salicylates*

hyaluronic acid
Hyaluronan

Used in skin-care products as a moisturizer and humectant, hyaluronic acid occurs naturally throughout the body and is an important component of connective tissue. The synthetic nature-identical version used in cosmetics provides little more than a temporary boost to aging skin. It appears to be safe, although it has not been fully evaluated for safety in humans.

hydramethylnon

An insecticide used to kill insects both indoors and outdoors, this is a skin and eye irritant. Long term exposure in animals has produced liver damage and accumulation of the chemical in the testicles. It is also highly toxic to fish.

hydrated silica
amorphous silica

A silica gel comprising *crystalline silica* in a watery matrix, hydrated silica is used in pharmaceutical and personal-care products as a carrier for active ingredients, a dispersant for colors and dyes, and as an anticaking agent. It is also used as an abrasive and stain remover in toothpastes and in some household cleaning products.

While it's the crystalline form of silica that is considered carcinogenic when inhaled, wet formulations contain these same particles. Used on teeth, it can weaken tooth enamel and damage gums. In rare cases, the silica can build up under the gum margins, causing inflammation that mimics gingivitis. The safety of ingested silica has not been adequately proven, and some observers have linked it with Crohn's disease, although this claim remains unsubstantiated. (See also *silica*.)

hydrochloric acid
E507

A caustic and acidity regulator commonly found in toilet-bowl cleaners, metal polishes, bathroom cleaners, and lime scale and rust removers. In foods, it is used as a solvent, as a modifier for starch, and in the manufacture of *monosodium glutamate* and gelatin. In cosmetics, it is used in hair bleaches to speed up oxidation and remove color. Fumes are irritating to the eyes, nose, and throat, and it can cause side effects, such as wheezing, sneezing, and a feeling of being suffocated. It can dissolve and destroy skin tissue, so splashes and spills can result in burns, permanent scarring, and, if in contact with the eyes, blindness.

hydrochlorofluorocarbons
HCFCs

These synthetic industrial gases, primarily used in refrigeration and semiconductor manufacturing, are also found in household products, where they are used as propellants. Although introduced primarily as substitutes for ozone-depleting *chlorofluorocarbons* (CFCs), HCFCs remain in the atmosphere for decades to centuries, and are themselves damaging greenhouse gases that are hastening the phenomenon of global climate change.

hydrofluoric acid

Commonly found in rust removers and aluminum cleaners, this agent easily penetrates the skin and body tissues—and may even reach the bone. This is a dangerous acid that, due to its anesthetic effects, causes no warning signs of pain.

hydrofluorocarbons
HFCs

Used as refrigerants, cleaning solvents, and propellants, HFCs are promoted by industry as replacements for *CFCs* and *HCFCs* (see below). While they pose no direct threat to the ozone layer, they are still very powerful global warming gases and environmentally destructive chemicals.

hydrogen chloride
See *chlorine*

hydrogen peroxide

A disinfectant, bleaching, and oxidizing agent found in toiletries (such as hair dyes) and household cleaners, it irritates the eyes, skin, and mucous membranes, is carcinogenic in animals and mutagenic in laboratory tests.

hydrogenated castor oil

This is castor oil that has been thickened with the addition of hydrogen atoms. It improves the feel of cosmetic products, such as body lotions, but can be a contact allergen.

CHEMICALS: A TO Z   291

hydrogenated vegetable oil

This is vegetable oil to which hydrogen has been added to thicken it. Widely used in margarines and spreads, and in snack foods, such as chips and baked goods, hydrogenation is a process that can promote the formation of free radicals in oils. Free radicals are highly reactive molecules that can damage and age the skin and body tissues. Hydrogenated oils are also high in unhealthy trans fats, the consumption of which is linked to a higher risk of heart disease, high cholesterol, preeclampsia, and ulcerative colitis. Complete hydrogenation converts unsaturated fatty acids to saturated ones. In practice, the process is not usually carried to completion, which is why this type of oil is often listed on the label as "partially hydrogenated vegetable oil." Since there is no safe level of trans fats, partially hydrogenated fats are no healthier than hydrogenated ones.

hydroprene

An insecticide used to control cockroaches, beetles, and moths, it is a hormone-disrupting chemical. Although animal studies suggest it is generally low in toxicity, the data are both incomplete and poor, and no human studies have been conducted on this chemical to rule out harmful effects due to long-term exposure.

hydroquinone

This agent inhibits melanin production when applied to the skin, and so is used in many skin-lightening creams and gels to remove freckles, age spots, and other hyperpigmented areas of skin. It is also found in some pesticide formulations. It is a severe skin, eye, and respiratory tract irritant and allergen as well as a suspected carcinogen.

hydroxycaprilic acid
See *alpha-hydroxy acids*

hydroxycitronellol

A synthetic floral fragrance, it is also a contact allergen, and skin, eye, and lung irritant.

imidazolidinyl urea

A broad-spectrum antibacterial preservative with particularly good activity against *pseudomonas* species. This, after *parabens*, is the most commonly used cosmetic preservative. It is found in baby shampoos, personal-care products, and fragrances, and is a sensitizing agent and a primary cause of contact dermatitis. It can release *formaldehyde* into the formulation and is most dangerous when used in combination with ethanolamines (any ingredient names containing the acronyms DEA, MEA, or TEA).

iodofenphos

An organophosphate insecticide found in a variety of commercial products used to control cockroaches, lice, flies and mosquitoes, fleas, mites, and ticks, the data on toxicity in humans are lacking. In common with other organophosphates, however, exposure may cause headache, nausea, sweating, altered heart rate, salivation, fatigue, and anxiety.

iso e super

This synthetic floral, woody fragrance is similar in structure to synthetic musk compounds and may have similarly devastating, hormone-disrupting health effects. It has been poorly studied for safety. For that reason, the U.S. National Toxicology Program has recently called for more and better data to be provided for this chemical.

isobutane
E943b

A propellant used in cosmetics, household and garden products, and foods, chronic exposure can produce a range of central-nervous-system symptoms, such as headache, breathing difficulties, mood swings, nausea, vomiting, dizziness, and symptoms mimicking drunkenness.

Isobutane is a highly flammable volatile organic chemical (VOC) popular with solvent abusers because it produces a quick high—however, it can also result in convulsions, coma, and rapid death. VOCs also accumulate in human breast milk. While it doesn't damage the earth's ozone layer, it does contribute to the formation of ground-level ozone, or smog, which can cause serious breathing problems. See also *butane* and *propane*.

isobutylparaben
See *parabens*

isocyanates

Plasticizers found in paints and packaging materials, isocyanates can cause asthma and other lung problems, even with very low exposure levels. They can also irritate your eyes, nose, throat, and skin.

isoeugenol
See *eugenol*

isomalt
See *sugar alcohols*

isopentane
methylbutane, 2-methylbutane
A solvent and propellant, and a major component of gasoline vapor, this chemical relative of *isobutane* can produce such symptoms as breathing difficulties, dry skin, contact dermatitis, altered heart rhythms, dizziness, and headaches. It also has an anesthetic effect on the skin.

isophorone
An industrial solvent found in some printing inks, paints, lacquers, and adhesives, this is also used in some herbicide and pesticide formulations. Fumes can cause irritation of the skin, eyes, nose, and throat, as well as dizziness and fatigue. Animal studies suggest that chronic exposure to isophorone vapors may cause kidney damage and birth defects, and slow the growth of offspring. Ingestion has been linked to an increase in tumors of the kidneys and liver as well as the lymph and reproductive glands.

isopropanol
See *isopropyl alcohol*

isopropylthioxanthone
IXT
A food-packaging chemical found in aseptic or Tetra Paks, it can leach into fatty foods and beverages (such as milk). It is poorly studied in terms of how safe or otherwise it is for humans to consume or be exposed to. Sunlight appears to activate this chemical, and human data suggest that topical exposure plus sunlight can cause skin rashes.

isopropyl alcohol
A solvent found in glass cleaners and windshield-wiper solutions, this chemical irritates the eyes and mucous membranes, and causes central-nervous-system depression. Prolonged contact can cause eczema and sensitization. Animal studies show that inhalation can damage the liver; ingestion results in drowsiness, unconsciousness, and death.

isopropyl palmitate
palmitic acid, hexadecanoic acid
Used in cosmetics as a thickening agent and emollient, this can be synthetic or derived from the palmitic acid in coconut oil. It is often used in moisturizers, where it forms a thin layer and easily penetrates the skin. It can clog pores.

isotridecyl salicylate
See *salicylates*

isoxaben
A broad-spectrum herbicide found in garden weed-control products, its fumes can cause eye and respiratory irritation. Based on animal data, it is a potential carcinogen and reproductive toxin, and is able to cause detrimental changes in blood chemistry if ingested.

Kathon CG
A preservative compound widely used in cosmetics, this is a mixture of two synthetic chemicals, *methylchloroisothiazolinone* and *methylisothiazolinone*. It is a contact allergen and sensitizer. Methylisothiazolinone has recently been identified as a neurotoxin that can damage nerve endings with repeated exposure.

kerosene
mineral spirits
This is a neurotoxic solvent found in all-purpose cleaners, furniture polishes, and waxes. An eye and skin irritant, it can damage lung tissues, and may contain the carcinogen *benzene*.

lactic acid
E270, butyl lactate, ethyl lactate
Used in a variety of food products as an acidity regulator and flavoring, this is generally considered safe to consume. In cosmetics, it can often be found in antiaging products, where it is used as an *alpha-hydroxy acid*.

lambda cyhalothrin
A synthetic pyrethroid insecticide used to control cockroaches, mosquitoes, ticks, flies, and aphids, this agent is a powerful neurotoxin that can provoke tingling, burning, or numbness (particularly at the point of skin contact), tremors, muscle incoordination, paralysis or other disrupted motor functions, and confusion or loss of consciousness. It is also highly toxic to many fish, aquatic invertebrate species, and bees.

lanolin
Derived from wool fat, and used as an emollient and thickener in a wide range of cosmetics, hair products, ointments, and lotions, lanolin itself is nontoxic and unlikely to cause adverse effects, but impurities mixed in with it can cause allergic skin rashes in some people. Cosmetic-grade lanolin can be contam-

inated with toxic pesticides, such as *DDT*, *dieldrin*, and *lindane*, which are carcinogenic, and *diazinon*, which is neurotoxic. These chemicals can enter the bloodstream through the skin. Labels do not disclose which lanolin-based ingredients are pure.

lauramide DEA
See *diethanolamine*

laureth compounds
Such ingredients as laureth-7, laureth-10, and laureth-23 are commonly used as emulsifiers in cosmetic products. These compounds are known as ethoxylated alcohols and, due to the way they are processed, can be contaminated with the carcinogen 1,4-*dioxane*.

lauric acid
dodecanoic acid

The major fatty acid found in coconut oil or palm-kernel oil, lauric acid is a common ingredient in many cosmetics, soaps, and detergents. In foods, it is used in the manufacture of various flavorings for beverages, desserts, baked goods, and puddings, and is generally regarded as safe.

lilial
A synthetic fragrance known to cause sensitization when applied topically, this can cause immune suppression after inhalation.

limonene
This synthetic citrus fragrance is found in perfumes, colognes, personal-care products, household cleaners, and air fresheners, and is a common pesticide in flea-control products. It can cause skin and eye irritation, and may trigger asthma attacks. It is a powerful sensitizer, and can produce tumors, reproductive abnormalities, and delayed growth in some animals.

linalool
A synthetic herbal/woody fragrance found in perfumes, colognes, personal-care products, household cleaners, and air fresheners, it is also a common pesticide in flea-control products. Able to cause skin, eye, and respiratory irritation, it has a narcotic effect in high doses, and has been shown to cause central-nervous-system disorders in animals. Symptoms include altered mood, poor muscle coordination, and reduced spontaneous motor activity. Exposure can cause fatal respiratory disturbances. It attracts bees, and thus poses a threat to people who are allergic to bee stings.

lindane

An organochlorine insecticide and fumigant used to control a wide range of soil-dwelling and plant-eating insects, this is also used in some lotions, creams, and shampoos for the control of lice and mites in humans. Readily absorbed through the skin, its toxic effects include central-nervous-system stimulation (usually developing within an hour), mental and motor impairment, excitation, clonic (intermittent) and tonic (continuous) convulsions, increased respiratory rate and/or failure, pulmonary edema, and dermatitis. In animals, it has been shown to damage the liver, kidneys, pancreas, testes, and immune system, and to produce a variety of tumors.

lye
See *sodium hydroxide*

magnesium oxide
E530

An anticaking and firming agent, and pH adjuster in foods, inhalation of this agent can cause fevers in humans. In animals, ingestion of magnesium oxide has produced tumors.

malathion

An organophosphate insecticide used for the control of garden pests as well as mosquitoes, flies, animal parasites, and head and body lice, this is easily absorbed through the skin. Acute exposure can produce symptoms of numbness, tingling sensations, incoordination, headache, dizziness, tremor, nausea, abdominal cramps, sweating, blurred vision, difficulty breathing or respiratory depression, and slow heartbeat. Very high doses may result in unconsciousness or incontinence. In test animals, malathion has caused reproductive abnormalities, and damaging effects to the central nervous and immune systems, adrenal glands, liver, and blood.

maltitol
See *sugar alcohols*

maneb

An ethylene(bis)dithiocarbamate (EBDC) fungicide used in a variety of garden products, this is irritating to the skin, eyes, and respiratory tract. Acute exposure to it may result in effects such as hyperactivity and incoordination, loss of muscle tone, nausea, vomiting, diarrhea, loss of appetite, weight loss, headache, confusion, and drowsiness. In the body, it targets the thyroid, kidneys, and heart, and, in animals, has been shown to cause increased rates of stillbirth.

mannitol

See *sugar alcohols*

mcpp

mecoprop

A phenoxy herbicide found in weed-and-feed products, mecoprop is irritating to the skin and eyes. It causes redness and swelling, and can cause cloudy vision. Human studies suggest exposure can cause cancer of soft tissues and non-Hodgkin's lymphoma. Animal data show it may increase the risk of miscarriage.

methanol

methyl alcohol, wood alcohol

A solvent and denaturant, this is a systemic poison easily absorbed through all routes of exposure, and a neurotoxin that can produce symptoms of headache, dizziness, confusion, abdominal pain, and weakness. Ingestion can damage the eyes and cause blindness. Methanol is one of the toxic breakdown products of the artificial sweetener *aspartame*.

methoprene

This hormone-disrupting insecticide is used to control mosquitoes and several types of ants, flies, lice, moths, beetles, and fleas. It is also used in animal feeds or mineral blocks for cattle. Data on its toxicity are incomplete. In the body, it primarily targets the liver.

methyl alcohol

See *methanol*

methyl anthranilate

Derived from *coal tar* and used as a synthetic grape flavoring agent in foods and beverages, this is also found in perfumes and fruit-essence aromas, and, occasionally, as a sunscreening agent in cosmetics. It can irritate the skin. Used in agriculture to repel animals, it may be present as a coating on fruit and vegetables. Toxicity data in humans are almost nonexistent. In animals, it targets the kidneys and liver.

methyl bromide

Used primarily as a pesticide to fumigate soil and buildings, inhalation causes dizziness, headache, vomiting, abdominal pain, confusion, and convulsions. Chronic exposure can cause central-nervous-system depression and kidney injury.

methyl cellulose

Used as a thickener in sauces and salad dressings, and as a thickener and sta-bilizer in ice creams, where it prevents ice crystals from forming during freezing, this is a bulk laxative and eating large amounts can cause flatulence, distention of the abdomen, or intestinal obstruction. It may also affect the absorption of min-erals. Methyl cellulose is used in cosmetics as a viscosity adjuster and in laundry detergents as an anti-redisposition agent (in other words, it keeps dirt from being redeposited on clothes during the wash). It is generally regarded as safe when used topically.

methyl heptine carbonate

A synthetic fragrance used in perfumes and air fresheners to impart a fresh, sweet, green, fruity scent, it is a cause of skin sensitization and may trigger breathing difficulties.

methylchloroisothiazolinone

This cosmetic preservative is usually combined with *methylisothiazolinone* (a combination also known as *Kathon CG*). It is a strong allergen that binds quickly to the skin, remaining there long after use. Laboratory studies suggest it is a po-tential mutagen, and a suspected carcinogen due to its corrosive action.

methylene chloride

Used as an industrial solvent and a paint stripper, this may also be found in some aerosol and pesticide products. Harmful if swallowed, inhaled, or absorbed through skin, it is a potential carcinogen that affects the central nervous system, liver, cardiovascular system, and blood, and causes irritation to the skin, eyes, and respiratory tract.

methylisothiazolinone

This cosmetic preservative is usually combined with *methylchloroisothiazoli-none* (in a combination known as *Kathon CG*). It is a strong allergen that binds quickly to the skin and remains there long after use. Laboratory studies suggest this substance causes nerve damage. It is also a potential mutagen, and a sus-pected carcinogen due to its corrosive action on the skin.

methylparaben
See *parabens*

microban
See *triclosan*

mineral oil
See *parafinnum liquidum*

monoethanolamine
2-aminoethanol

A surfactant found in wash-off toiletries, it is a relative of *diethanolamine*. Often denoted by the prefix or suffix MEA, as in cocamide MEA, linoleamide MEA, or stearamide MEA, it is a skin and eye irritant. Inhaling MEA can irritate the lungs and trigger asthma attacks. It is also a gastrointestinal, liver, and nervous system toxin.

monosodium glutamate
E621, MSG

This controversial flavor enhancer is contained in gelatin, textured protein, autolyzed yeast, monopotassium glutamate, yeast extract, and any kind of hydrolyzed protein. MSG is a neurotoxin that causes adverse reactions, including migraine headache, asthma, nausea and vomiting, fatigue, tightness in the chest, a burning sensation in the forearms and back of the neck, disorientation, and depression. Recent studies suggest long-term eye damage as a result of its use, including retinal lesions, thinning of the retina itself, and macular degeneration.

morpholine
A contaminant found in the waxy coatings used to preserve fruit and vegetables, this is toxic on inhalation, ingestion, and skin contact. The World Health Organization reports the morpholine can turn into the carcinogen *N*-nitrosomorpholine during storage.

muriatic acid
See *hydrochloric acid*

myristaminde DEA
See *diethanolamine*

n-butane
See *butane*

naphthas
A collective term for solvents derived from both petroleum distillation and *coal tar*, these can normally be found in dry-cleaning fluids and industrial-strength cleaners. Petroleum naphtha has a lower order of toxicity than coal-tar

naphtha; however, overexposure to either type may cause central-nervous-system depression, with symptoms of inebriation followed by headache and nausea. Naphthas can enter into your system through inhalation of their vapors, ingestion, and eye and skin contact. They are irritating to the skin, eyes, and upper respiratory tract. Skin chapping and sensitivity to light may develop after repeated contact.

naphthalene

A *coal-tar* derivative that is poisonous to humans and a potential carcinogen, this is one of a number of possible petroleum distillates that may be present in air fresheners. It is also a solvent, and pesticide, insecticide, and fungicide. It is used in the manufacture of lacquers and varnishes. Like all petroleum distillates, it is irritating to the skin, eyes, mucous membranes, and upper respiratory tract. Exposure can cause nausea, vomiting, and profuse sweating. Prolonged exposure is known to cause damage to the kidneys, liver, and red blood cells, and is thought to possibly cause cancer.

neotame

A close chemical relative of *aspartame*, this artificial sweetener is a staggering seven thousand to thirteen thousand times sweeter than ordinary sugar. Since it is made from the same chemicals as aspartame, there is no reason, and no independent evidence, to suggest that it is any safer, though the manufacturers say it is more heat stable than its predecessor. In animal studies, neotame ingestion increased weight gain beyond what would normally be expected from the given amount of food, suggesting an effect on the body that is potentially dangerous.

nitrate

This is a naturally occurring form of nitrogen found in soil. Nitrogen is essential to all life. Most crop plants require large quantities to sustain high yields, and, in moderate amounts, nitrate is a harmless constituent of food and water. In children and adults who have insufficient stomach acid, excessive nitrate ingestion can cause methaemoglobinaemia, the most obvious symptom of which is a bluish color of the skin, especially around the eyes and mouth. Nitrate in food and drinking water can be converted into toxic *nitrites* in the body.

nitrites

The collective term for potassium and sodium nitrite used in smoked and cured meats, such as bacon, salami, frankfurters, and sausages, nitrite preservatives greatly delay the development of botulinum toxin (causing botulism, a fatal food poisoning) in meat. It is used to develop a cured meat flavor and color, retards rancidity during storage, and preserves the flavor of spices and smoke. Nitrites are also used as preservatives in other foods, such as beer, fish and fish by-products, and some cheeses. Nitrites combine with chemicals naturally present in foods and in the gastrointestinal tract to form powerful carcinogens known as nitrosamines. (The same carcinogens can also form in cosmetics; see chapter 6.) There is no safe dose of nitrosamines.

nitrobenzene

A highly toxic solvent used in metal and shoe polishes, and many other products, this can enter your body through inhalation, skin and eye contact, and ingestion, and lead to spleen and liver damage. It also affects the central nervous system, producing headache, fatigue, weakness, vertigo, and, in some cases, severe depression, unconsciousness, and coma. Drinking alcohol increases its toxic effects. Nitrobenzene quickly crosses the placenta and can cause birth defects.

2-nitro-p-phenylenediamine
See *phenylenediamines*

nitrophenylenediamine
See *phenylenediamines*

octafluorocyclobutane
946

A refrigerant and propellant used in sprayed food products, it can irritate the skin, eyes, nose, and throat, and cause respiratory distress.

octocrylene
See *cinnamates*

octyl methoxycinnamate
See *cinnamates*

octyl salicylate
See *salicylates*

oleamide dea
See *diethanolamine*

oleic acid

Derived from various animal and vegetable fats, this is used in the food industry to make synthetic butters and cheeses. It is also used to flavor baked goods, sweets, ice creams, and sodas. In cosmetics, it is an emollient and emulsifier. Although generally regarded as safe to ingest, because of its film-forming ability it can clog pores when applied topically.

olestra

A synthetic fat substitute used in snack and convenience foods, it has no calories and cannot be digested; however, it is not healthy because it attaches to valuable nutrients known as carotenoids and flushes them out of the body. Carotenoids protect against diseases, such as lung cancer, prostate cancer, heart disease, and macular degeneration. The Harvard School of Public Health states that "the long-term consumption of olestra snack foods might therefore result in several thousand unnecessary deaths each year from lung and prostate cancers and heart disease and hundreds of additional cases of blindness in the elderly due to macular degeneration. Besides contributing to disease, olestra causes diarrhea and other serious gastrointestinal problems, even at low doses."

Olestra is banned in Canada.

oleth

Cosmetic emulsifiers and surfactants denoted by names such as oleth-5 and oleth-2, they can produce allergic skin reactions, and, because they are in the same family as PEG compounds, they may also contain impurities linked to breast cancer (for example, 1,4-*dioxane*, *ethylene oxide*). They are toxic to aquatic organisms.

optical brighteners

Used in laundry detergents and carpet and upholstery cleaners, these compounds put a thin chemical film on your clothes that converts ultraviolet light to visible blue light, making clothes look brighter. Like thousands of minuscule mirrors, they reflect light back to the eye, giving the impression that the cleaning product has worked better than it has. Optical brighteners belong to a family of agents that were once used in food products like flour and sugar to make them look whiter. They have long since been banned for this purpose. As they are used today, they can cause skin sensitization and allergic reactions.

ortho-aminophenol

Found in hair dyes, it imparts a light brown color to hair. This is a derivative of p-phenylenediamine (see *phenylenediamines*).

ortho-phenylenediamine

See *phenylenediamines*

oxalic acid

A poisonous organic compound commonly used in household cleaners, this is also used for cleaning car radiators and other metals. Oxalic acid can damage the kidneys and liver, irritate the eyes and respiratory tract, and is corrosive to the mouth and stomach.

oxybenzone

See *benzophenones*

PABA

para-aminobenzoic acid

PABA and its related compounds, which include ethyl dihydroxypropyl PABA, padimate-O (ocyl dimethyl PABA), padimate-A, and glyceryl PABA, are used as sunscreening agents. Applied topically, they can cause skin irritation and sensitization, as well as lead to light sensitivity (with blistering and peeling skin) in some individuals. PABAs are *formaldehyde*-forming chemicals that can form carcinogenic nitrosamines when combined with amines, such as DEA, TEA, and MEA. PABAs can cause skin irritation, and are relatives of the cosmetic preservatives *parabens*. In addition to being irritating to the skin, they are also thought to be estrogenic.

padimate-A

amyl dimethylaminobenzoate

See *PABA*

padimate-O

octyl dimethyl PABA

See *PABA*

palmitic acid

An emollient, moisturizer, and emulsifier found in a wide range of cosmetics, this can cause contact dermatitis in some individuals.

para-aminobenzoic acid

See *PABA*

para-aminophenol

This reddish brown color found in hair dyes must be mixed with an oxidizing agent (for example, *hydrogen peroxide*, *resorcinol*) to produce the required color. It can trigger moderate-to-severe skin reactions in some individuals. Once in the body, it can cause kidney damage.

parabens
butylparaben, ethylparaben, isobutylparaben, methylparaben, propylparaben

The most widely used group of preservatives found in cosmetics, it is estimated that more than 90 percent of all cosmetic products contain some form of parabens. They are also used in foods as a preservative, such as in dried meats, cereals, and snack foods.

Applied topically, they can cause skin irritation, contact dermatitis, and contact allergies. Animal and laboratory studies have long shown that parabens have a weak estrogenic activity. Butylparaben and isobutylparaben have the strongest hormonal effects, followed by propylparaben, ethylparaben, and methylparaben. Whether that poses any health risk for humans is still unclear. In animal studies, ingested parabens can induce cell proliferation (often a precursor of cancer) in the fore-stomach, and birth defects in mice and rats. Recently, when scientists conducted an analysis of breast-cancer tissue, they found accumulated parabens in every sample examined. The researchers suggested that parabens in deodorants and antiperspirants could be the cause.

Our bodies are exposed to estrogens from many sources, and it is possible that regularly ingesting or absorbing weak estrogens from a number of different sources may add up to a strong estrogenic effect in the body. Too much estrogen in the body is a trigger for estrogen-dependent cancers of the breast, ovary, uterus, and testicles, and may even have effects on fetal development. Although parabens are used in small amounts in individual products, they are widely used in all toiletries and cosmetics—usually in products that are left on for long periods of time. It is likely that we absorb parabens from each of the products we use. Thus, parabens need to be viewed in the light of the larger problem of exposure to environmental estrogens.

paradichlorobenzenes
PDCBs

Paradichlorobenzenes are neurotoxic solvents commonly found in toilet fresheners, mothballs, room deodorants, and industrial-strength odor controllers and moth-repellents, as well as in general insecticides and mildew-control agents. They replaced the older chemical *naphthalene*, a suspected carcinogen. Symptoms of exposure to PDCB fumes include eye and nose irritation, drowsiness, weakness, headache, swollen eyes, stuffy head, loss of appetite, nausea, vomiting, and throat and eye irritation. They are particularly toxic to small children and infants, who have experienced severe toxic reactions on being dressed in clothing stored in mothballs.

paraffinum liquidum
905a, mineral oil, baby oil

A transparent, odorless, and colorless oil derived from petroleum, this is used in foods as a glazing agent, release agent, and sealing agent. In cosmetics, it is an emollient and film former. Ingested, it can inhibit the absorption of essential fats and have a mild laxative effect. This is also a human carcinogen and reproductive toxin if inhaled.

In cosmetics, it is used as an emollient to produce a temporary moisturising effect; however, prolonged use destroys the natural oily barrier of the skin, leading to more persistent dryness. By destroying the protective oily barrier of the skin, mineral oil also acts like a penetration enhancer, allowing other chemicals to be more easily absorbed into the skin and bloodstream. In addition, mineral oil can be contaminated with *polycyclic aromatic hydrocarbons* (PAHs). The U.S. National Toxicology Program recognizes some PAHs as potential human carcinogens. Studies link them with an increased risk of breast cancer. If inhaled, it can cause fatal pneumonia and, in the United States, products containing mineral oil are obliged to carry a warning and have childproof caps.

Manufacturers have slowly been replacing the mineral oil in their products with other synthetics, such as *silicones*.

para-phenylenediamine
p-phenylenediamine
The black color found in hair dyes, this must be mixed with an oxidizing agent (for example, *hydrogen peroxide*, *resorcinol*) to produce the required color. It can trigger moderate-to-severe skin reactions in some individuals. Once in the body, it can cause kidney damage. See also *phenylenediamines*.

para-toluenediamine
p-toluenediamine
The brown color found in hair dyes, this must be mixed with an oxidizing agent (for example, *hydrogen peroxide*, *resorcinol*) to produce the required color, and can trigger moderate-to-severe skin reactions in some individuals. Once in the body, it can cause liver damage. It belongs to a family of dyes and intermediaries known as *diaminotoluenes*.

pareth
This surfactant belongs to the same family as *polyethylene glycol*.

parfum
perfume, fragrance
"Parfum" is the collective name given to hundreds of different chemicals used to produce a fragrance in cosmetics and toiletries, pesticides, household cleaners, air fresheners, foods, and cigarettes (where it is called an *aroma*). Per-

fumes contain every kind of poison known to man, which is why many perfume ingredients double up as pesticides. Most, for instance, are solvents, and, as such, are neurotoxic. Many are persistent (that is, they don't break down in the environment, and they accumulate in human tissue and breast milk) and can cause birth defects. Artificial musks, a common ingredient in fragrances and toiletries, are hormone-disrupting and cancer-causing. Immediate reactions to parfum include headache, mood swings, depression, forgetfulness, and irritation. It is also a major trigger of attacks in asthmatics.

Of the twenty most common perfume ingredients, four—*acetone*, ethanol, *ethyl acetate*, and *methylene chloride*—are classified as hazardous waste by the U.S. Environmental Protection Agency.

Other commonly used chemicals in perfume include *propylene glycol*; cyclohexanol, a central-nervous-system depressant; *linalool*, which can provoke depression, loss of equilibrium, and respiratory disturbances; methyl ethyl ketone, which is toxic to the liver and kidneys, and irritating to the eyes, nose, and throat; and *formaldehyde*, a known carcinogen. Spray formulations mean you inhale more of these toxic chemicals.

partially hydrogenated vegetable oil
See *hydrogenated vegetable oil*

PEG
polyethylene glycol
Polyethylene glycol (PEG) compounds are derived from natural gas and have numerous functions in toiletries, including as moisturizers, emulsifiers, emollients, and antioxidants, as well as plasticizers, solvents, and softeners. Adding PEG to a product will also prevent moisture loss during storage.

On the ingredients label, PEGs are usually listed followed by a number (for example, PEG-4 or PEG-350) that refers to their molecular weight. These numbers represent the liquidity of the compound: the higher the number, the more solid it is. PEG compounds can be contaminated with the carcinogen 1,4-*dioxane*. They can also form carcinogens when mixed with DEA and TEA compounds. (See also chapter 6.)

pendimethalin
An herbicide used to control grasses and weeds, this can be irritating to the skin and lungs; it is toxic to the liver with long-term use.

pentachloronitrobenzene
PCNB, quintozene
An organochlorine fungicide, very high doses can induce fatigue, possible dizziness, and lethargy. Long-term exposure is toxic to the liver.

pentachlorophenol
PCP

A reproductive toxin found in products like laundry starch, it is associated with fetal abnormalities and birth defects.

pentane

Often found in dryer sheets and fabric softeners, this is irritating to the eyes and can cause skin rashes. Its vapors may cause headache, nausea, vomiting, dizziness, drowsiness, irritation of the respiratory tract, and loss of consciousness. Prolonged and repeated inhalation of vapors may cause central-nervous-system depression.

pentasodium disodium edta
See *disodium EDTA*

perchloroethylene
PERC, tetrachloroethylene, ethylene tetrachloride

A solvent commonly found in dry-cleaning fluids and spot removers, PERC is fat-soluble and so collects in the tissues of living organisms and accumulates in the environment. Its vapors are irritating to the skin, eyes, and upper respiratory tract, and can produce giddiness, headache, inebriation, nausea, vomiting, and sinus inflammation. Chronic inhalation can cause serious depression of the central nervous system as well as kidney and liver damage.

Long-term exposure can cause liver and central-nervous-system damage. It is a proven carcinogen in animals and suspected human carcinogen.

permethrin

A synthetic pyrethroid insecticide used against a variety of pests, including flies and cockroaches, this compound can cause irritation to the skin and eyes. Human studies are lacking, but animal studies suggest it can suppress the immune system and is toxic to the liver.

petrolatum
petroleum jelly, Vaseline

This chemical lubricant derived from petroleum is used to make skin creams feel smoother. It can provoke allergic skin reactions and, over time, will destroy the natural oily barrier on the skin, leaving it more prone to drying, flaking, and cracking.

phenol
carbolic acid

The largest single use of phenol is in resins used in the plywood, adhesive, construction, automotive, and appliance industries. It is also used as an intermediate in the production of caprolactam, which is used to make nylon and other synthetic fibers, and *bisphenol A*, which is used to make epoxy and other resins. In household products, phenol is used as a disinfectant—for instance, in bathroom and toilet cleaners—and as an anesthetic in medicinal preparations, including ointments, ear and nose drops, cold-sore lotions, throat lozenges, and antiseptic lotions. Exposure to its fumes can irritate the eyes, nose, and throat, and cause sweating, pallor, weakness, headache, dizziness, muscle ache and pain, tremors and twitches, ringing in the ears, shock, and, in extreme cases, a profound fall in body temperature.

phenoxyethanol

This is a cosmetic preservative that can cause skin irritation, contact dermatitis, and contact allergies.

phenoxyisopropanol

A preservative and solvent found in acne treatments, shampoos, and facial cleansers, this is a strong irritant that can only be used in wash-off products. Skin reactions are likely.

phenylenediamines

A family of dyes commonly found in permanent and semipermanent hair colors, they can damage the skin, cause allergic reactions (sometimes fatal ones), and are irritating to the eyes. Phenylenediamines are also carcinogenic, and can cause immune system dysregulation as well as kidney and liver damage. They are toxic to wildlife and soil. The type of phenylenediamine used depends on the end color, thus:

- para-phenylenediamine (black)

- para-toluenediamine (brown)

- ortho-phenylenediamine (brown)

- para-aminophenol (reddish-brown)

- ortho-aminophenol (light brown)

phenylmercuric acetate
PMA

An organomercury compound used as a fungicide and herbicide, mercury is a neurotoxin and there is no safe dose. It is corrosive to the skin and eyes, and animal studies suggest it is a reproductive and developmental toxin.

2-phenylphenol

o-Phenylphenol, 2-biphenylol, o-hydroxybiphenyl

A fungicide and disinfectant of the phenol family, this is found in household disinfectant sprays and wood treatments. It's also used as a postharvest fungicide for vegetables and fruits, especially citrus, and as an antimicrobial preservative in cosmetics and a flavoring in food. A recognized carcinogen and suspected hormone disrupter, neurotoxin, and reproductive toxin implicated in liver and kidney damage, exposure can cause skin and respiratory irritation. Common symptoms include headache, giddiness, nervousness, blurred vision, weakness, nausea, cramps, diarrhea, and discomfort in the chest. Rarely, when used in cosmetics, it can cause skin depigmentation and photoallergy (light sensitivity).

phenyl-p-phenylenediamine

See *phenylenediamines*

phospholipids

Fat substances found in all living cells, phospholipids are critical building blocks for all body cells. Lecithin, found in soybeans and other seeds as well as in eggs, contains several phospholipids, such as phosphatidylcholine, phosphatidylethanolamine, phosphatidylinositol, or phosphatidylserine. In cosmetics, they are extracted from natural sources or synthesized in the lab to be used as emollients, moisturizers, emulsifiers, dispersants, wetting agents, and stabilizers. They are generally regarded as safe.

phosphoric acid

A common ingredient in metal cleaners and rust removers, this is irritating to the skin and lungs. Phosphoric acid is also used to acidify foods and beverages, such as various colas. Ingesting high levels of this leaches essential calcium from the bones, and raises the risk of brittle bones and fractures. Children consuming at least six cups of phosphoric acid–containing soft drinks daily have more than five times the risk of developing low blood levels of calcium compared with children who don't drink sodas.

phthalates

Phthalates are a class of widely used industrial compounds that have become ubiquitous, not just in the products in which they are intentionally used, but also as contaminants in almost everything. They can be used as softeners in plastics, oily substances in perfumes, and additives to hairsprays, lubricants, and wood finishers. Phthalates are estrogen mimics that can easily leach out of products in our homes. Animal studies show that exposure to very low levels of the phthalates dibutyl phthalate (DBP) and diethylhexyl phthalate (DEHP) in the womb caused demasculinization of male fetuses and increased the rate of reproductive disorders, such as hypospadias (where the urethra opens on the underside of the penis). Phthalate exposure is also linked to reduction in sperm quality.

pine oil

A common antimicrobial component of household cleaning solutions, its fumes are irritating to the mucous membranes and gastrointestinal tract. Large exposures can cause severe respiratory distress, cardiovascular collapse, severe central-nervous-system effects, and kidney failure.

piperonyl butoxide

This is a synergist that is used in a wide variety of insecticides. Synergists are chemicals that, while lacking killing properties of their own, enhance the pesticidal properties of other active ingredients. Piperonyl butoxide is used in conjunction with insecticides, such as *pyrethrins*, pyrethroids, *rotenone*, and carbamates.

pirimiphosmethyl

An organophosphate insecticide that is irritating to the eyes, respiratory system, and skin, high exposure can result in headache, nausea, vomiting, abdominal cramps, diarrhea, dizziness, sweating, extreme weakness, blurred vision, muscle tremors, and tightness in the chest.

polychlorinated biphenyls
PCBs

Related to *DDT* and *dioxins*, PCBs were once used extensively in transformers, for insulating cooling equipment, and in hydraulic fluids, lubricants, and other electrical components. Banned since the 1970s, they are still present in many older electrical installations. PCBs resist biodegradation, are fat-soluble, and tend to accumulate in animals higher up the food chain. PCBs are both antiestrogens and antiandrogens (in other words, they disrupt signaling from both female and male hormones). Exposure to PCBs in food has been linked to delayed brain development and reduced IQ in children. PCBs can still be found as contaminants in plastics, dyes, inks, older types of carbonless copy paper, adhesives, wood treatments, and pesticides. They have also been detected as contaminants in such foods as meat and fish, waterfowl, poultry, eggs, and milk.

polycyclic aromatic hydrocarbons

Polycyclic aromatic hydrocarbons (PAHs) are a group of over one hundred different chemicals created by incineration of plastic waste, such as polyvinyl chloride (PVC), high-density polyethylene (HDPE), and polypropylene, as well as other industrial waste; large quantities are released during natural events, such as volcanic eruptions and forest fires, but also by many human activities, such as burning coal, oil, and wood for heat, smoking cigarettes, frying food, and gas-powered motor travel. They are found in asphalt, creosote, coal-tar pitch, roofing tar, coal, and crude oil. A few PAHs are used in such products as medicines, plastics, dyes, and pesticides.

Animal studies have also shown that PAHs can have harmful effects on the skin, body fluids, and immune system after both short- and long-term exposure. Mice exposed to high levels of PAHs during pregnancy had difficulty reproducing, as did their offspring. These offspring also had higher rates of birth defects and lower body weights. In laboratory animals, PAHs produced a variety of cancers.

polyethylene glycol
See *PEGs*

polyoxyethylene alkyl ethers
This family of detergents, surfactants, and wetting agents is found in household cleaning products and cosmetics. Lauryl alcohol and cetyl alcohol, as well as sorbitan, are polyoxyethylene compounds found in cosmetics and in toiletries as emulsifying agents. In household cleaning compounds like nonyl phenol, these are used because of their strong degreasing effects. Some polyoxyethylene compounds are also used as fabric softeners and antistatic agents. They are mostly nonirritating, but can be contaminated with the carcinogen 1,4-*dioxane*.

polysorbates
Emulsifiers and surfactants used in foods and cosmetics, these belong to a large group of chemicals known as *polyoxyethylene alkyl ethers*, and can be contaminated with the carcinogen 1,4-*dioxane*.

polytetrefluoroethylene
PTFE, Teflon
See *Teflon*

polyvinylpyrrolidone
E1201
A clarifying additive in wine, beer, and vinegar, and used in the production of dietary supplements, PVP compounds can also be found in some hairstyling products, especially hairsprays. Inhalation of PVP damages the lungs; animal studies suggest that when ingested, it is associated with damage to the kidneys and liver as well as an increased risk of cancer.

potassium benzoate
See *benzoates, sodium benzoate*

potassium hydroxide
E525, caustic potash, lye
A harsh alkali used as an intermediate in soap production and as a neutralizer in food production, this is also found in nail-cuticle softeners and depilatories. It is corrosive to the eyes, mucous membranes, and skin, and can cause dermatitis and burns even in dilute solutions.

potassium nitrite
E249
See *nitrites*

PPG-3 methyl ether
See *propylene glycol*

PPG-14 butyl ether
Used primarily in cosmetics as a preservative, the solvent PPG-14 butyl ether is a relative of *propylene glycol*. In addition to being a skin irritant and neurotoxin, it is potentially toxic to the kidneys and liver. In the United States, it is a pesticide component used in sprays to protect animals from flies, gnats, and mosquitoes. It is poisonous in high concentrations and can enhance the skin penetration of other, more toxic chemicals.

pronamide
An herbicide used either before weeds emerge (preemergence) and/or after weeds come up, it controls a wide range of annual and perennial grasses, as well as certain annual broadleaf weeds.
Pronamide has caused liver tumors in mice after two years at high doses, suggesting that it could be carcinogenic in humans exposed to sufficient quantities. Target organs identified in animal studies include the liver and the thyroid, adrenal, and pituitary glands. It is poorly studied in humans.

propane
A petroleum-derived propellant for aerosol sprays, especially after the ban of *chlorofluorocarbons* (CFCs), skin contact may result in frostbite and burns. A central-nervous-system toxicant, it can produce such symptoms as rapid breathing, incoordination, rapid fatigue, excessive salivation, disorientation, headache, nausea, and vomiting.

propoxur

Used to control a variety of insect pests, including ants, cockroaches, crickets, flies, and mosquitoes, signs of propoxur intoxication over the short or long term include nausea, vomiting, abdominal cramps, sweating, diarrhea, excessive salivation, weakness, imbalance, blurring of vision, breathing difficulty, increased blood pressure, incontinence, and death. Animal studies suggest it can reduce birth weight, retard the development of some reflexes, and impair the central nervous system.

propyl gallate
E310

An antioxidant used in such foods as fats, oils, mayonnaise, shortening, baked goods, sweets, dried meat, fresh pork sausage, and dried milk to keep oils and fats in products from turning rancid, it is usually found in combination with another antioxidant, ascorbyl palmitate, as each enhances the effect of the other. It is also used in cosmetics, hair products, adhesives, and lubricants. It has low toxicity, but can cause contact dermatitis in those who are exposed to it regularly.

propylene glycol
PPG, 1,2-propanediol

This is a solvent, humectant, and wetting agent found in foods, cosmetics, and household products. In foods, it is used as an emulsifier and viscosity adjuster for confectionery, chocolate products, ice creams, beverages, and baked goods. Irritating to the eyes, skin, and respiratory tract, applied topically it acts as a penetration enhancer, altering skin structure, thereby allowing other, more toxic chemicals to penetrate deeply into the skin and eventually the bloodstream.

PVP
See *polyvinylpyrrolidone*

pyrethrins

Pyrethrins are natural insecticides produced by certain species of the chrysanthemum plant. The flowers of the plant are harvested shortly after blooming, and are either dried and powdered, or the oils within the flowers are extracted with solvents. The active insecticidal components in these dusts and extracts are collectively known as pyrethrins. Synthetic pyrethrins are usually referred to as pyrethroids, and the term "pyrethrum" is a general name covering both compounds.

Pyrethrums have been used primarily to control human lice, mosquitoes, cockroaches, beetles, and flies. They are contact poisons that quickly penetrate the nervous system of the insect. Synthetic pyrethroids are considered more powerful toxins than their natural counterparts. Inhaling high levels of pyrethrum may bring about asthmatic breathing, sneezing, nasal stuffiness, headache, nausea, incoordination, tremors, convulsions, facial flushing, and swelling, burning, and itching sensations. At high doses, pyrethrum can be damaging to the central nervous system and the immune system. When the immune system is attacked by pyrethrum, allergies can be worsened. Animals fed large doses of pyrethrins may experience liver damage.

quaternary ammonium compounds

This large family of strong disinfectants and surfactants is found in household cleaners, but also in medications, such as ophthalmic preparations and in cosmetics. Highly toxic and implicated in the rise of drug-resistant bacteria in homes and hospitals, in eyedrops, they can damage eyes on contact. Examples of quaternary ammonium compounds include *benzalkonium chloride*, alkyl triethanol ammonium chloride, benzethonium chloride, and cetrimide (cetyltrimethylammonium bromide).

In cosmetics, they are used as preservatives, examples of which include quaternium-15, quaternium-18, and quaternium-80. Applied to the skin, they can be irritating and, because they are *formaldehyde*-forming compounds, they can produce carcinogenic nitrosamines when mixed with DEA and TEA. (See also chapter 6.)

red petrolatum

A reddish brown, greaselike petroleum jelly, its natural pigments are effective in blocking the sun's ultraviolet rays. During World War II, red petrolatum was extensively used by the military. It has largely fallen out of fashion, but is still used as a sunblocker in some products.

resmethrin

A synthetic pyrethroid used to control flying and crawling insects in homes and greenhouses, this is also used for fabric protection, pet sprays, and shampoos. Symptoms of exposure by any route may include incoordination, twitching, loss of bladder control, and seizures. Dermal exposure may lead to local numbness, itching, burning, and tingling sensations near the site of exposure. In animal studies, it damaged the liver, decreased blood glucose levels, and increased the rate of stillbirth. It is also highly toxic to bees and fish.

resorcinol
1,3-benzenediol, m-dihydroxybenzene, resorcin

An oxidizing agent commonly found in permanent and semipermanent hair dyes, this is also used as an antidandruff agent in shampoo and in sunscreen products, as well as in pesticide formulations. Resorcinol fights fungal and bacterial organisms, and promotes softening, dissolution, and peeling of the skin; it is sometimes used to treat acne, eczema, psoriasis, corns, calluses, warts, and other skin conditions. Irritating to eyes and skin, it can cause contact allergies. Resorcinol may be absorbed into the body through the skin and into the bloodstream, where it acts like a hormone disruptor. It has been linked to reproductive effects, thyroid damage, and central-nervous-system effects, such as dizziness, nausea, altered heartbeat, and restlessness.

rotenone

Rotenone is used in home gardens for insect control and lice and tick control on pets. Local effects on the body include conjunctivitis, dermatitis, sore throat, and congestion. Ingestion produces effects ranging from mild irritation to nausea and vomiting. Growth retardation and vomiting in rats and dogs resulted from chronic exposures. In female rats, it reduced fertility. Chronic exposure may produce changes in the liver and kidneys, as also indicated by the animal studies cited above.

s-bioallethrin
See *bioallethrin*

s methoprene
See *methoprene*

saccharin
Hermesetas, Sweetex (EU), Sweet'N Low (U.S.),
Sucaryl, Sugar Twin, and Sweet Magic

The grandfather of artificial sweeteners, saccharin was discovered in 1879 and was widely used during both world wars, compensating for sugar shortages. It is two hundred to three hundred times sweeter than sugar, but tends to have a bitter or metallic aftertaste. Saccharin is still ubiquitous today, as it is cheap, has a long shelf life, and is heat-resistant. It is thus often added to baked goods, jams, and processed fruits, but it also crops up in salad dressings and sauces.

In the 1970s, it was found to cause bladder cancer in rats. The U.S. Food and Drug Administration (FDA) all but banned it outright, but reprieved it in 1991, while requiring the label to declare it to be potentially carcinogenic. Canadian authorities banned it outright until 1997. In the U.K., it has never been prohibited.

Although saccharin is still widely used, the U.S. government's National Toxicology Program classifies it as an anticipated carcinogen. In 2002, a group of

Canadian scientists concluded that there was "ample evidence" that it can cause bladder cancer in laboratory animals and possibly in humans at high doses.

salicylates

This is a vast range of chemicals that can be used as flavorings and aromas in foods (for example, amyl, phenyl, menthyl, and glyceryl salicylate), and as perfume ingredients in fragranced cosmetics and household products (for example, benzyl salicylate, CIS-3-hexenyl salicylate). One of their most widespread uses is in cosmetics as sunscreening agents (for example, homosalate, ethylhexyl salicylate, octyl salicylate, isotridecyl salicylate, and trolamine salicylate). People who are sensitive to aspirin may develop allergic-type reactions after ingesting salicylates or applying them to the skin. In addition, salicylates are penetration enhancers that allow other chemicals in the product to get deeper into the bloodstream; research also shows that some salicylates used in suncreams are estrogenic.

salicylic acid

Used as a preservative in food products and cosmetics, this is also a common dandruff treatment in shampoos. In antiaging creams, salicylic acid is a *beta-hydroxy acid*, used as a chemical peel to dissolve and remove the outermost layer of skin. Because of its exfoliating action, salicylic acid can increase photosensitivity of the skin and cause contact dermatitis. (See also *salicylates*.)

selenium sulphide

An antidandruff agent that is irritating to the skin and eyes, it is best to avoid contact of this agent with broken skin.

semicarbazide
SEM

A breakdown product of azodicarbonamide, a chemical used in the plastic seals for jars and other types of food packaging, this is a contaminant that leaches into foods from the plastic gaskets used to seal glass jars with metal twist-off lids. SEM has been detected at low levels in a number of such food products, including baby foods. It has also been detected in seaweed-derived products (for example, *carrageenan*), used widely in food production. In addition, azodicarbonamide is also approved as a food additive in a number of countries for use as a bleaching agent in cereal flour and as a dough conditioner. Azodicarbonamide is also used in certain pesticide formulations and industrial applications. Animal studies show that semicarbazide is carcinogenic.

siduron

An herbicide used in weed-control products, this is moderately irritating to the skin, eyes, and mucous membranes.

silica

A natural mineral (silicon dioxide) used as an anticaking agent in salts and salt substitutes and other dry food items; in cosmetics, it is used as an abrasive, absorbent, and viscosity adjuster. Inhaling silica dust is a risk factor in developing lung cancer. (See *crystalline silica, hydrated silica*.)

silicates

This is a family of naturally occurring, quartz-containing minerals (for example, *silica*). In dry form, they are used in powder bases for cosmetics, such as face powder, eyeshadow, or blusher.

Magnesium silicate, or *talc*, is a good example of a silicate used for this purpose. Other types of powdered silicates are used as abrasives in toothpastes and household cleaners. Inhaling silica dust is a risk factor in developing lung cancer.

silicones

A group of semisynthetic fluid oils, rubbers, and resins derived from silica (for example, *dimethicone, simethicone*), these are widely used in cosmetics as film formers, skin-conditioning agents, and water repellents. They are generally considered safe, though they are poorly studied with regard to toxicity in humans.

simethicone

This synthetic silicone-based moisturizer and film former is used in cosmetics. Film formers trap other substances (including other ingredients in the product) beneath them. Because they do not allow the skin to breathe, they may exacerbate skin irritation caused by sweat or other substances.

sodium benzoate

This preservative is used in such foods as margarines, soft drinks, pickles, jellies, and jams. Ingestion has caused birth defects in experimental animals. Currently, there is concern that sodium benzoate and its salts react with ascorbic acid (vitamin C) in soft drinks to form the carcinogen *benzene*.

sodium bicarbonate
baking soda

Often used as a flour treatment agent and baking aid in bakery goods and in toothpastes as a whitening/bleaching agent, this can be a harsh abrasive if used in concentrated form; however, it is generally regarded as safe.

sodium bisulphate
sulphuric acid
A strong deodorizer that is corrosive and irritating to the skin and eyes, if ingested it can damage body tissues. Its fumes are a trigger of asthma attacks.

sodium carbonate
E500, soda ash, washing soda
A strong alkali used as a neutralizer in dairy products, cocoa products, and in the canning of olives, ingesting large amounts can cause gastrointestinal upset and even damage. Sodium carbonate can be found in more concentrated forms in household cleaners as a disinfectant and bleaching agent. It can be irritating to the skin and may produce sensitivity reactions.

sodium chloride
salt
Simple table salt can be added as a water softener to help products rinse better in hard water. It is used in cosmetics and household cleaners as a viscosity adjuster (thickener).

sodium cocoate
A detergent derived from coconut oil, this is generally considered mild and safe.

sodium cocoyl isethionate
This detergent/surfactant made from entirely synthetic sources can be irritating to the skin.

sodium dodecylbenzenesulphonate
A harsh detergent commonly found in car and wheel shampoos, metal polishes, dish and laundry detergents, and even foaming bath products, sodium dodecylbenzenesulphonate can produce skin irritation.

sodium fluoride
See *fluoride*

sodium hydroxymethylglycinate
A broad-spectrum antimicrobial that is active against a variety of bacteria, yeasts, and molds, this is used as a preservative in toiletries and household cleaners. It is a *formaldehyde*-forming ingredient that can mix with other ingredients to form carcinogenic nitrosamines. (See *diethanolamine*; see also chapter 6.)

sodium hydroxide
lye, caustic soda

This caustic bleaching/cleaning agent, commonly found in bathroom cleaners, toilet-bowl cleaners, oven cleaners, and drain cleaners, is also used in the manufacture of soaps.

In its pure form, lye will quickly eat through skin and body tissue. Mixed with acids, it will release harmful vapors. It is also corrosive, alkaline, and poisonous. If accidentally splashed in the eyes, it will cause blindness.

sodium hypochlorite
bleach

An effective disinfectant and bleaching agent commonly found in cleaners, disinfectants, laundry products, toilet bowl cleaners, and tub and tile cleaners, bleach is one of the household cleaners most frequently implicated in household poisonings. It can irritate the skin and respiratory tract, and if ingested can damage the mouth, esophagus, and stomach.

sodium isethionate

A detergent made from entirely synthetic sources, this can be irritating to the skin.

sodium laureth sulphate
SLES

A detergent and foaming agent found in bath foams, bubble baths, and shampoos, this can be irritating to eyes and skin. Laureth compounds can be contaminated with the carcinogen 1,4-*dioxane*.

sodium lauryl sulphate
SLS

A detergent and foaming agent found in bath foams, bubble baths, shampoos, and toothpastes, SLS is not carcinogenic, but can nevertheless be damaging. It is so harsh that it is used in medical research to induce a kind of benchmark skin irritation against which all other potential skin irritants are measured. Used in toothpastes, it can damage the delicate mucosal lining of the mouth and, if it gets into the eyes during shampooing, it can damage the cornea. Because it strips the protective oily layer from the skin, it can also act as a penetration enhancer, making it easier for other toxic chemicals to be absorbed into the body.

As new detergents have been invented, the popularity of SLS among manufacturers has waned, but it is still found in many products. Often, its presence is a good indicator of other undesirable ingredients, including *formaldehyde-*

containing preservatives (for example, *imidazolidinyl urea*) and nitrosamine-forming agents (for example, *cocamide DEA*, *triethanolamine*), as well as a long list of skin and hair conditioners necessary to repair some of the initial damage it causes.

sodium lauroamphoacetate
This detergent/surfactant is found in body washes and shampoos. It is comparatively mild, so is often found in sensitive or "no tears" baby shampoos.

sodium metabisulphite
E223
A preservative and bleaching agent found in alcoholic beverages, juices, and dried fruits, ingestion can trigger asthma attacks. It is also used in cosmetics as a preservative, where it can cause skin irritation. (See *sulphites*.)

sodium monofluorophosphate
See *fluoride*

sodium palm kernelate
A detergent syntheszsed from the oil of palm kernels, it is usually found in soap and bath bars, and is generally thought to be nontoxic.

sodium palmate
A detergent synthesized from the oil of palm kernels, this is usually found in soap and bath bars, and is generally considered to be nontoxic.

sodium silicate
A commonly used corrosion inhibitor found in laundry detergents, it is a strong alkali; inhalation is irritating to the lungs and mucous membranes.

sodium stearate
Found in shampoos and facial washes, this is a fatty acid added as a skin softener to replace the oils that are stripped away from the skin by detergents in these products.

sodium sulphite
See *sulphites*

sodium tallowate
A detergent synthesized from animal fats found in facial and bath soaps, this is generally nontoxic.

sodium tripolyphosphate

With various applications, such as a preservative for seafood, meats, poultry, and pet foods, this agent is also used in toothpaste, and as a builder and water softener in household cleaners and laundry detergents, improving their cleansing ability. It is a caustic that can be irritating to the skin.

solvents

The solvents used in household products are called organic—not because they are free from harmful chemicals, but because they contain the carbon atoms common to all life on earth.

All organic solvents are hazardous. They are easily absorbed through the skin and via their fumes. Solvents have been associated with liver and kidney problems, birth defects, and nervous system disorders. Most recently, solvent exposure has been linked to an increased risk of developing Parkinson's disease. Many of these problems develop slowly over time and are thought to be the result of chronic low-level exposure to solvents, such as *isopropanol*, *propylene glycol*, and *ethanol*.

sorbitan laurate

An emulsifier and surfactant used in cosmetics, this is generally mild, but it can cause skin irritation in some.

sorbitan oleate

Used in cosmetics as an emulsifier and surfactant, this is synthesized from olive oil. Generally mild, it can nevertheless cause skin irritation in some.

sorbitan stearate

A modified fatty acid derived from beef tallow, it is used as an emulsifier, stabilizer, and surfactant in cosmetics. Generally mild, it can cause blackheads in some individuals.

sorbitol

Used in foods and some toiletries as a sweetener and tartar-control agent, as well as a humectant (to keep the product moist), sorbitol is an alcohol-derived sugar that tastes sweet, but only breaks down in the gut. If swallowed, sorbitol can cause gastrointestinal cramps and bloating. Because of its laxative effects, the use of gel toothpastes (which can contain up to 70 percent sorbitol) by small children should be supervised, and possibly even discouraged, by parents. See also *sugar alcohols*.

soytrimonium chloride

A *quaternary ammonium compound* used as a surfactant and detergent in foaming bath products and shampoos, this is toxic by all routes of exposure. Skin and airways irritation are common. Depending on the concentration, quaternary compounds may also produce nausea, vomiting, abdominal pain, anxiety, restlessness, coma, convulsions, and respiratory muscle paralysis.

stannous chloride
tin dichloride
An antioxidant found in sodas and canned asparagus, this may be irritating to the skin and mucous membranes.

stearalkonium chloride
Originally developed by the fabric industry as a softener, it is commonly found in hair conditioners and creams, and may cause allergic reactions.

stearamide MEA
See *monoethanolamine*

stearamidopropyl dimethylamine
Part of a larger group of *glycol ethers* (the same family as *propylene glycol* and *polyethylene glycol* compounds), stearamidopropyl dimethylamine is a solvent and wetting agent that is quickly absorbed into the skin. In the body, it is a reproductive toxin.

steareth
Waxy compounds (for example, steareth-2 and steareth-21) used as emulsifiers, they are part of a larger group of ethoxylated alcohols that are toxic and potentially carcinogenic, and may also be contaminated by the carcinogen 1,4-*dioxane*.

stearic acid
A lubricant and emulsifier derived from both animal and vegetable sources, this is a fatty acid added as a skin softener. Found in shampoos and facial washes, it replaces the oils stripped away from the skin by the mix of detergents. It can be irritating to the skin, eyes, and respiratory tract.

stearyl alcohol
An emollient, moisturizer, and stabilizer derived from animal fats, this is also used as a lubricating agent to help the product go on more smoothly. It is thought to be nontoxic, but can cause mild skin irritation and even contact dermatitis.

stevia
A natural sweetener derived from the shrub Stevia rebaudiana, stevia has been used for centuries in South America, Japan, China, and Korea; however, it is

not a permitted food additive in either the EU or the United States on the basis of insufficient safety data.

Fears have been raised that stevia may be carcinogenic, damage DNA, and affect fertility, but a 2003 review of all the evidence by J. M. Geuns titled "Stevioside" concluded that the plant is, in fact, of "very low toxicity" and that it is "safe when used as a sweetener." It also has the added advantage of reducing blood pressure in people with hypertension.

The main concern is that the plant is a source of phytosterols that may cause reproductive abnormalities in men; however, official concern as to the toxicity of plant sterols seems to be a moveable feast. All over the Western world, men and women gulp down plant estrogens and sterols in the form of soy supplements that have been approved as safe. Likewise, we are encouraged to eat sterol-containing spreads and yogurt drinks to lower cholesterol on the basis that these are healthy. The concern is legitimate, and better research is needed to show to what extent sterols in all these foods may have an estrogenic effect in humans.

Stevia, which can have a slight licorice flavor and a bitter aftertaste if not processed correctly, is available as a nutritional supplement in the United States, but not in Europe.

strontium chloride

Added to some toothpastes to reduce periodontal disease, this is also found in some treatment shampoos and facial washes. Considered toxic, it can be irritating to the skin and mucous membranes.

sucralose
Splenda

One of the few sweeteners to be derived from sugar itself, sucralose tastes more like sugar than other artificial sweeteners and contains about one-eighth the calories and carbohydrates of sugar. It is produced by chlorinating sugar.

Animal studies, conducted by the manufacturers, have found a range of problems at high doses, including shrunken thyroid glands, and kidney and liver problems. Human studies suggest that a dose at half the current approved level for six months could raise blood-glucose levels. It is widely used in soft drinks, desserts, and confectionery, and as a tabletop sweetener; consumer reports suggest a wide range of adverse effects from regular ingestion of sucralose, including gastrointestinal upsets, cramping, and bladder problems.

sugar alcohols
sorbitol, xylitol, lactitol, mannitol, maltitol, isomalt,
hydrogenated starch hydrolysates (HSH)

Though not technically artificial sweeteners, these are lower-calorie sweeteners derived from sugar alcohol. Sugar alcohols have fewer calories than sugar and are claimed not to promote tooth decay or cause sudden increases in glucose in diabetics. They have a pleasant sweet taste similar to sucrose, and are often used in sweets, cookies, and chewing gum.

The regulatory authorities classify sugar alcohols as GRAS (generally recognized as safe), but they may cause diarrhea, bloating, and stomach pain in high doses (over 1 gram). This is because they are more slowly digested and remain longer in the intestinal tract, rather than being absorbed into the blood. The nonabsorbed carbohydrates create an osmotic effect that pulls water into the intestines. Also, when the nonabsorbed carbohydrates reach the colon, normal bacteria metabolize them into gases and short-chain fatty acids.

sulisobenzone
This is a sunscreening agent. See *benzophenones*

sulphites
A class of chemical preservatives used widely in food production, they can keep cut fruit and vegetables looking fresh, preventing discoloration in apricots, raisins, and other dried fruits. They can also control "black spot" in freshly caught shrimp, and prevent discoloration, bacterial growth, and fermentation in wine. Until the early 1980s, they were considered safe, but research now shows they can provoke sometimes severe allergic reactions, especially in asthmatics. In 1995, the U.S. Food and Drug Administration banned sulphites from most (but not all) commercially prepared fruit and vegetables. They are still widely used elsewhere, however.

sulphur dioxide
Used to bleach vegetable colors, and preserve fruits and vegetables, this is an antioxidant and preservative found in a wide variety of foods, including wines, beverages, soups, and condiments. Poisonous and highly irritating, it also destroys the vitamin content of foods. This is on the U.S. Environmental Protection Agency's list of extremely hazardous substances.

sulphuric acid
A cleaner and disinfectant used in toilet-bowl cleaners and metal polishes, this can produce severe skin burns even when diluted. Also, it is very dangerous when splashed in the eyes, and has been known to cause blindness.

talc
magnesium silicate
Talc is made up of finely ground particles of stone. It is used widely in powdered cosmetics and is an absorbent on its own. As it originates in the ground and

is a mined product, it can be contaminated with other substances. Asbestos is a good example, and recent reports of the talc used in crayon manufacture being contaminated with this poisonous substance have caused alarm to every parent whose child has ever chewed on a crayon.

Regular use is also associated with respiratory problems in adults and children. Because it comprises finely ground stone, it can lodge in the lungs and never leave. In women, its use in the genital area has been linked to ovarian cancer; it is now estimated that women who frequently use talc have three times the risk of developing ovarian cancer compared with nonusers.

TEA lauryl sulphate
See *triethanolamine*

TEA-sodium lauryl sulphate
See *triethanolamine*

Teflon
polytetrafluoroethylene, PTFE

This is the nonstick coating found on cookware, and in the packaging of such fast and microwaveable foods as french fries, popcorn, and pizza, as well as in candy wrappers and other products. As a waterproof coating on fabrics, it is known as Stainmaster, Gore-Tex, and Scotchgard. It's also frequently used as a film former in cosmetics.

According to the U.S. Environmental Protection Agency, one of the breakdown products of Teflon, known as PFOA (perfluorooctanoic acid), is an expected human carcinogen. PFOA can be released when Teflon is heated and can cause severe respiratory distress (and is deadly to pet birds). It is a persistent chemical pollutant found in almost every animal on the planet, including humans. As evidence of PFOA's toxicity continues to accumulate, some observers believe that its effect on humans may yet make *DDT* look almost safe by comparison.

tetramethrin
A synthetic pyrethroid insecticide used to control wasps, ants, and other garden insects, this is a skin, eye, and respiratory irritant, neurotoxin, and suspected carcinogen.

tetrasodium EDTA
tetrasodium ethylenediaminetetraacetic acid

A cosmetic preservative used in soaps and other toiletries, it helps to isolate impurities, such as metals, that cause the mixture to degrade. It can cause skin, mucous membrane, and eye irritation, as well as contact dermatitis and contact allergies, and also acts as a penetration enhancer. Environmentally persistent, it binds with heavy metals in lakes and streams, aiding their reentry into the food chain.

tetrasodium etidronate
A synthetic preservative used to stop impurities, such as metals, from making the product deteriorate, it can be irritating to the skin.

thimerosal
This mercury-containing preservative is found in certain cosmetics, such as mascara, as well as in ophthalmic preparations. Highly toxic and damaging to the eyes, it may add to the body's burden of the neurotoxin mercury.

titanium dioxide
E171
Titanium dioxide is extracted from the naturally occurring mineral ilmenite. It is used in such foods as cottage and mozzarella cheese, horseradish cream and sauces, lemon curd, in sweets, where it is often used to provide a barrier between different colors, and in sauces to increase their opacity. It is also found in tablets and capsules, and is used as a coloring, opacifier, and sunscreening agent in cosmetics. Thought not to be easily absorbed and generally considered safe when used in topical formulations, ingestion can produce detectable amounts in the blood, brain, and glands, with the highest concentrations being in the lymph nodes and lungs. It is banned in Germany.

toluene
toluol, methylbenzene
This and its chemical cousin *xylene* are *aromatic hydrocarbons* used primarily as *solvents*. Commonly found in dry-cleaning solutions and perfume, toluene easily enters the body through inhalation and ingestion, but is poorly absorbed via the skin. Irritating to the skin and respiratory tract, it can cause damage to several organs, including the eyes, liver, kidneys, and the central nervous system (where it acts like a narcotic). Symptoms of chronic exposure include fatigue, weakness, confusion, headache, watery eyes, muscular fatigue, insomnia, dermatitis, and photosensitivity.

2,4-toluenediamine
4-methyl-m-phenylenediamine
See *phenylenediamines*

triadimefon
A triazole fungicide used to control powdery mildews, rusts, and other fungal pests in turf, shrubs, and trees, it is irritating to the lungs. Long-term exposure can produce pathological changes in red blood cell counts, increase blood cholesterol levels, and damage the liver. Animal studies indicate that it may have reproductive effects, such as causing more neonatal deaths and lower birth weights in offspring.

tributyltin oxide
TBT
A fungicide used as a wood treatment and preservative, it can cause irritation of the skin, eyes, and respiratory tract. It is a central nervous system toxin that can produce headache, nausea, vomiting, dizziness, breathing difficulties, and flu-like symptoms. It is also a suspected reproductive toxin and carcinogen, based on limited animal data.

1,1,2-trichloroethane
A solvent for chlorinated rubbers, fats, oils, waxes, and resins, this is common in household products, such as typewriter correction fluid, paint removers, adhesives, and spot removers, and can cause stinging and burning sensations on the skin. It is poorly studied for its potential capacity to cause cancer, reproductive defects, and central-nervous-system damage.

trichloroethane
TCA
A solvent and cleaning agent commonly found in spot removers, metal polishes and fabric cleaners, film cleaner, insecticides, paint and varnish removers, and degreasers, it is also used as an aerosol propellant.

It is absorbed into the body by inhalation and ingestion, is an irritant to the eyes and nose, and can result in central-nervous-system depression, and liver and kidney damage, if ingested.

trichloroethylene
TCE
Found in spot cleaners and dry-cleaning fluids, TCE is another commonly used solvent. It is a suspected carcinogen. When inhaled, it can cause dizziness and sleepiness and, in some cases, memory loss. Irritating to the eyes and nose, it can cause skin to become dry and flaky, and may produce rashes. It is associated with central-nervous-system disorders and damage to vital organs, such as the kidneys and liver. It can also cause cardiac failure.

Trichloroethylene can persist on fabrics long after its application. It is also a common groundwater contaminant that easily works its way back into the food chain and water supply.

trichlorphon

An organophosphate insecticide used to control cockroaches, crickets, silverfish, bedbugs, and fleas, long-term exposure can provoke impaired memory and concentration, disorientation, severe depression, irritability, confusion, speech difficulties, delayed reaction times, nightmares, sleepwalking, and drowsiness or insomnia. This is a highly toxic substance that is a reproductive toxin, carcinogen, and mutagen, and toxic to birds and fish.

triclopyr

An herbicide that is irritating to the skin and eyes, and may damage the liver and kidneys.

triclosan
2,4,4'-trichloro-2'-hydroxy diphenyl ether

An antibacterial agent found in household cleaners, toothpastes, mouthwashes, face washes, and bath products, it is used as a coating on plastics (for example, cutting boards and storage containers), and it is known as Microban. Applied to the skin, it can cause allergic reactions and ulceration. In the mouth, it kills both good and bad bacteria, and makes users more vulnerable to infection. It can also cause premature cell death in the gingival tissues, resulting in gum damage. It's easily absorbed into the body via the mouth, and has been associated with liver damage and eye irritation. A chlorinated aromatic compound, triclosan is molecularly similar to *dioxins*, *PCBs*, and Agent Orange. Indeed, the manufacturing process of triclosan can release dioxins—powerful hormone disrupters—into the environment. It is also a chlorophenol, a class of chemicals that can cause cancer in animals. Commonly used as a pesticide, the widespread use of triclosan in commercial products is also implicated in our increasing rates of bacterial resistance.

triethanolamine
TEA

A surfactant, emulsifier, dispersant, and pH adjuster commonly used in shampoos and foaming bath products, this can be irritating to the skin and eyes. More worrisome, it may—during storage, on the skin, or in the body after absorption—mix with *formaldehyde*-forming chemicals in the product to form carcinogenic compounds called nitrosamines. (See also chapter 6.) TEA is a suspected endocrine disrupter. Animal studies have demonstrated liver and kidney damage due to chronic exposure.

triethanolamine lauryl sulphate
See *triethanolamine*

trifluralin
An herbicide used to control many annual grasses and weeds, ingestion of this agent can cause nausea and severe gastrointestinal discomfort. Inhalation may cause irritation of the lining of the mouth, throat, or lungs. Animal studies suggest that long-term exposure can reduce red blood cell counts and raise cholesterol levels, as well as lead to malignant tumors in the kidneys, bladder, and thyroid.

triisopropanolamine
TIPA

This alkanolamine (the same family as *diethanolamine*, *triethanolamine*, and *monoethanolamine*) is a hormone-disrupting solvent and surfactant.

tripolyphosphate
Used as a water softener and emulsifier, it may cause esophageal stricture and violent vomiting if swallowed.

trisodium edta
See *tetrasodium EDTA*

urea
E927b, carbamide

Naturally found in urine and other body fluids, today it is synthesized from ammonia and carbon dioxide and used as a fertilizer. In foods, it can be used as a texturizer in chewing gum and, in skin-care products, it is used to moisturize hardened skin. Generally regarded as safe, although regular topical applications can cause thinning of the skin.

VA/vinyl butyl benzoate/crotonates copolymer
A petroleum-based vinyl acetate that forms a thin plasticlike film on the hair that aids styling, it can cause mild skin irritation.

vinyl acetate/acrylic copolymer
A petroleum-based chemical that forms a thin plasticlike film on the hair that aids styling, it can cause mild skin irritation.

xylene
xylol, dimethylbenzene

A chemical cousin of *toluene* and one of the *aromatic hydrocarbons* used primarily as a *solvent*, this is commonly found in dry-cleaning solutions and perfume.

Xylene easily enters the body through inhalation and ingestion, but is poorly absorbed via the skin. It is irritating to the skin and respiratory tract, and can cause damage to the eyes, liver, kidneys, and central nervous system. Symptoms of chronic exposure include fatigue, weakness, confusion, headache, watery eyes, insomnia, dermatitis, and photosensitivity.

xylitol
See *sugar alcohols*

zinc oxide
This popular mineral-based sunblocker is generally considered safe and effective, although, in some individuals, it can cause skin irritation.

zinc stearate
Found in shampoos and facial washes, this is a fatty acid added as a skin softener to replace the oils stripped away from the skin by detergents.

ziram
A carbamate fungicide, also used as a bird and rodent repellent, it is irritating to the skin, eyes, and mucous membranes. Animal studies indicate it can reduce fertility, delay development in offspring, and cause chromosomal damage and cancer. In humans it can cause nerve and visual disturbances, chromosomal damage, and enlarged thyroid glands.

AFTERWORD: PICK YOUR POISON

We are both passive and direct recipients of pollution. Reading through this book, you may find yourself becoming dismayed at the overwhelming number of ways in which the products you use every day can affect your health, but don't give up and don't get discouraged.

In an ideal world, the absolute best way to stay healthy is to avoid being exposed to chemical toxins altogether. But this is not realistic. Given how badly we have polluted our planet and our home environments, none of us can avoid all the known poisons that are threatening our day-to-day health and well-being. But you do have more power than you think and you can, to a very large and influential extent, learn to pick your poisons.

One way to do this is to be aware of what your particular weak spots are. These may be genetic vulnerabilities, or weak spots developed in your own lifetime. For instance, if you have a family history of cancer, it makes sense to avoid carcinogenic chemicals and metals as much as possible. If your family has a history of neurological disorders (for instance, multiple sclerosis) or autoimmune diseases (such as arthritis), you should be on the lookout for neurotoxic and immunotoxic chemicals. If you suffer from menstrual problems, chemicals that disrupt your hormones may play a part. Get to know what these chemicals are and learn to avoid them.

It may also mean making the occasional compromise. If there is something you absolutely can't live without, then keep using it. But try to make "chemical savings" elsewhere in your life by, for instance, saving perfume or makeup for special occasions only, using a fluoride-free toothpaste, cutting down on the number of other largely unnecessary toiletries you use, getting rid of toxic air fresheners, making use of some of the suggestions in this book for chemical-free cleaning or pest control, or seeking out paints and other home decoration supplies that are low in toxic ingredients.

By doing this, you are protecting yourself as well as your children—who are the most vulnerable to the effects of chemical exposures—and ensuring that they have a healthy future to look forward to.

You are in control, you do have the power, and it is your responsibility.

Appendix

A Complete Guide to Common Food Additives

Foods sold in the European Union (EU) have had full ingredient labeling since the mid-1980s. For ease of reference and to help avoid the problems of translating them into the wide range of languages used in Europe, many of these ingredients are abbreviated as "E numbers." In Australia and New Zealand, these same numbers are used but without the E prefix.

This simple numbering system for food additives is now being adapted for international use by the Codex Alimentarius Commission, an organization created in 1963 by the Food and Agriculture Organization (FAO) of the United Nations and the World Health Organization (WHO). When this system is finally adopted, it will be known as the International Numbering System (INS), and will use mostly the same numbers (but without the E prefix). While the number system has not been adopted in the United States just yet, the list of common food additives below is a useful reference when scanning food labels for harmful ingredients. Until the number system is implemented in the United States, look for ingredients on labels by their full names.

As the table below shows, the list of food additives is simply staggeringly long. Many of these additives began life as naturally derived substances; however, most are now prepared or produced in the lab, as synthetically produced compounds are often less expensive than the natural product.

While the E numbering system may seem dense and impenetrable, there is a logic to it. Each group of numbers represents a particular type or group of additive:

- E100s are colors

- E200 to E282 are preservatives and acids

- E300 to E341 are antioxidants and acid regulators

- E400s include emulsifiers, stabilizers, thickeners, anticaking agents, release agents, and bulking agents

- E500s are mineral salts and anticaking agents

- E620 to E640 are flavor enhancers

- E900 and upward are additives that don't fall into any of the above categories

The list is constantly being updated and changed, which makes it hard for conscientious shoppers to keep track of it. The list below gives an overview of the additives currently permitted in the EU. Most of these are permitted elsewhere, but, in the United States for instance, they are known by their chemical names. Those additives in the table without an E prefix are unique to Australia and New Zealand. Remember, not all additives have been fully tested for safety, so it is impossible to say categorically which ones are safe and which ones are not. Likewise, some individuals may be more sensitive than others to the effects of certain additives, such as colors and sulphites.

Colors

Alkanet (E103)
Natural "port-wine" color from A. tinctoria plant. Banned in the United States; not approved in Europe.

Allura Red AC (E129)
Suspected carcinogen. Prohibited throughout the EU. Synonyms: FD&C Red 40.

Aluminum (E173)
Suspected neurotoxin, linked to osteoporosis.

Amaranth (E123)
Associated with birth defects and fetal deaths. Can cause urticaria and liver problems. Suspected carcinogen. Banned in Austria, Japan, Norway, Russia, Sweden, and the United States. Synonyms: FD&C Red 2, CI Acid Red 27, CI Food Red 9.

Ammonia caramel (E150c)
See *Plain caramel (E150a)*

Annatto (E160b)
Can cause urticaria and flare-ups of angioneurotic edema, asthma, and hyperactivity. Synonyms: bixin, norbixin.

Anthocyanins (E163)
Violet, red, blue color matter of flowers, buds, and plants. No known adverse effects.

Beet Red, Betanin (E162)
Purple color derived from beets. No known adverse effects.

Beta-apo-8'-carotenal (C 30) (E163e)
Natural orange color. No known adverse effects.

Brilliant Black BN (E151)
Can trigger asthma attacks and hyperactivity in asthmatics, as well as urticaria and rhinitis. Also known to interfere with some digestive enzymes. Banned in Denmark, Australia, Belgium, France, Germany, Switzerland, Austria, the United States, and Norway, and greatly restricted in Sweden. Synonyms: Black PN, CI Food Black 1.

Brilliant Blue FCF (E133)
Can cause hyperactivity, skin rashes, bronchoconstriction (when combined with Erythrosine [E127] and Indigotine [E132]). Linked with chromosomal damage. Banned in Austria, Belgium, France, Germany, Norway, Switzerland, and Sweden. Synonyms: FD&C Blue 1, CI Acid Blue 9, CI Food Blue 2, CI Pigment Blue 24.

Brown FK (E154)
Potential carcinogen. Banned in Austria, Australia, Japan, New Zealand, Switzerland, the United States, and all EU countries except the U.K. Synonyms: Kipper Brown, Food Brown.

(Chocolate) Brown HT (E155)
Can provoke asthmatic reactions, hyperactivity, and skin sensitivity. Suspected carcinogen. Banned in Austria, Belgium, Denmark, France, Germany, Norway, Switzerland, Sweden, and the United States.

Calcium carbonate (E170)
Mineral salt; may be derived from rock mineral or animal bones. High doses create mineral imbalance and many other physical problems, such as hemorrhoids, kidney stones, abdominal pain, and confused behavior.

Carmoisine (E122)
Can trigger asthmatic reactions and hyperactivity, urticaria, and edema. Suspected carcinogen. Banned in Austria, Japan, Norway, Sweden, and the United States. Synonym: Azo rubine.

Carotene (alpha-, beta-, gamma-) (E160a)
Natural orange/yellow color; human body converts it to vitamin A in the liver; found in carrots and other yellow or orange fruits and vegetables.

Caustic sulphite caramel (E150b)
See *Plain caramel (E150a)*

Chlorophylis, chlorophyllins (E140)
Generally harmless, although an excess can cause sensitivity to light.

Cochineal (E120)
Can promote hyperactivity, rhinitis, urticaria (hives), and asthma. Banned in the United States.

Copper complexes of chlorophyll and chlorophyllins; copper phaeophytins (E141)
No adverse effects are known.

Curcumin (E100)
Derived from the root of the curcuma plant, but can be artificially produced. No known adverse effects.

Erythrosine (E127)
Linked with sensitivity to light and learning difficulties; can increase thyroid hormone levels and lead to hyperthyroidism; was shown to cause thyroid cancer in rats. As a pesticide, kills maggot larvae and flies. Banned in Norway. Synonym: FD&C Red 3.

Ethyl ester of beta-apo-8'-carotenic acid (C 30) (E160f)
Natural orange color. No known adverse effects.

Fast Yellow AB (E105)
Effects unknown.

Gold (E175)
Rarely used. Adverse effects unknown.

Green S (E142)

May cause asthma, rashes, and hyperactivity. Mutagenic in animal tests. Banned in Canada, Japan, Sweden, the United States, and Norway. Synonyms: CI Acid Green 50, CI Food Green 4.

Indigotine, Indigo Carmine (E132)

Can cause nausea, vomiting, high blood pressure, skin rashes, breathing problems, and allergic reactions. Suspected carcinogen. Banned in Norway. Synonyms: FD&C Blue 2.

Iron oxides and hydroxides (E172)

High doses can create mineral imbalances.

Latolrubine BK (E180)

Probable cause of rashes and hyperactivity, and potentially dangerous to asthmatics. Banned in Australia and New Zealand.

Lycopene (E160d)

Can be derived from GM sources. Banned in some countries, including Australia.

Paprika extract, capsanthin, capsorubin (E160c)

Natural colors derived from fruit pods of the red pepper. No known adverse effects.

Patent Blue V (E131)

May cause dermatitis and purpura. Banned in Australia, Norway, Japan, New Zealand, and the United States.

Plain caramel (E150a)

Plain caramel is mostly naturally derived. Other forms, such as those made with ammonia, are toxic and can provoke hyperactivity. Some caramels may damage genes, slow down growth, cause enlargement of the intestines and kidneys, and may destroy vitamin B.

Ponceau 4R (E124)

Carcinogenic in animals, can trigger asthma and allergic reactions. Banned in Canada, Norway, and the United States (in 1976 for cancer-causing agents). Restricted in Sweden. Synonym: Cochineal Red A.

Quinoline Yellow (E104)

May cause asthma, rashes, and hyperactivity. Aspirin-sensitive people must avoid it. Banned in Japan, the United States, Norway, and Australia. Synonyms: FD&C Yellow 10.

Red 2G (E128)

Should be avoided by hyperactive people, asthmatics, and aspirin-sensitive people. Suspected carcinogen. Banned in Australia, Austria, Belgium, Denmark, Germany, Japan, Switzerland, New Zealand, and the United States.

Riboflavin, riboflavin-5'-phosphate (E101)

Doubles as color and added nutrient. Synonyms: Vitamin B_2.

Riboflavin-5'-[sodium phosphate] (E106)

Doubles as a color and added nutrient. Synonyms: Vitamin B_5.

Silver (E174)

No adverse effects known, but high doses can lead to bluish gray skin (cyanosis). Banned in Australia.

Sulphite ammonia caramel (E150d)

See *Plain caramel (E150a)*

Sunset Yellow FCF, Orange Yellow S (E110)

Can provoke allergic reactions, abdominal pain, hyperactivity, hives, nasal congestion, bronchoconstriction. Suspected carcinogen. Has been linked to growth retardation, severe weight loss, and increased incidence of tumors in animals. Banned in Finland, Norway, and the U.K. Synonyms: FD&C Yellow 6, CI Food Yellow 3.

Tannic acid, tannins (E181)

Clarifying agent in alcoholic drinks; derived from the nutgalls and twigs of oak trees; occurs naturally in tea. May cause gastric irritation.

Tartrazine (E102)

Known to provoke asthma attacks and skin rashes, altered states of perception and behavior, and hyperactivity. Suspected carcinogen. Inhibits zinc metabolism and interferes with digestive enzymes. Banned in Norway, Austria, and Finland. Restricted use in Sweden and Germany. Synonyms: FD&C Yellow 5, CI Acid Yellow 23, CI Food Yellow 4.

Titanium dioxide (E171)
No known adverse effects.

Vegetable carbon (E153)
Suspected carcinogen due to impurities. Banned in the United States.

Xanthophylls (E161)
Natural yellow color derived from plants and animals, naturally found in green leaves, marigolds, and egg yolk. No known adverse effects.

Xanthophylls (canthaxanthin) (E161g)
Yellow color possibly derived from animal sources, such as shellfish, fish, and flamingo feathers. No known adverse effects.

Xanthophylls (lutein) (E161b)
See *Xanthophylls (E161)*

Yellow 2G (E107)
May cause asthma, rashes, and hyperactivity. People sensitive to aspirin should avoid it. Banned in Australia, Austria, Belgium, Denmark, France, Germany, Japan, Norway, Sweden, Switzerland, and the United States. Synonyms: Acid Yellow 17, CI Food Yellow 5.

Preservatives

acetic acid (E260)
No known adverse effects.

ammonium acetate (E264)
Can cause nausea and vomiting.

benzoic acid (E210)
Obtained from benzoin, a resin exuded by trees native to Asia. Can cause hyperactivity and asthma, especially in those using steroid asthma medications. Also reputed to cause neurological disorders and to react with sulphur bisulphite (E222). Synonyms: flowers of benzoin, phenlycarboxylic acid, carboxybenzene.

biphenyl, diphenyl (E230)
A constituent of the wood preservative creosote. Banned in Australia.

boric acid (E284)
Suspected neurotoxin often used as a pesticide.

calcium acetate (E263)
No known adverse effects.

calcium benzoate (E213)
See *potassium benzoate* (E212)

calcium formate (E238)
Banned in Australia. See *formic acid (E236)*

calcium hydrogen sulphite (E227)
May cause an allergic reaction. Banned in Australia.

calcium propoionate (E282)
Can cause symptoms similar to a gallbladder attack. See also *propionic acid (E280)*

calcium sorbate (E203)
See *sorbic acid (E200)*

calcium sulphite (E226)
May cause asthma. A gastric irritant. Destroys vitamins B and E. Banned in Australia.

carbon dioxide (E290)
Suspected neurotoxin.

dimethyl dicarbonate (E242)
Effects unknown.

ethyl p-hydroxybenzoate (E214)
Banned in France and Australia. See *benzoic acid (E210)*

formic acid (E236)
Cumulative tissue poison with risk of acidosis (disturbance in the body's acid-base balance). Banned in Australia.

hexamethylene tetramine (E239)
Obtained by reacting ammonia with formaldehyde. Not recommended for children. Banned in Australia.

lactic acid (E270)
No known adverse effects.

methylparaben (E218)
Suspected hormone disrupter; allergen. Synonym: Methyl p-hydroxyben-zoate.

natamycin (E235)
Can cause nausea, vomiting, anorexia, diarrhea, and skin irritation.

nisin (E234)
Antibiotic derived from bacteria. Effects unknown.

orthophenyl phenol (E231)
Toxic antifungal; not recommended for consumption by children. Banned in Australia.

potassium acetate (E261)
Should be avoided by people with impaired kidney function.

potassium benzoate (E212)
Can provoke allergic reactions.

potassium hydrogen sulphite (E228)
Synonym: potassium bisulphite. See *sulphur dioxide (E220)*

potassium metabisulphite (E224)
See *sulphur dioxide (E220)*

potassium nitrate (E252)
May provoke hyperactivity and other adverse reactions. Suspected carcino-gen. Restricted in many countries. See *potassium nitrite (E249)*

potassium nitrite (E249)
Nitrites can affect oxygen-carrying capacity, resulting in shortness of breath, dizziness, and headaches; potential carcinogen; not permitted in foods for infants and young children.

potassium propionate (E283)
See *propionic acid (E280)*

potassium sorbate (E202)
See *sorbic acid (E200)*

potassium sulphite (E225)
See *sulphur dioxide (E220)*

propionic acid (E280)
Propionates are linked with migraine headaches.

propylparaben (E216)
Suspected hormone disrupter, allergen. Synonym: Propyl p-hydroxyben-zoate.

sodium acetate and anhydrous, sodium diacetate (E262)
No known adverse effects.

sodium benzoate (E211)
Causes nettle rash and aggravates asthma. Suspected neurotoxin.

sodium ethyl p-hydroxybenzoate (E215)
Banned in Australia. See *benzoic acid (E210)*

sodium formate (E237)
Banned in Australia. See *formic acid (E236)*

sodium hydrogen sulphite (E222)
Synonym: sodium bisulphite. See *sulphur dioxide (E220)*

sodium metabisulphite (E223)
See *sulphur dioxide (E220)*

sodium methyl p-hydroxybenzoate (E219)
Banned in France and Australia. See *benzoic acid (E210)*

sodium nitrate (E251)
See *sodium nitrite (E250)*

sodium nitrite (E250)
May provoke hyperactivity and other adverse reactions. Suspected carcino-gen.

sodium orthophenyl phenol (E232)
See *orthophenyl phenol (E231)*

sodium propionate (E281)
See *propionic acid (E280)*

sodium propyl p-hydroxybenzoate (E217)
Banned in France and Australia. See *benzoic acid (E210)*

sodium sorbate (E201)
See *sorbic acid (E200)*

sodium sulphite (E221)
See *sulphur dioxide (E220)*

sorbic acid (E200)
Either obtained from berries or synthesized from ketene; possible skin irritant, and may cause rashes, asthma, and hyperactivity. Inhibits yeast and bacteria growth.

sulphur dioxide (E220)
Can provoke gastric irritation, nausea, diarrhea, skin rash, asthma attacks; difficult to metabolize for those with impaired kidney function. Also destroys vitamin B_1, and should be avoided by anyone suffering from conjunctivitis, bronchitis, emphysema, bronchial asthma, or cardiovascular disease.

thiabendazole (E233)
High regular doses associated with anorexia, nausea, vomiting, and vertigo.

Acids, Antioxidants, Mineral Salts

1,4-heptonolactone (E370)
Poorly studied. Banned in Australia.

adipic acid (E355)
Only a small amount can be metabolized by humans. Possible teratogen (fetal toxin).

alpha-tocopherol (E307)
See *tocopherols (E306)*

ammonium ferric citrates (E381)
Unsafe in large amounts.

ammonium lactate (E328)
See *sodium lactate (E325)*

ammonium phosphates (340)
No known adverse effects.

ascorbic acid (E300)
Very large doses can cause dental erosion, vomiting, diarrhea, and dizziness. Take under medical advice if you have kidney stones, gout, or anemia. Synonym: Vitamin C.

ascorbyl palmitate, ascorbyl stearate (E301)
See *ascorbic acid (E300)*

butylated hydroxyanisole (BHA) (E320)
Not permitted in infant foods; can provoke an allergic reaction, hyperactivity. Suspected carcinogen and hormone disrupter.

butylated hydroxytoluene (BHT) (E321)
See *butylated hydroxyanisole (E320)*

calcium ascorbate (E301)
See *ascorbic acid (E300)*

calcium citrates (E333)
No known adverse effects.

calcium disodium, ethylenediamine tetraacetic acid (EDTA) (E385)
Causes mineral imbalance. Known enzyme and blood-coagulant inhibitor. Gastrointestinal disturbances, blood in urine, kidney damage, and muscle cramps are side effects. Banned in Australia.

calcium fumarate (E367)
No known adverse effects.

calcium lactate (E327)
See *sodium lactate (E325)*

calcium malates (E352)
No known adverse effects. Synonym: D, L-Calcium malate.

calcium phosphates (E341)
No known adverse effects.

calcium tartrate (E354)
No known adverse effects.

citric acid (E330)
No known adverse effects.

delta-tocopherol (E309)
See *tocopherols (E306)*

dodecyl gallate (E312)
See *propyl gallate (E310)*

erythorbic acid (E315)
No known adverse effects.

fumaric acid (E297)
No known adverse effects.

gamma-tocopherol (E308)
See *tocopherols (E306)*

lecithin (E322)
No known adverse effects.

magnesium lactate (E329)
See *sodium lactate (E325)*

magnesium phosphates (E343)
No known adverse effects.

malic acid, D, L-malic acid (E296)
No known adverse effects.

metatartaric acid (E353)
No known adverse effects.

niacin (E375)
No known adverse effects. Synonym: Vitamin B$_3$.

octyl gallate (E311)
See *propyl gallate (E310)*

phosphoric acid (E338)
Too much leads to the loss of calcium in bones and the onset of osteoporosis.

potassium adipose (E357)
No known adverse effects.

potassium ascorbate (E301)
See *ascorbic acid (E300)*

potassium citrates (monopotassium, tripotassium) (E332)
No known adverse effects.

potassium fumarate (E366)
No known adverse effects.

Potassium lactate (E326)
See *sodium lactate (E325)*

potassium malate (E351)
No known adverse effects.

potassium phosphates (340)
See *phosphoric acid (E338)*

potassium tartrates (E336)
See *sodium tartrates (E335)*

propyl gallate (E310)
May cause gastric or skin irritation; not permitted in foods for infants and small children because it is known to cause the blood disorder methaemoglobinaemia.

sodium ascorbate (E301)
See *ascorbic acid (E300)*

sodium citrates (E331)
No known adverse effects.

sodium erythorbate (E316)
See *erythorbic acid (E315)*

sodium erythorbin (E318)
See *erythorbic acid (E315)*

sodium fumarate (E365)
No known adverse effects.

sodium lactate (E325)
No known adverse effects. See *lactic acid (E270)*

sodium malates (sodium hydrogen malate) (E350)
No known adverse effects.

sodium phosphates (E339)
See *phosphoric acid (E338)*

sodium potassium tartrate (E337)
See *sodium tartrates (E335)*

sodium tartrates (E335)
People with cardiac failure, high blood pressure, damaged liver or kidneys, and fluid retention may wish to avoid this additive.

succinic acid (E363)
Large doses associated with stomach upsets. Banned in Australia.

tartaric acid (E334)
No known adverse effects.

tert-butylhydroquinone (E319)
May cause nausea, vomiting, delirium.

tocopherols (concentrate, mix) (E306)
No known adverse effects. Synonym: Vitamin E.

tri-ammonium citrate (E380)
May interfere with liver and pancreas function.

Vegetable Gums, Emulsifiers, Stabilizers, and Others

acacia (E414)
Derived from the sap of Acacia senegal; possible allergen.

agar (E406)
No known adverse effects.

alginic acid (E400)
No known adverse effects.

amidated pectin (E440b)
No known adverse effects.

ammonium alginate (E403)
See *alginic acid (E400)*

ammonium phosphatides (E442)
No known adverse effects.

calcium alginate (E404)
See *alginic acid (E400)*

calcium stearoyl-2-lactylate (E482)
No known adverse effects.

carboxy methyl cellulose, sodium carboxy methyl cellulose (E466)
No known adverse effects.

carrageenan (E407)
Known adverse effects include gastrointestinal ulcers (but it is also used to treat ulcers in humans), liver damage, and effects on the immune system; it is suspected to cause cancer.

cellulose (E460)
No known adverse effects.

dioctyl sodium sulphosuccinate (E480)
No known adverse effects.

diphosphates (E450)
High intakes may upset the calcium/phosphate balance.

esters of glycerides of fatty acids (E472)
No known adverse effects.

ethyl methyl cellulose (E4120)
Effects unknown.

gelatine (E441)
Possible allergen.

glycerol (E422)
Large quantities can cause headaches, thirst, nausea, and high blood sugar.

guar gum (E412)
Derived from the seeds of Cyamopsis tetragonolobus; can cause nausea, flatulence, and cramps.

hydroxypropyl cellulose (E463)
Effects unknown. Banned in some countries.

hydroxypropyl methyl cellulose (E464)
Effects unknown.

karaya gum (E416)
Derived from the tree Sterculia urens; possible allergen.

locust bean gum (E410)
Mild laxative effect.

mannitol (E421)
Possible allergen; not permitted in infant foods due to its ability to cause diarrhea and kidney dysfunction; also may cause nausea and vomiting.

methyl cellulose (E461)
Can cause flatulence, distention, intestinal obstruction.

mono and diglycerides of fatty acids (E471)
No known adverse effects.

pectin (E440a)
Large quantities may cause temporary flatulence or intestinal discomfort.

polyglycerol esters of fatty acids (E475)
No known adverse effects.

polyglycerol polyricinoleate (E476)
No known adverse effects.

polysorbate 20 (E432)
Banned in some countries.

polysorbate 40 (E434)
Avoid it; banned in some countries.

polysorbate 60 (E435)
See *polysorbate 80 (E433)*

polysorbate 80 (E433)
May increase the absorption of fat-soluble substances.

polysorbate 120 (E436)
See *polysorbate 80 (E433)*

potassium alginate (E402)
See *alginic acid (E400)*

propylene glycol alginate (E405)
No known adverse effects.

propylene glycol esters of fatty acids (E477)
No known adverse effects.

sodium alginate (E401)
See *alginic acid (E400)*

sodium caseinate (E469)
No known adverse effects.

sodium stearoyl-2-lactylate (E481)
No known adverse effects.

sodium, potassium, and calcium salts of fatty acids (E470)

In large amounts can interfere with intestinal function. Banned in some countries.

sorbitan monolaurate (E493)

May be harmful or act as an irritant; effects largely uninvestigated. Banned in some countries.

sorbitan monooleate (E494)

No known adverse effects.

sorbitan monopalmitate (E495)

Effects unknown.

sorbitan monostearate (E491)

No known adverse effects.

sorbitan tristearate (E492)

May increase the absorption of fat-soluble substances.

sorbitol (E420)

Can cause stomach upset.

stearyl tartrate (E483)

Suspected carcinogen. Banned in some countries.

sucroglycerides (E474)

Effects unknown. Banned in some countries.

sucrose esters of fatty acids (E473)

No known adverse effects.

tara gum (E417)

Derived from the tara bush, Caesalpinia spinosa; no known adverse effects.

thermally oxidized soya bean oil interacted with mono- and diglycerides of fatty acids (E497b)

In laboratory tests, oxidized and heated (modified) fats fed in very large amounts to test animals can produce toxic symptoms, including liver and thyroid changes, and the development of tumors. May be GM-derived.

tragacanth (E413)
Resin from the tree Astragalus gummifer; possible allergen.

xanthan gum (E415)
No known adverse effects.

Mineral Salts and Anticaking Agents

aluminum silicate (E559)
Synonym: Kaolin. See *sodium aluminum silicate (E554)*

ammonium carbonates (503)
Irritant to mucous membranes, alters pH of urine, and may cause loss of calcium and magnesium.

ammonium chloride (E510)
Should be avoided by people with impaired liver or kidney function.

ammonium hydroxide (E527)
Dilute household ammonia. Banned in Australia.

ammonium polyphosphates (E545)
Banned in Australia. See *calcium polyphosphates (544)*

ammonium sulphate (E517)
White solid; used in water purification.

bentonite (E558)
No known adverse effects.

bone phosphate, edible bone phosphate (E542)
No known adverse effects.

calcium aluminum silicate (E556)
See *sodium aluminum silicate (E554)*

calcium chloride (E509)
No known adverse effects.

calcium gluconate (E578)
See *sodium gluconate (E576)*

calcium hydroxide (E526)
No known adverse effects.

calcium oxide (E529)
No known adverse effects.

calcium polyphosphates (544)
May cause enzyme blocking in the digestive system and cause calcium phosphorus imbalance. Banned in Australia.

calcium silicate (E552)
No known adverse effects.

calcium sulphate (E516)
No known adverse effects.

copper sulphate (E519)
High doses of copper can act as a cumulative poison.

dicalcium diphosphate (E540)
Unknown effects. Banned in Australia.

ferrous gluconate (E579)
In small amounts it is safe, but may cause gastrointestinal stress.

ferrous lactate (E585)
Effects unknown.

glucono delta-lactone (E575)
No known adverse effects.

hydrochloric acid (E507)
Suspected teratogen (fetal toxin) and cocarcinogen when mixed with formaldehyde. Safe in small quantities.

magnesium carbonate (E504)
No known adverse effects.

magnesium chloride (E511)
No known adverse effects.

magnesium hydroxide (E528)
Laxative effects. Banned in Australia.

magnesium oxide (E530)
Laxative effects. Banned in Australia.

magnesium silicate (synthetic) (E553i)
No known adverse effects.

magnesium stearate (572)
No known adverse effects.

magnesium sulphate (E518)
Dangerous to people with kidney problems and possible teratogen (fetal toxin). Synonym: Epsom salts.

magnesium trisilicate (E553ii)
No known adverse effects.

potassium carbonates (E501)
No known adverse effects.

potassium chloride (E508)
Large quantities can cause gastric ulceration.

potassium ferrocyanide (E536)
Reduces oxygen transport in the blood, which may cause breathing difficulties, dizziness, or headache. Banned in the Uuited States.

potassium gluconate (E577)
See *sodium gluconate (E576)*

potassium hydroxide (E525)
Caustic. Banned in Australia.

potassium sulphates (E515)
No adverse effects known, but large doses can cause severe gastrointestinal bleeding.

silicon dioxide (E551)
No known adverse effects.

sodium aluminum phosphate, acidic (E541i)

A risk to babies, the elderly, and people suffering from kidney and heart complaints. Possible links with osteoporosis, Parkinson's, and Alzheimer's disease.

sodium aluminum phosphate, alkaline (E541ii)

Aluminum compounds are potentially neurotoxic. Banned in Australia.

sodium aluminum silicate (E554)

Aluminum is known to cause placental problems in pregnancy and has been linked with Alzheimer's, Parkinson's, and bone loss.

sodium carbonates (E500)

No known adverse effects.

sodium ferrocyanide (E535)

No known adverse effects.

sodium gluconate (E576)

Concentrated traces of heavy metals in the product. Banned in Australia.

sodium hydroxide (E524)

Caustic. Banned in Australia. Synonym: Lye.

sodium sulphates (E514)

May upset water balance.

stearic acid (E570)

No known adverse effects.

sulphuric acid (E513)

Teratogenic (fetal-toxic) properties. Banned in Australia.

talc (E553iii)

No known adverse effects.

Flavor Enhancers

calcium di-L-glutamate (E623)

Possible problems for asthmatics and aspirin-sensitive people. See *monosodium L-glutamate (MSG) (E621)*

calcium guanylate (E629)
Effects unknown.

disodium 5'-ribonucleotide (E635)
Made from disodium guanylate (E627) and disodium inosinate (E631). Associated with itchy skin rashes for up to thirty hours after ingestion.

disodium guanylate (E627)
Not permitted in foods for infants and young children. Those with gout, hyperactivity, asthma, and aspirin sensitivity should avoid it.

disodium inosinate (E631)
Frequently contains monosodium L-glutamate (MSG) (E621).

ethyl maltol (E637)
See *maltol (E636)*

glutamic acid (E620)
Can cause similar problems to monosodium L-glutamate (MSG) (E621).

glycine (and its sodium salts), glycol, amino acetic acid (E640)
Mildly toxic if ingested.

guanylic acid (E626)
No known adverse effects.

inosinic acid (E630)
Effects unknown.

magnesium di-L-glutamate (E625)
See *monosodium L-glutamate (MSG) (E621)*

maltol (E636)
In large quantities, it can help aluminum pass into the brain, so is potentially linked to Alzheimer's disease. Some countries ban it for babies and young children.

monoammonium L-glutamate (E624)
See *monosodium L-glutamate (MSG) (E621)*

monopotassium L-glutamate (E622)

Can cause nausea, vomiting, diarrhea, and abdominal cramps. Not for babies under twelve months old or for people with impaired kidneys. See *monosodium L-glutamate (MSG) (E621)*

monosodium L-glutamate (MSG) (E621)

Neurotoxin linked with headaches and migraines, and also such diseases as Huntington's, Alzheimer's, and Parkinson's. Children, pregnant women, hypoglycemics, asthmatics, the elderly, and those with heart disease may be particularly sensitive.

Miscellaneous

acesulfame potassium (E950)

Possible carcinogen in humans (caused cancer in test animals). Synonym: Acesulfame K.

acetylated distarch adipate (E1422)

No known adverse effects.

acetylated distarch phosphate (E1414)

No known adverse effects.

acetylated oxidized starch (E1451)

No known adverse effects.

acetylated starch (E1420)

No known adverse effects.

acid-treated starch (1401)

No known adverse effects.

alitame (956)

Unknown effects, but possibly similar to aspartame (E951).

alkaline-treated starch (1402)

No known adverse effects.

amylase (1100)

Effects unknown.

argon (E938)
Effects unknown.

aspartame (E951)
Carcinogenic neurotoxin; linked to reproductive disorders.

azodicarbonamide (E927)
Effects unknown. Banned in Australia.

beeswax (white and yellow) (E901)
No known adverse effects.

benzoyl peroxide (E928)
Similar effects to benzoic acid (E210).

benzyl alcohol (E1519)
Consumption of large doses may cause vomiting, diarrhea, and central-nervous-system depression.

bleached starch (1403)
Effects unknown.

candelilla wax (E902)
No known adverse effects.

carbamide (E927b)
Potential allergen.

carnauba wax (E903)
Occasionally causes allergic reactions and is a possible carcinogen.

chlorine (E925)
Destroys nutrients, known carcinogen.

chlorine dioxide (E926)
See *chlorine (E925)*

choline salts and esters (1001)
Effects unknown.

cyclamic acid (E952)

Known to cause migraines and other reactions; can be carcinogenic; found to be a reproductive toxin in animal tests. Banned in the United States and U.K.

dextrin roasted starch (1400)

Effects unknown.

dimethyl polysiloxane (E900)

No known adverse effects.

distarch phosphate (E1412)

No known adverse effects.

enzyme-treated starch (1405)

No known adverse effects.

ethanol, ethyl alcohol (E1510)

Suspected neurotoxic hazard; may provoke symptoms in people with candida and allergies.

glucose oxidase (1102)

Effects unknown.

glycerol diacetate (E1517)

May cause headaches, nausea, vomiting, dehydration, diarrhea, thirst, dizziness, and mental confusion.

glycerol triacetate, triacetin (E1518)

Binder for solid rocket fuels. Fungicide, humectant, and solvent. Effects unknown.

helium (E939)

Effects unknown.

hydroxypropyl distarch phosphate (E1442)

No known adverse effects.

hydroxypropyl starch (E1440)

No known adverse effects.

invertase (E1103)
Effects unknown.

isomalt, isomaltitol (E953)
Can cause softer than normal stools and intestinal gas. Not permitted in infant foods.

lactitol (E966)
Stomach upsets; laxative in high concentrations.

lanolin (E913)
No known adverse effects. Synonym: hydrous wool fat.

l-cysteine (E921)
See *l-cysteine monohydrochloride (E920)*

l-cysteine monohydrochloride (E920)
A known neurotoxin.

lipases (1104)
Effects unknown.

lysozyme (E1105)
Effects unknown.

maltitol, hydrogenated glucose syrup (E965)
Stomach upsets; laxative in high concentrations.

mineral oil (white) (905a)
Listed as having teratogenic (fetal-toxic) properties; linked with bowel cancer.

monostarch phosphate (E1410)
No known adverse effects.

montanic acid esters (E912)
Effects unknown.

neohesperidine DC (E959)
Effects unknown.

nitrogen (E931)
Effects unknown.

nitrogen (E941)
Effects unknown.

nitrous oxide (E932)
Safe in small quantities. Long exposure has been linked to liver and kidney disease and cancer.

oxidized polyethylene wax (E914)
Effects unknown.

oxidized starch (E1404)
Effects unknown.

oxygen (E948)
No known adverse effects.

paraffins, microcrystalline wax (E905)
Possible link with bowel cancer.

petrolatum (petroleum jelly) (905b)
May inhibit absorption of fats and fat-soluble vitamins. Is a mild laxative. Suspected teratogen (fetal toxin).

phosphated distarch phosphate (1413)
No known adverse effects.

polydextrose (E1200)
No known adverse effects.

polyethylene glycerol 8000 (1521)
Effects unknown.

polyvinylpolypyrrolidone (PPVP) (E1202)
May cause damage to kidneys and stay in the system for up to a year.

polyvinylpyrrolidone (E1201)
Made from formaldehyde. Excess may cause damage to the lungs or kidneys, gas, and fecal impaction. Suspected carcinogen.

potassium bromate (E924)
Large quantities can cause nausea, vomiting, diarrhea, abdominal pain, kidney damage, and failure. The WHO classifies it as a possible carcinogen.

propylene glycol (E1520)
Large doses can cause central-nervous-system depression and kidney damage.

proteases (papain, bromelain, ficin) (1101)
Effects unknown.

quillaia extract (E999)
Effects unknown.

refined microcrystalline wax (E907)
Effects unknown.

saccharine (E954)
Interferes with normal blood coagulation, blood-sugar levels, and digestive function. Potential carcinogen. Banned in France, Germany, Hungary, Portugal, and Spain. Banned as food additive in Malaysia and Zimbabwe. Banned as a beverage additive in Fiji, Israel, Peru, and Taiwan.

shellac (E904)
Derived from the lac insect of India; occasionally causes skin irritation.

starch acetate esterified with vinyl acetate (1421)
No known adverse effects.

starch sodium octenyl succinate (E1450)
No known adverse effects.

sucralose (955)
Can cause bloating, gas, nausea. In animal tests before being accepted in Australia, this showed detrimental effects to the thalamus glands, liver and kidney enlargement, and renal mineralization. Synonym: trichlorogalactosucrose.

thaumatin (E957)
Effects unknown.

triethyl acetate or citrate (E1505)
No known adverse effects.

xylitol (E967)
Stomach upsets; laxative in high concentrations.

Foods That Fight Toxic Damage

A good diet can go a long way toward keeping you healthy. Along with essential nutrients, many foods also contain important cofactors, enzymes, and fiber that turn them into what are known as functional foods—that is, foods that bring extra bonuses that go beyond basic nutrition, such as helping the body to eliminate chemical toxins. Consider these simple kitchen-cupboard solutions to keeping your body free from chemical toxins:

- **Garlic and onions** contain powerful antioxidants that aid the body's natural day-to-day efforts to detox. Use these liberally in cooking. Other sulphur-rich foods, such as broccoli, and bile stimulants, such as lemon and bitter greens, also assist in detoxification.

- **Peas, beans, and lentils** also contain unique antioxidants, and are high in fiber, which can bind to toxins and aid their removal from the body. Legumes are a good alternative source of protein, so consider substituting a couple of meat meals each week with one based on (organic) legumes.

- **A high-fiber diet** in general is useful for trapping toxins and assisting in the elimination of heavy metals. Fiber helps reduce intestinal permeability, sometimes known as a leaky gut—a condition that can sometimes lead to allergies and toxic buildup in the bloodstream. It also prevents deactivated estrogens from being reactivated and reabsorbed. Consider adding water-soluble mucilaginous fibers, such as psyllium seeds and flaxseeds, to your diet. These can be ground up, and sprinkled onto cereals, soups, and baked foods.

- **Pectin**, found in apple and pear seeds, can protect your body from damage by toxic metals. It works by blocking the absorption of toxins while aiding detoxification. Try making apples or pears stewed with their seeds a regular feature of your diet.

- **Bananas** have antioxidant qualities that help to fight chemical damage.

- **Eggs** protect against lead and mercury contamination.

- **All leafy dark green vegetables**, especially cruciferous vegetables (belonging to the cabbage family), can inhibit the carcinogenic effects of chemicals. Try to include plenty of kale, spinach, broccoli, and brussels sprouts in your diet. Other green foods that contain chlorophyll are also natural chelators that can draw heavy metals out of the system. Herbs like cilantro are a good choice. A good way to have your greens is to buy a juicer and use it to make vegetable juices—they are not as sweet as fruit juices, but they pack more punch in the detox stakes.

• **Seaweeds**, which, along with alginates, can bind to heavy metals. There is evidence, for instance, that the freshwater green algae chlorella can draw persistent chemicals, such as PCBs, out of the system. Similarly, research stretching back several decades shows that Arctic seaweeds are an aid to detoxification. These can be taken as supplements or added to your diet.

• **Black and green teas** are packed with antioxidants that may provide some protection from heavy-metal toxicity.

• **Forget your fat phobia**, because increasing your intake of healthy fats is important to maintaining good health. Good fats, such as omega-3 and -6, can help leach toxins out of your system, prevent inflammation, and protect the gut from toxic damage. Modern diets are particularly low in omega-3 fatty acids. The best natural sources of these are flaxseed, hempseed, canola, soybean and walnut oils, dark-green leaves, and coldwater fish, such as salmon, mackerel, and sardines. The best natural sources of omega-6 are safflower, sunflower, hemp, soybean, walnut, pumpkin, sesame and flax oils, as well as borage seed, blackcurrant seed, and evening primrose oil. To get your daily dose of good fats, include more of the following foods in your diet:

For omega-3 fats
1 tablespoon hempseed oil; 1 tablespoon flaxseed oil; 2 tablespoons flaxseeds; 4 tablespoons pumpkinseeds; 1,000 mg EPA/DHA supplement.

For omega-6 fats
1 tablespoon hempseeds; 1 tablespoon sunflower seeds; 2 tablespoons pumpkinseeds; 1½ tablespoons sesame seeds; 1,000 mg evening primrose oil; 500 mg borage oil.

Choose one source of omega-3 and omega-6 from each list to achieve a good intake of essential fatty acids (EFAs). Another good source of both types of fatty acids is dried beans, such as kidney, haricot, and soy. Regularly including these in your diet will ensure your good fat needs are met.

• **Juice**. Fruit juices—even freshly squeezed ones—are tasty, but full of sugar; when it comes to detoxing, they cannot compare with the powerful effect of vegetable juices. Having said that, you need to be choosy about which vegetables you select. Veggie juices made from carrots and beets taste good, but are as full of sugar as most fruit juices. Mild detox drinks can be made from such greens as celery, fennel, and cucumber. This is a good way to introduce yourself to the taste and effects of veggie juices if you've never had them before.

The dark-green leafy vegetable juices, though sometimes less palatable, will benefit you the most. This is partly because of their chlorophyll content and partly because of their high antioxidant content. Once you get used to the milder juices, you can introduce more powerful mixtures made from lettuces, such as red leaf, green leaf, romaine, and endive, as well as other greens like escarole, spinach, cabbage, and Chinese cabbage, or bok choy.

Adding herbs like parsley and cilantro to the juices will add flavor as well as further detoxification benefits. Start with small amounts and monitor your body's responses.

Other types of greens you can use (but sparingly, as they are very bitter) include kale, collard greens, dandelion greens, and mustard greens.

Make sure you wash all your greens thoroughly before juicing, and, where possible, buy organic for even more health benefits.

Better Buying

Below is a brief list of companies that specialize in producing or recommending less-toxic products. However, with a few rare exceptions, it is impossible to unreservedly recommend every product that these companies produce. Instead, it is advised that consumers ask questions, read labels, and choose for themselves the products with which they feel safe.

Food and Drink

Organic Buying Guides

Coop Directory Service
www.coopdirectory.org

Eat Well Guide
www.eatwellguide.org

Eat Wild
www.eatwild.com

LocalHarvest
www.localharvest.org

Mail-Order/Wholesalers

All Natural Distributors
(800) 666-2225
Foxboro, MA

Co-opportunity
www.cooportunity.com

Diamond Organics
www.diamondorganics.com

Earthbound Farm
www.ebfarm.com

Food for Thought, Inc.
www.foodforthought.net

My Organic Market
www.myorganicmarket.com

Beer, Wine, and Spirits

Etica
www.eticafairtrade.com

Frey Premium Organic & Biodynamic Wines
www.freywine.com

New Belgium Brewing Company
www.newbelgium.com

Organic Vintners
www.organicvintners.com

Coffee and Tea

A&E Custom Coffee Roastery
www.aeroastery.com

Caffe Ibis Coffee Roasting Co.
www.caffeibis.com

Honest Tea
www.honesttea.com

Beauty

Bodycare Products

Avalon
www.avalonnaturalproducts.com

The Body Shop
www.thebodyshop.com

Burt's Bees
www.burtsbees.com

Dr. Bronner's Magic Soaps
www.drbronner.com

Sanitary Products

Glad Rags
www.gladrags.com

NatraCare
www.natracare.com

Baby and Child

Baby Basics

Babyworks
www.babyworks.com

EcoBaby
www.ecobaby.com

Mommas Baby
www.mommasbaby.com

Clothing

Baby Naturopathics
www.babynaturopathics.com

EthicBaby
www.ethicbaby.com

Green for Baby
www.greenforbaby.com

Pure Beginnings
www.purebeginnings.com

Cloth Diapers

Diaperaps, Ltd.
www.diaperaps.com

Lil Diaper Depot
www.lildiaperdepot.com

Swaddlebees
www.swaddlebees.com

Household

Cleaning Products

American Formulating and Manufacturing
www.afmsafecoat.com

Earth Friendly Products
www.ecos.com

Ecover, Inc.
www.ecover.com

Green Clean, Inc.
www.greenclean.biz

Paints

AURO USA
www.aurousa.com

EnvironSafe Paint Co.
www.envirosafepaint.com

Green Planet Paints
www.greenplanetpaints.com

Decorating

Design Solutions
www.sfdesignsolutions.com

Earth Friendly Interior Design
www.earthfriendlyinteriordesign.com

Harmonious Environment
www.harmoniousenvironment.com

Gardening

East Coast Organics, Inc.
www.eastcoastorganics.com

Gardener's Supply
www.gardeners.com

Harmony Farm Supply & Nursery
www.harmonyfarm.com

Select Bibliography

An enormous amount of research has formed the background to this book, so these pages represent only a selection of the papers and books that readers may find of interest.

Papers and Reports

General

M. B. Abou-Donia, et al., "Neurotoxicity Resulting from Coexposure to Pyridostigmine Bromide, DEET, and Permethrin: Implications of Gulf War Chemical Exposures," *Journal of Toxicology and Environmental Health* 48, no. 1 (1996), pp. 35–56.

S. F. Arnold, et al., "Synergistic Activation of Estrogen Receptors with Combinations of Environmental Chemicals," *Science* 272 (1996), pp. 1489–92.

C. F. Bearer, "How Are Children Different from Adults?" *Environmental Health Perspectives* 103, suppl. 6 (1995), pp. 7–12.

S. K. Brown, "Exposure to Volatile Organic Compounds in Indoor Air: A Review," *Proceedings of the International Clean Air Conference of the Clean Air Society of Australia and New Zealand* 1 (1992), pp. 95–104.

S. K. Brown, "Volatile Organic Pollutants in New and Established Buildings in Melbourne, Australia," *Indoor Air* 12 (2002), pp. 55–63.

D. O. Carpenter, et al., "Human Health and Chemical Mixtures: An Overview," *Environmental Health Perspectives* 106, suppl. 6 (1998), pp. 1263–70.

"Chemical Hazard Data Availability Study: What Do We Really Know About the Safety of High Production Volume Chemicals?" U.S. Environmental Protection Agency, 1998.

T. Colbin, et al., "Our Stolen Future"; available online at www.ourstolenfuture.org. Accessed September 2007.

S. D. Cooper, et al., "Identification of Polar Organic Compounds Found in Consumer Products and Their Toxicological Properties," *Journal of Exposure Analysis and Environmental Epidemiology* 5 (1995), pp. 57–75.

W. J. Crinnion, "Environmental Medicine, Part 1: The Human Burden of Environmental Toxins and Their Common Health Effects," *Alternative Medicine Review* 5 (2000), pp. 52–63.

"Crisis in Chemicals: The Threat Posed by the 'Biomedical Revolution' to the Profits, Liabilities and Regulation of Industries Making and Using Chemicals," Friends of the Earth, May 2000.

"Draft Risk Assessment of the Potential Human Health Effects Associated with Exposure to Perfluorooctanoic Acid and Its Salts," U.S. Environmental Protection Agency, January 4, 2005; available online at www.epa.gov/oppt/pfoa. Accessed September 2007.

K. K. Eaton and H. M. Anthony, "Multiple Chemical Sensitivity Recognition and Management: A Document on the Health Effects of Everyday Chemical Exposures and Their Implications," Third Scientific Report of the British Society for Allergy, Environmental and Nutritional Medicine (BSAENM), March 2000.

"11th Annual Report on Carcinogens, National Toxicology Program," U.S. Department of Health and Human Services, Public Health Service.

"Environmental Diseases from A to Z," Publication no. 96-4145, National Institutes of Health, U.S. Department of Health and Human Services, 1997.

S. Epstein, et al., "Synergistic Toxicity and Carcinogenicity of 'Freons' and Piperonyl butoxide," *Nature* 214 (1967), pp. 526–28.

"Estimate of Risk of Skin Cancer from Dislodgeable Arsenic on Pressure Treated Wood Playground Equipment," Consumer Product Safety Commission (Washington, D.C., 1990).

K. Fujii and S. Epstein, "Effects of Piperonyl Butoxide on the Toxicity and Hepatocarcinogenicity of 2-acetylaminofluorene and 4-acetylaminobiphenyl, and Their N-hydroxylated Derivatives, Following Administration to Newborn Mice," *Oncology* 36 (1979), pp. 105–12.

C. Harris, et al., "The Estrogenic Activity of Phthalate Esters In Vitro," *Environmental Health Perspectives* 105 (1997), pp. 802–11.

"Health-Hazard Information," U.S. Environmental Protection Agency, 1991.

"How Chemical Exposures Affect Reproductive Health: Patient Fact Sheet," Greater Boston Physicians for Social Responsibility (GBPSR), 1996.

"Identification of Polar Volatile Organic Compounds in Consumer Products and Common Microenvironments," U.S. Environmental Protection Agency, 1991.

D. Kolpin, et al., "Pharmaceuticals, Hormones, and Other Organic Wastewater Contaminants in U.S. Streams, 1999–2000: A National Reconnaissance," *Environmental Science and Technology* 36 (2002), pp. 1202–11.

P. Lichtenstein, et al., "Environmental and Heritable Factors in the Causation of Cancer: Analyses of Cohorts of Twins from Sweden, Denmark, and Finland," *New England Journal of Medicine* 343 (2000), pp. 78–85.

R. D. Masters, "Biology and Politics: Linking Nature and Nurture," *Annual Review of Political Science* 4 (2001), pp. 345–69.

W. J. Meggs, "Neurogenic Inflammation and Sensitivity to Environmental Chemicals," *Environmental Health Perspectives* 101 (1993), pp. 234–38.

W. J. Meggs, "Neurogenic Switching: A Hypothesis for a Mechanism for Shifting the Site of Inflammation in Allergy and Chemicals Sensitivity," *Environmental Health Perspectives* 103 (1995), pp. 54–56.

"National Report on Human Exposure to Environmental Chemicals," Centers for Disease Control and Prevention (Atlanta, Ga.), March 2001; available online at www.cdc.gov/ exposurereport. Accessed September 2007.

"Neurotoxins: At Home and the Workplace," Report by the Committee on Science and Technology, U.S. House of Representatives, September 15, 1986, no. 99–827.

N. Pearce and P. Bethwait, "Increasing Incidence of Non-Hodgkin's Lymphoma: Occupational and Environmental Factors," *Cancer Research* 52, suppl. 19 (1992), pp. 5496S–5500S.

"PFCs: A Family of Chemicals That Contaminate the Planet," Environmental Working Group (EWG), April 2003.

"Second National Report on Human Exposure to Environmental Chemicals," Centers for Disease Control and Prevention (Atlanta, Ga.), March 2003; available online at www .cdc.gov/exposurereport. Accessed September 2007.

J. Tickner, et al., "The Precautionary Principle in Action: A Handbook," Science and Environmental Health Network, 1998.

"Toxic Alert: A Survey of High-Street Companies and Their Approach to Suspect Chemicals," Friends of the Earth, October 2000.

"Toxic Nation: A Report on Pollution in Canadians," Environmental Defence, Canada, November 2005; available online at www.environmentaldefence.ca. Accessed September 2007.

L. Wallace, "Identification of Polar Volatile Organic Compounds in Consumer Products and Common Microenvironments," EPA, 1991.

M. Warhurst, "Introduction to Hormone Disrupting Compounds"; available online at http://website.lineone.net/~mwarhurst. Accessed September 2007.

Food

J. A. Brotons, et al., "Xenoestrogenestrogens Released from Lacquer Coatings in Food Cans," *Environmental Health Perspectives* 103 (1995), pp. 608–12.

"Children's Drinks Contain Ingredients That Can Form Benzene: FDA Silent Despite Knowledge of the Problem," Environmental Working Group press release, February 28, 2006.

P. Cressey, et al., "1997–98 New Zealand Total Diet Survey, Part 1: Pesticide Residues," Ministry of Health, 2000.

"CSPI's Guide to Food Additives," Center for Science in the Public Interest; available online at www.cspinet.org/reports/chemcuisine.htm. Accessed September 2007.

"Eating Oil: Food in a Changing Climate," Sustain/Elm Farm Research Centre Report, 2001.

"Feeding Minds: The Impact of Food on Mental Health," Mental Health Foundation, Winter 2005; available online at www.mentalhealth.org.uk. Accessed September 2007.

"Genetic Engineering and Human Health," Soil Association, February 2005.

J. M. Geuns, "Stevioside," *Phytochemistry* 64, no. 5 (November 2003), pp. 913–21.

E. L. Gunderson, "FDA Total Diet Study, April 1982–April 1984: Dietary Intakes of Pesticides, Selected Elements, and Other Chemicals," *Journal of the Association of Official Analytical Chemists* 71 (1988), pp. 1200–1209.

K. Lau, et al., "Synergistic Interactions Between Commonly Used Food Additives in a Developmental Neurotoxicity Test," *Toxicological Sciences* 90, no. 1 (2006), pp. 178–87.

M. E. P. Lucas and C. Hines, "Stopping the Great Food Swap: Relocalising Europe's Food Supply," The Green Party, 2001.

A. M. Mayer, "Historical Changes in the Mineral Content of Fruits and Vegetables: A Cause for Concern?" *British Food Journal* 99 (1997), pp. 207–11.

R. A. McCance and E. M. Widdowson, "The Chemical Composition of Foods," 1st ed., Special Report Series no. 235, U.K. Royal Society of Chemistry/MAFF, 1940.

R. A. McCance and E. M. Widdowson, "The Composition of Foods," 5th ed., U.K. Royal Society of Chemistry/MAFF, 1991.

"Nanotechnology in Food and Food Processing Industry Worldwide," Helmut Kaiser Consultancy, 2004.

"The 19th Australian Total Diet Survey," Australia New Zealand Food Authority, April 2001.

"Organic Food: Facts and Figures 2005," Soil Association, December 2005.

"Pesticide Residues Monitoring: Second Quarter Results April to June 2003," Pesticide Residues Committee, December 3, 2003; available online at www.pesticides.gov.uk/prc_home.asp. Accessed September 2007.

J. N. Pretty, et al., "Farm Costs and Food Miles: An Assessment of the Full Cost of the UK Weekly Food Basket," *Food Policy* 30 (2005), pp. 1–19.

D. Thomas, "Mineral Depletion in Foods Over the Period 1940 to 1991," *Nutrition Practice* 2 (2001), pp. 27–29.

"The Total Diet Study: Summary of Residues Found Ordered by Food, Market Baskets, 91-3-99-1," Food and Drug Administration, September 2000.

C. Van der Weyer, "Changing Diets, Changing Minds: How Food Affects Mental Well Being and Behaviour," Mental Health Foundation/Sustain, Winter 2005; available online at www.sustainweb.org. Accessed September 2007.

"Vegetables without Vitamins," Life Extension, March 2001; available online at www.lef.org/magazine/mag2001/mar2001_report_vegetables.html.

"What's Wrong With Supermarkets?" 4th ed., Corporate Watch, April 2004; available online at www.corporatewatch.org.uk. Accessed September 2007.

A. White, "Pesticides in Food: Why Go Organic?" Pesticide Action Network NZ/Safe Food Campaign NZ, New Zealand, 1999.

R. Wiles, "EWG Letter to the FDA Re: Benzene," Environmental Working Group, February 28, 2006. Available online at www.ewg.org/node/22007. Accessed September 2007.

"Working Party on Pesticide Residues—1999 Report" (London: MAFF Publications), 1999.

V. Worthington, "Nutritional Quality of Organic Versus Conventional Fruits, Vegetables and Grains," *Journal of Alternative and Complementary Medicine* 7, no. 2 (2001), pp. 161–73.

Beauty

R. C. Anderson and J. H. Anderson, "Acute Toxic Effects of Fragrance Products," *Archives of Environmental Health* 53 (1998), pp. 138–46.

L. M. Brown, et al., "Hair Dye Use and Multiple Myeloma in White Men," *American Journal of Public Health* 82 (1992), pp. 1673–74.

G. Buchbauer, et al., "Fragrance Compounds and Essential Oils with Sedative Effects upon Inhalation," *Journal of Pharmacological Science* 82 (1993), pp. 660–64.

K. P. Cantor, et al., "Hair Dye Use and Risk of Leukemia and Lymphoma," *American Journal of Public Health* 78 (1988), pp. 570–71.

T. H. Connor, et al., "Mutagenicity of Cosmetic Products Containing Kathon," *Environmental and Molecular Mutagens* 28 (1996), pp. 127–32.

L. S. Cook, et al., "Hair Product Use and the Risk of Breast Cancer in Young Women," *Cancer Causes Control* 10 (1999), pp. 551–59.

D. W. Cramer, et al., "Genital Talc Exposure and Risk of Ovarian Cancer," *International Journal of Cancer* 81 (1999), pp. 351–56.

P. D. Darbre, et al., "Concentrations of Parabens in Human Breast Tumours," *Journal of Applied Toxicology* 24, no. 1 (2004), pp. 5–13.

C. Daughton and T. Ternes, "Pharmaceuticals and Personal Care Products in the Environment: Agents of Subtle Change?" *Environmental Health Perspectives* 107, suppl. 6 (1999), pp. 907–38.

G. Eisenbrand, et al., "N-Nitrosoalkanolamines in Cosmetics in Relevance to Human Cancer of N-nitroso Compounds, Tobacco Smoke and Mycotoxins," International Agency for Research on Cancer (IARC), 1991.

P. J. Frosch, et al., "Patch Testing with Fragrances: Results of a Multicentre Study of the European Environmental and Contact Dermatitis Research Group with 48 Frequently Used Constituents of Perfumes," *Contact Dermatology* 33 (1995), pp. 333–42.

D. M. Gertig, et al., "Prospective Study of Talc Use and Ovarian Cancer," *Journal of the National Cancer Institute* 92 (2000), pp. 249–52.

A. B. Graves, et al., "The Association Between Aluminum-Containing Products and Alzheimer's Disease," *Journal of Clinical Epidemiology* 43 (1990), pp. 35–44.

F. Grodstein, et al., "A Prospective Study of Permanent Hair Dye Use and Hematopoietic Cancer," *Journal of the National Cancer Institute* 86 (1994), pp. 1466–70.

B. L. Harlow and B. S. Weiss, "A Case-control Study of Borderline Ovarian Tumors: The Influence of Perineal Exposure to Talc," *American Journal of Epidemiology* 130 (1989), pp. 390–94.

L. Hastings, et al., "Olfactory Primary Neurons as a Route of Entry for Toxic Agents into the CNS," *Neurotoxicology* 12 (1991), pp. 707–14.

D. S. Heller, et al., "The Relationship Between Perineal Cosmetic Talc Usage and Ovarian Talc Particle Burden," *American Journal of Obstetries and Gynecology* 74 (1996), pp. 1507–10.

E. A. Holly, et al., "Hair-Color Products and Risk for Non-Hodgkin's Lymphoma: A population-based Study in the San Francisco Bay Area," *American Journal of Public Health* 88 (1998), pp. 1767–73.

P. Kumar, et al., "Inhalation Challenge Effects of Perfume Scent Strips in Patients with Asthma," *Annals of Allergy, Asthma & Immunology* 75 (1995), pp. 429–33.

R. Lawson, "Have You Met This Syndrome?" *Medical Monitor* (September 4, 1996), p. 66.

S. Mauller, et al., "Occurrence of Nitro and Non-Nitro Benzenoid Musk Compounds in Human Adipose Tissue," *Chemosphere* 33 (1996), pp. 17–28.

E. Millqvist and O. Lowhagen, "Placebo-Controlled Challenges with Perfume in Patients with Asthma-like Symptoms," *Allergy* 51 (1996), pp. 434–39.

P. C. Nasca, et al., "Relationship of Hair Dye Use, Benign Breast Disease, and Breast Cancer," *Journal of the National Cancer Institute* 64 (1980), pp. 23–28.

E. J. Routledge, et al., "Some Alkyl Hydroxy Benzoate Preservatives (Parabens) Are Estrogenic," *Toxicology and Applied Pharmacology* 153 (1998), pp. 12–19.

M. Schlumpf, et al., "In Vitro and In Vivo Estrogenicity of UV Screens," *Environmental Health Perspectives* 109 (2001), pp. 239–44.

N. Shafer and R. W. Shafer, "Potential of Carcinogenic Effects of Hair Dyes," *New York State Journal of Medicine* 76 (1976), pp. 394–96.

R. E. Shore, et al., "A Case-Control Study of Hair Dye Use and Breast Cancer," *Journal of the National Cancer Institute* 62 (1979), pp. 277–83.

J. D. Shulman and L. M. Wells, "Acute Fluoride Toxicity from Ingesting Home-Use Dental Products in Children, Birth to 6 Years of Age," *Journal of Public Health Dentistry* 57 (1997), pp. 150–58.

P. S. Spencer, et al., "Neurotoxic Fragrance Produces Ceroid and Myelin Disease," *Science* 204 (1979), pp. 633–35.

P. S. Spencer, et al., "Neurotoxic Properties of Musk Ambrette," *Toxicology and Applied Pharmacology* 75 (1984), pp. 571–75.

M. J. Thun, et al., "Hair Dye Use and Risk of Fatal Cancers in U.S. Women," *Journal of the National Cancer Institute* 86 (1994), pp. 210–15.

H. Weibel, et al., "Penetration of the Fragrance Compounds, Cinnamaldehyde and Cinnamyl Alcohol, Through Human Skin In Vitro," *Contact Dermatology* 34 (1996), pp. 423–26.

G. M. Whitford, "Fluoride in Dental Products: Safety Considerations," *Journal of Dental Research* 66 (1987), pp. 1056–60.

Household

R. C. Anderson and J. H. Anderson, "Toxic Effects of Air Freshener Emissions," *Archives of Environmental Health* 52 (1997), pp. 433–41.

R. C. Anderson, "Toxic Emissions from Carpets," *Journal of Nutrition and Environmental Medicine* 5 (1995), pp. 375–86.

"Exercise Caution When Using 'Nano-Sealing Sprays' Containing a Propellant!" Federal Institute for Risk Assessment, March 31, 2006, press release; available online at www .bfr.bund.de/cms5w/sixcms/detail.php/7699. Accessed September 2007.

H. Guo and F. Murray, "Determination of Total Volatile Organic Compound Emissions from Furniture Polishes," *Clean Products and Processes* 3, no. 1 (2001), pp. 42–48.

C. Hertzman, et. al., "Mortality and Cancer Incidence Among Sawmill Workers Exposed to Chlorophenate Wood Preservatives," *American Journal of Public Health* 87, no. 1 (1997), pp. 71–79.

J. A. Hoppin, et al., "Occupational Chlorophenol Exposure and Soft Tissue Sarcoma Risk Among Men Aged 30–60 Years," *American Journal of Epidemiology* 148, no. 7 (1998), pp. 693–703.

W. Karmaus and N. Wolf, "Reduced Birthweight and Length in the Offspring of Females Exposed to PCDFs, PCP, and Lindane," *Environmental Health Perspectives* 103, no. 12 (1995), pp. 1120–25.

E. L. Larson, "Effect of Antibacterial Home Cleaning and Handwashing Products on Infectious Disease Symptoms: A Randomized, Double-Blind Trial," *Annals of Internal Medicine* 140, no. 5 (2004), pp. 321–29.

W. R. Ott and J. W. Roberts, "Everyday Exposure to Toxic Pollutants," *Scientific American* (Feb. 1998), pp. 86–91.

P. Thomas, "Dawn of the Domestic Superbug," *Ecologist* (July/August 2005), pp. 42–48.

L. A. Wallace, et al., "Personal Exposure, Indoor-Outdoor Relationships, and Breath Levels of Toxic Air Pollutants Measured for 355 Persons in New Jersey," Environmental Protection Agency 0589, presented at the Annual Meeting of the Air Pollution Control Association, San Francisco, CA, June 25, 1984.

L. A. Wallace, et al., "Personal Exposure, Indoor-Outdoor Relationships, and Breath Levels of Toxic Air Pollutants Exposures, Outdoor Concentrations, and Breath Levels of Toxic Air Pollutants Measured for 425 Persons in Urban, Suburban and Rural Areas," EPA 0589, presented at the Annual Meeting of the Air Pollution Control Association, San Francisco, CA, June 25, 1984.

A. M. Warhurst, "An Environmental Assessment of Alkylphenol Ethoxylates and Alkylphenols," Friends of the Earth, London, 1995.

R. F. White and S. P. Proctor, "Solvents and Neurotoxicity," *Lancet* 349 (1997), pp. 1239–43.

Pesticides

"The Secret Hazards of Pesticides: Inert Ingredients," Office of the Attorney General of New York State, Environmental Protection Bureau, February 1996.

"Chemical Trespass: A Toxic Legacy," World Wildlife Fund (WWF-UK), 1999.

J. R. Davis, et al., "Family Pesticide Use and Childhood Brain Cancer," *Archives of Environmental Contamination and Toxicology* 24 (1993), pp. 87–92.

"European Workshop on the Impact of Endocrine Disrupters on Human Health and

Wildlife," December 2–4, 1996, Weybridge, U.K. Proceedings, Report No. EUR 17549, Copenhagen, Denmark: European Commission DG XII, April 1997.

P. T. C. Harrison, "Endocrine Disrupters and Human Health," *British Medical Journal* 323 (2001), pp. 1317–18.

P. T. C. Harrison, et al., "Reproductive Health in Humans and Wildlife: Are Adverse Trends Associated with Environmental Chemical Exposure?" *Science of the Total Environment* 205 (1997), pp. 97–106.

"Hormonally Active Agents in the Environment," Committee on Hormonally Active Agents in the Environment, National Research Council, National Academy of Sciences, 2000.

"Intolerance Risk: Pesticides in Our Children's Food," Natural Resources Defense Council, Washington, D.C., 1989.

R. Lowengart, et al., "Childhood Leukemia and Parents' Occupational and Home Exposure," *Journal of the National Cancer Institute* 79 (1987), pp. 39–46.

"Gardening for Health," Pesticide Action Network UK; available online at www.pan-uk .org/info/gardening.htm. Accessed September 2007.

L. Ritter, "Report of a Panel on the Relationship Between Public Exposure to Pesticides and Cancer," Ad Hoc Panel on Pesticides and Cancer, National Cancer Institute of Canada; *Cancer* 80 (1997), pp. 2019–33.

"Systematic Review of Pesticide Human Health Effects," Ontario College of Family Physicians, April 23, 2004. Available online at www.ocfp.on.ca/local/files/communications /current%20issues/pesticides/final%20paper%2023APR2004.pdf. Accessed September 2007.

Pest Control

"Least Toxic Pest Control Solutions and Products," Pesticide Action Network UK; available online at www.pan-uk.org. Accessed September 2007.

"Natural Insect Pest Control," Eartheasy; available online at www.eartheasy.com. Accessed September 2007.

Pets

G. M. Davenport, "The Impact of Nutrition on Skin and Hair Coat," presented at the 4th World Congress of Veterinary Dermatology, in Current Research in Canine Dermatology, the IAMS Company, Dayton, Ohio, 2000.

B. J. Hawkins, "Periodontal Disease in Dogs and Cats," Proceedings of the North American Veterinary Conference, Orlando, Fla., 1996.

K. C. Hayes, et al., "An Ultrastructural Study of Nutritionally Induced and Reversed Retinal Degeneration in Cats," *American Journal of Pathology* 78 (1975), p. 505.

R. G. Lewis, et al., "Evaluation of Methods for Monitoring the Potential Exposures of

Small Children to Pesticides in the Residential Environment," *Archives of Environmental Contamination and Toxicology* 26 (1994), pp. 37–46.

A. N. Martin, " 'Mad Pet' Disease: Mad Cow Disease Is Killing Europe's Pets," in *Nutrient Requirements of Cats*, National Research Council (Washington, D.C.: National Academy Press, 1986).

J. G. Morris and Q. R. Rogers, "Assessment of the Nutritional Adequacy of Pet Foods Through the Life Cycle," *Journal of Nutrition* 124 (1994), pp. S2520–34.

J. Neff, "Dog Eat Dog & Cats? Fur Flies as Charges of Canine Cannibalism and Willful Malnourishment Roil Pet Industry," *Food Processing*, March 2002.

National Research Council, *Nutrient Requirements of Dogs* (Washington, D.C.: National Academy Press, 1985).

W. Pollak, "The Effects of a Natural vs. Commercial Pet Food Diet on Wellness of Common Companion Animals"; available online at www.healthyvet.com. Accessed September 2007.

A. D. Shojaim, "How Cat Litter Is Made," *Cat Fancy Magazine*, October 1994, pp. 12–19.

D. Wallinga and L. Greer, "Poisons on Pets: Health Hazards from Flea and Tick Products," Natural Resources Defense Council, November 2000.

R. Williams, "Safe Flea Control and Organic Labelling," *Townsend Letters for Doctors and Patients*, April 1, 2003.

"What Vets Don't Tell You: Special Report," London, UK: WDDTY, 2003; available online at www.wddty.co.uk. Accessed September 2007.

"What's Really in Pet Food?" Animal Protection Institute, 2001; available online at www .api4animals.org. Accessed September 2007.

Books

S. Antczak and G. Antczak, *Cosmetics Unmasked* (New York: Thorsons, 2001).

N. Ashford and C. Miller, *Chemical Exposures: Low Levels and High Stakes* (New York: Wiley-Interscience, 2001).

J. Blythman, *Shopped! The Shocking Truth about British Supermarkets* (New York: Harper-Perennial, 2005).

R. Bowlby, *Carried Away: The Invention of Modern Shopping* (New York: Columbia University Press, 2001).

F. M. Bradley and B. W. Ellis, *Rodale's All-New Encyclopedia of Organic Gardening: The Indispensable Resource for Every Gardener* (New York: Rodale Books, 1993).

M. Bremner, *Enquire Within*, 3rd ed. (London: Helicon, 1994).

S. A. Briggs and the Staff of the Rachel Carson Council, *Basic Guide to Pesticides* (Washington, D.C.: CRC, 1992).

R. Carson, *Silent Spring*, reprint ed. (New York: Mariner Books, 1994).

T. Colborn, et al., *Our Stolen Future: How We Are Threatening Our Fertility, Intelligence and Survival* (New York: Plume, 1997).

P. Cox and P. Brusseau, *Secret Ingredients* (New York: Bantam Books, 1997).

C. Engel, *Wild Health: How Animals Keep Themselves Well and What We Can Learn from Them* (New York: Houghton Mifflin, 2002).

S. Epstein, et al., *The Breast Cancer Prevention Program* (New York: Macmillan, 1997).

R. E. Gosselin, et al., *Clinical Toxicology of Commercial Products*, 5th ed. (Philadelphia: Williams & Wilkins, 1984).

J. Harte, et al., *Toxics A to Z: A Guide to Everyday Pollution Hazards* (Los Angeles: University of California Press, 1991).

F. Lawrence, *Not on the Label* (New York: Penguin, 2004).

W. Lijinsky, *Chemistry and Biology of N-nitroso Compounds* (Cambridge: Cambridge University Press, 1990).

K. Logan, *Clean House, Clean Planet* (New York: Pocket Books, 1997).

A. Lopez, *Natural Pest Control: Alternatives to Chemicals for the Home and Garden*, rev. ed. (Harmonious Technologies, 1998).

A. N. Martin, *Foods Pets Die For: Shocking Facts about Pet Food*, 2nd ed. (Troutdale, Ore.: NewSage Press, 2003).

G. Monbiot, *Captive State: The Corporate Takeover of Britain* (London: Pan Books, 2001).

K. Mumby, *The Complete Guide to Food Allergies and Environmental Illness* (New York: HarperCollins, 1993).

Neal's Yard Remedies, *Make Your Own Cosmetics* (London: Aurum Press, 1997).

W. Olkowski, *Common Sense Pest Control: Least-toxic Solutions for Your Home, Garden, Pets and Community* (New Town, Conn.: Taunton Press, 1991).

B. Pagram, *Natural Housekeeping* (London: Gaia, 1997).

R. J. Palma, *The Complete Guide to Household Chemicals* (New York: Prometheus, 1995).

C. Robbins, *Poisoned Harvest: A Consumer's Guide to Pesticide Use and Abuse* (London: Victor Gollancz, 1992).

R. J. Roberts, "Overview of Similarities and Differences Between Children and Adults: Implications for Risk Assessment," in P. S. Guzelian, et al., eds., *Similarities and Differences Between Children and Adults* (Washington, D.C.: ILSI Press, 1992).

G. Ross Lewis, *1001 Chemicals in Everyday Products*, 2nd ed. (New York: Wiley-Interscience, 1999).

D. Sarjeant and K. Evans, *Hard to Swallow: The Truth about Food Additives* (Burnaby, B.C.: Alive Books, 1999).

T. Schettler, et al., *Generations at Risk: Reproductive Health and the Environment* (Cambridge, Mass.: MIT Press, 2000).

E. Schlosser, *Fast Food Nation: The Dark Side of the American Meal* (New York: HarperPerennial, 2001).

A. Seth and G. Randall, *The Grocers* (London: Kogan Page 1999).

D. Steinman and S. Epstein, *The Safe Shopper's Bible: A Consumers Guide to Nontoxic Household Products* (New York: Wiley, 1995).

D. Steinman and R. M. Wisner, *Living Healthy in a Toxic World* (New York: Perigee, 1996).

P. Thomas, *Cleaning Yourself to Death* (Dublin: New Leaf, 2001).

P. Thomas, *Living Dangerously* (Dublin: New Leaf, 2003).

J. Tickner, et al., *The Precautionary Principle in Action: A Handbook* (Ames, Iowa: Science and Environmental Health Network, 1998).

A. Ursell, *L Is for Labels* (Carlsbad, Calif.: Hay House, 2004).

R. Whitehead, ed., *The UK Pesticide Guide 2000* (Wallingford, Oxon: CABI Publishing, CAB International).

R. Winter, *A Consumer's Dictionary of Food Additives* (New York: Three Rivers Press, 2004).

V. A. Wormwood, *The Fragrant Pharmacy* (New York: Bantam, 1992).

W. Young, *Sold Out: The True Cost of Supermarket Shopping* (London: Fusion Press, 2004).

Index

Patricia Thomas is a journalist and author in the field of alternative and environmental health. She is the health editor for the *Ecologist* magazine, where she writes the regular column Behind the Label. She is the author of the bestselling *Cleaning Yourself to Death* as well as *Living Dangerously: Are Everyday Toxins Making You Sick?* A former radio producer and broadcaster, Thomas is a regular contributor to newspapers and appears frequently on TV and radio.